AF575189

Carel L Davidson and Ivar A. Mjör

Advances in Glass-Ionomer Cements

Advances in Glass-Ionomer Cements

Edited by

Carel L. Davidson, PhD
Professor and Chairman
Department of Dental Materials Science
Academic Centre for Dentistry
University of Amsterdam
Amsterdam, The Netherlands

Ivar A. Mjör, BDS, MSD, MS, Dr Odont
Professor Academy 100 Eminent Scholar
College of Dentistry, University of Florida
Gainesville, Florida

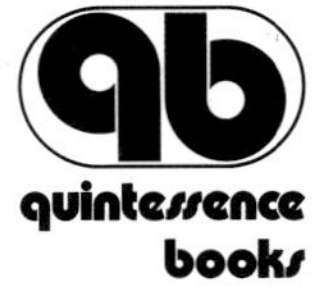

Quintessence Publishing Co, Inc

Chicago, Berlin, London, Tokyo, Paris, Barcelona,
São Paulo, Moscow, Prague, and Warsaw

Library of Congress Cataloging-in-Publication Data

Advances in glass-ionomer cements / edited by Carel L. Davidson, Ivar A. Mjör
p. cm.
Includes bibliographical references and index.
ISBN 0-86715-360-1
1. Dental glass ionomer cements. 2. Prosthodontics.
I. Davidson, C. L. II. Mjör, Ivar Andreas, 1933-
[DNLM: 1. Glass Ionomer Cements. 2. Cementation—methods.
3. Dental Restoration, Permanent—methods. WU 190 A244 1999]
RK652.8.G55A35 1999
617.6'95—dc21
DNLM/DLC
for Library of Congress 99-22881
CIP

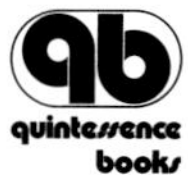

Quintessence Publishing Co, Inc
551 Kimberly Drive
Carol Stream, IL 60188

Lithography: Fotolito Veneta, Verona
Typesetting: Satzstudio L, Strausberg
Printing and Binding: Jütte Druck GmbH, Leipzig

Printed in Germany

ISBN 0-86715-360-1

Contents

Foreword

There has been much progress in recent years in the formulation and understanding of glass-ionomer cements, and many questions about the efficacy of the newer polyacid-modified resin materials are covered in this book. The editors are to be congratulated on their choice of authors, who clearly understand the problems associated with these. At the same time, they take a constructive approach to the potential and immediate benefits of such materials, in particular their use in developing countries where the materials need to be mixed on-site and can be used with simple instrumentation. Their conservative preparation in pedodontics is another area where glass-ionomer cements have made an invaluable contribution.

Several chapters cover the adhesion and fluoride release of these cements, including a very up-to-date assessment of how the cements attach to tooth structure and whether fluoride plays a role in the prevention of secondary caries around the restorations. The imaging of tooth tissue using confocal microscopy allows the examination of undisturbed structures below the section surface and has greatly assisted understanding of the adhesion processes. Indeed, enamel is not all it is cracked up to be. We should not expect too much of this fascinating material.

Resin-modified glass-ionomers have been critically evaluated, and setting contraction and water sorption remain controversial areas. The protection of the set surface with light-cured resins still appears to be mandatory, and the set polymeric matrix is not a barrier to salivary attack. The polyacid-modified materials have become very popular due to their excellent esthetics and ease of handling, but their adhesion mechanism has come under scrutiny and they do not appear to have the ion-exchange properties of the conventional glass-ionomer cement. It appears that as the glass-ionomer cements are modified their true adhesive properties decline with increasing resin content until they become indistinguishable from a resin composite.

The authors make it clear that at the present time glass-ionomer cements are not suitable for clinical use in high stress-bearing areas. However, their use in Class I, Class III, and Class V cavities is now well accepted. The controversial tunnel preparation has not become popular despite its obvious attractions as a conservative method of treating dental caries. Dentists would find this restoration easier if they approached it as an internal preparation, as described recently and in this text, because adequate access is vital to the success of the operation. The open "sandwich" technique also remains controversial but should not be abandoned in clinical research projects. More recently, Wassell and coworkers[1] have had some clinical success with this method in a study on direct composite inlays versus conventional composite restorations. The sealing of subgingival margins in the older patient could also prove useful for individuals with extensive caries where salivary control can be difficult.

The highly viscous glass-ionomers have been introduced as an alternative to amalgam alloys, but clinical trials are limited. I believe that surface wear of glass-ionomer cements will remain a problem due to fractures within the cement when it is placed under occlusal stress. The replacement of gold alloys and even amalgam alloys with these cements in the 21st century will need some imaginative improvements if the replacement materials are to maintain long-term occlusal stability. The authors of this book have the enthusiasm and intellectual gifts to meet this challenge, and this book will become an essential reference for all those engaged in clinical and laboratory research.

John W. McLean

Reference

1. Wassell RW, Walls AWG, McCabe JF. Direct composite inlays versus conventional composite restorations. Three-year clinical results. Br Dent J 1995;179:343–349.

Special Message

To be involved with exciting new materials is always a pleasure, particularly when such materials contribute to the well-being of patients.

So it was some 30 years ago that Dr Alan Wilson and Dr John McLean began the development of those very special materials that we now know as glass-ionomer cements. Coincidentally, at about the same time, dental materials research on the other side of the world were also trying to develop something special, using new ideas to extend the production technology of conventional dental cements.

With change, it usually takes considerable time to achieve significant results, but each year, more and more dental practitioners come to recognize the possibilities that glass-ionomers offer in almost every restorative situation. For example, glass-ionomer cements can be used as a base, cavity liner, bonding material, or restoration, or for pit and fissure protection; they can be used alone or in combination with other materials. Glass-ionomer cements are quite unique, providing chemical adhesion to the tooth and the benefits of fluoride release.

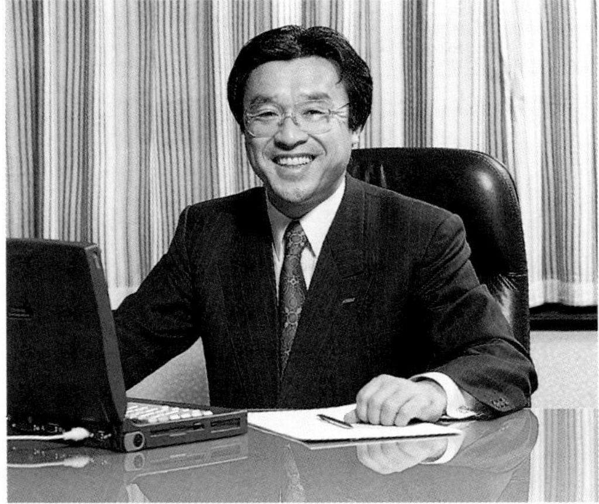

Today there are more exciting changes to look forward to. With the emphasis on minimum intervention and adhesive dentistry, glass-ionomer materials are especially appropriate for the future.

It has been our special pleasure to sponsor this publication and to cooperate with Prof Dr Carel L. Davidson and Prof Dr Ivar Mjör, who have produced this comprehensive publication which we hope you will enjoy reading.

Makoto Nakao
President and CEO
GC Corporation

Contributors

Eric Bonte, DSO
Associate Professor
Laboratory of Biology and Craniofacial Physiopathology
René Descartes University
Montrouge, France

Marc J. A. Braem, PhD
Professor, Department of Dental Materials
University of Anvers–RUCA
Anvers, Belgium

F. J. Trevor Burke, DDS, MSc, MDS, FDS, MGDSRCS (Edin), FDSRCPS (Glas)
Professor, University of Glasgow Dental School
Glasgow, United Kingdom

Xavier Daniau
Research Associate
Laboratory of Biology and Craniofacial Physiopathology
René Descartes University
Montrouge, France

Anton J. de Gee, PhD
Associate Professor
Department of Dental Materials Science
Academic Centre for Dentistry
University of Amsterdam
Amsterdam, The Netherlands

Michel Degrange, DDS, DSO
Professor and Head
Department of Biomaterials
Faculty of Dental Surgery
René Descartes University
Montrouge, France

George Eliades, DDS, Dr Odont
Head, Quality Control Section
Research Center for Biomaterials
Glyfada, Greece

Marco Ferrari, MD, DDS, PhD
Professor of Dental Materials
University of Siena, Italy
Research Professor, Tufts University
Boston, Massachusetts

Shimon Friedman, DMD
Professor and Head
Department of Endodontology
University of Toronto
Ontario, Canada

Michel Goldberg, DDS, DSO, DESN
Professor and Chairman
Laboratory of Biology and Craniofacial Physiopathology
René Descartes University
Montrouge, France

Reinhard Hickel, DDS, MS, PhD
Professor and Director
Polyclinic for Dentistry and Periodontology
Ludwig Maximilians University
Munich, Germany

Kazuo Hirota, Dr Eng
Director of Research and Development
GC Corporation
Tokyo, Japan

Pierre Jonas, DDS, DESN
Private Practice
Jouy en Josas, France

Jean-Jacques Lasfargues DDS, DSO
Professor and Head
Operative Dentistry and Endodontics
René Descartes University
Montrouge, France

Juergen Manhart, DDS, PhD
Polyclinic for Dentistry and Periodontology
Ludwig Maximilians University
Munich, Germany

Dorothy McComb, BDS, MScD, FRCD(C)
Professor and Head
Department of Restorative Dentistry
University of Toronto
Ontario, Canada

John W. McLean, OBE, FDSRCS (Eng), DSC, Odont Dr (Lund)
Consulting Professor in Fixed Prosthodontics and Biomaterials
Consultant Laboratory of the Government Chemist
London, United Kingdom

Graham J. Mount, AM, BDS, DDSc, FRACDS
Visiting Research Fellow
University of Adelaide
North Adelaide, South Australia

Dan Nathanson, DMD, MSD
Professor and Chairman
Department of Restorative Sciences and Biomaterials
Goldman School of Dental Medicine
Boston University
Boston, Massachusetts

Sueo Saito, DDS
Lecturer, Department of Operative Dentistry
Tokyo Medical and Dental University
Tokyo, Japan

Lena Stanislawski, INSERM CR1
Laboratory of Biology and Craniofacial Physiopathology
René Descartes University
Montrouge, France

Satoshi Tosaki, BS
Chief Researcher
Research and Development
GC Corporation
Tokyo, Japan

Timothy F. Watson, BSc, BDS, PhD FDSRCS
Senior Lecturer/Consultant
Division of Conservative Dentistry
King's College London, Guy's Hospital
London, United Kingdom

Nairn H. F. Wilson, PhD, MSc, BDS, FDS, FRDRCS (Edin), FDSRCS (Eng)
Professor, Department of Restorative Dentistry
University Dental Hospital of Manchester
Manchester, United Kingdom

Chapter 1

Characteristics of Glass-Ionomer Cements

Sueo Saito, Satoshi Tosaki, Kazuo Hirota

Different types of restorative materials and luting cements are currently used in daily dental practice. The most common are amalgam, composite resins, glass ionomers, dental casting alloys, and ceramics. Each material possesses advantages and disadvantages. Amalgam has a long history as a practical and relatively inexpensive restorative material and is still widely used. However, the toxicity controversy of the mercury is a disadvantage. Dental casting alloys have excellent physical properties, but the production process is costly and some components of the alloys may induce allergic reactions in patients. Moreover, amalgam and casting alloys are not tooth colored and the demand for more esthetic materials is increasing. Resin composites are the most esthetically acceptable of the available restorative materials with satisfactory physical properties. However, allergic problems have arisen and some concern about the estrogenic effects of bisphenol A as an environmental hormone has been indicated.[1] The glass-ionomer cements are more aesthetically pleasing than metallic restoratives, although less so than resin composites, and they are considered one of the safest restorative materials.

When reviewing the dental luting cements, glass-ionomers possess several advantages compared to the resin composite, zinc-phosphate, and other dental cements. The glass-ionomer cements can be used in a wide range of clinical applications. They also have an anticariogenic potential produced by incorporated fluorine,[2–8] good biocompatibility, good chemical adhesion to the tooth structure, well-balanced physical properties, and good manipulability.

The clinical applications of glass-ionomer cements are as luting agents, fillings for anterior and posterior teeth, linings, bases and cores, fissure protection materials for prevention of caries, sealants for patients with allergic reactions to resin-based materials, bonding agents for composite resin, root canal fillings, and adhesive cements for orthodontic brackets. The reason glass-ionomer cement is widely applicable is that it can exhibit varied physical properties by changing the powder–liquid ratio or the powder and liquid formulation. The large variety of glass-ionomer cements have different consistencies and can be designed for specific dental applications (Table 1-1). The ISO standard defines glass-ionomer

Table 1-1 Glass ionomer cement products

Clinical Application	Product	Classification	Manufacturer	Notes
Luting	Fuji I	Conventional	GC	
	Fuji I Capsule	Conventional	GC	Encapsulated
	Fuji Plus	Resin-modified	GC	
	Fuji Plus Capsule	Resin-modified	GC	Encapsulated
	Ketac-Cem Aplicap	Conventional	Espe	Encapsulated
	Ketac-Cem Maxicap	Conventional	Espe	Encapsulated
	Ketac-Cem Radiopaque	Conventional	Espe	
	Aquacem	Conventional	Dentsply	Water-activated
	Advance	Resin-modified	Dentsply	
	Vitremer Luting Cement	Resin-modified	3M	
	Hy-Bond Glas Ionomer CX	Conventional	Shofu	
Filling	Fuji II	Conventional	GC	
	Fuji Ionomer Type II–F	Conventional	GC	
	Fuji II Capsule	Conventional	GC	Encapsulated
	Fuji II LC	Resin-modified	GC	
	Fuji II LC Capsule	Resin-modified	GC	Encapsulated
	Fuji II LC Improved	Resin-modified	GC	
	Chelon-Fil	Conventional	Espe	
	Ketac-Fil Plus Aplicap	Conventional	Espe	Encapsulated
	Photac-Fil	Resin-modified	Espe	
	Photac-Fil Quick Aplicap	Resin-modified	Espe	Encapsulated
	Chem-Fil II	Conventional	Dentsply	Water-activated
	Chem-Fil II	Conventional	Dentsply	Encapsulated
	Chem-Fil Superior	Conventional	Dentsply	Water-activated
	Glas Ionomer F	Conventional	Shofu	
	Hy-Bond Glas Ionomer F	Conventional	Shofu	
	Vitremer	Resin-modified	3M	
	Alpha Fil	Conventional	DMG	
	Aqua Ionofil	Conventional	Voco	
Filling (highly viscous)	Fuji IX	Conventional	GC	
	Fuji IX GP	Conventional	GC	
	Fuji IX GP Capsule	Conventional	GC	Encapsulated
	Ketac-Molar	Conventional	Espe	
	Ketac-Molar Aplicap	Conventional	Espe	Encapsulated
	Ketac-Molar Maxicap	Conventional	Espe	Encapsulated
	Hi-Fi	Conventional	Shofu	

Clinical Application	Product	Classification	Manufacturer	Notes
Metal reinforced	Miracle Mix	Metal-reinforced	GC	
	Miracle Mix Capsule	Metal-reinforced	GC	Encapsulated
	Chelon-Silver	Metal-reinforced	Espe	
	Ketac-Silver Aplicap	Metal-reinforced	Espe	Encapsulated
	Ketac-Silver Maxicap	Metal-reinforced	Espe	Encapsulated
	Hi-Dense	Metal-reinforced	Shofu	
	Alpha Silver	Metal-reinforced	DMG	
	Aqua Silver	Metal-reinforced	Voco	
Base/liner	GC Lining Cement	Conventional	GC	
	Fuji Lining LC	Resin-modified	GC	
	GC Dentin Cement	Conventional	GC	
	Fuji II LC Core Material	Resin-modified	GC	
	Ketac-Bond	Conventional	Espe	
	Ketac-Bond Aplicap	Conventional	Espe	Encapsulated
	Photac-Bond Aplicap	Resin-modified	Espe	Encapsulated
	VitreBond	Resin-modified	3M	
	BaseLine	Conventional	Denstply	
	Base Cement	Conventional	Shofu	
	Hy-Bond Liner	Conventional	Shofu	
Fissure protection	Fuji III	Conventional	GC	
	Fuji III LC	Resin-modified	GC	
Bonding agent	Fuji Bond LC	Resin-modified	GC	
Root surface sealing	Cervical Cement	Conventional	GC	
Root canal sealing	Ketac-Endo Aplicap	Conventional	Espe	Encapsulated
Orthodontic bracket bonding	Fuji Ortho	Resin-modified	GC	
	Fuji Ortho LC	Resin-modified	GC	
	Fuji Ortho LC Capsule	Resin-modified	GC	Encapsulated
Orthodontic band bonding	Multi-Cure Glass-ionomer Orthodontic Band Cement	Resin-modified	3M Unitek	

cement as a polyalkenoate cement.[9] However, the term *glass-ionomer cement* has been more widely accepted by dental professionals and describes this material more accurately.

Traditional Glass-Ionomer Cements

Definition

The first glass-ionomer cement developed by Wilson and Kent[10,11] was a product of an acid-base reaction between basic fluoroaluminosilicate glass powder and polycarboxylic acid in the presence of water. The nature of the set cement comprised an organic-inorganic complex with high molecular weight. Therefore, glass-ionomer cement can be defined as a water-based material that hardens following an acid-base reaction between fluoroaluminosilicate glass powder and an aqueous solution of polyacid.

Composition and Structure of Filler Particles

The glass was developed on the basis of dental silicate cements and was prepared by melting alumina (Al_2O_3), silica (SiO_2), metal oxides, metal fluorides, and metal phosphates at temperatures higher than 1,100°C. The metal ions are usually selected from aluminum (Al), calcium (Ca), strontium (Sr), zinc (Zn), sodium (Na), potassium (K), and lanthanum (La). Phosphate and fluoride are used to decrease the melting temperature in the production process and are incorporated into the glass composition to modify the setting characteristics. Lanthanum oxide (La_2O_3) and strontium oxide (SrO) are incorporated to provide radiopaque cement. Barium sulfate ($BaSO_4$), La_2O_3, SrO, and zinc oxide (ZnO) also can be added to the glass powder, but not within the glass composition. The essential ingredients of the glass are aluminum oxide and silicon dioxide, which form the skeletal structure of the glass (Fig 1-1). The structure is a tetrahedron with a three-dimensional silicate glass structure. The aluminum ion may replace the silica ion in the center site of the tetrahedron[12] and has a four-coordinate number in the skeletal structure similar to that of the silicon ion. Because electric neutrality must be maintained in the total system, alkaline ions or alkaline earth ions (Na^+, K^+, Ca^{2+}, and Sr^{2+}) exist near the Al_3+ ion. These work as modifying ions and decrease the molecular weight of the silicate structure. The modified metal ions induce the high reactivity of the glass with the polyacid. Fluoride or phosphate ions also are present in the glass structure. These negatively charged ions are not included in the skeletal structure of the silicon tetrahedron.

The melted glass is crushed, milled, and powdered to fine particles. The particle size and distribution of the glass powder is of great importance for controlling the setting characteristics of the cement.[13] Fluoroaluminosilicate glass possesses a unique feature in that it releases fluorine without adding other fluoride compounds to the cement. The main source of this release from the set cement is thought to be the cement matrix; however, some of the fluorine is believed to originate in the glass core.

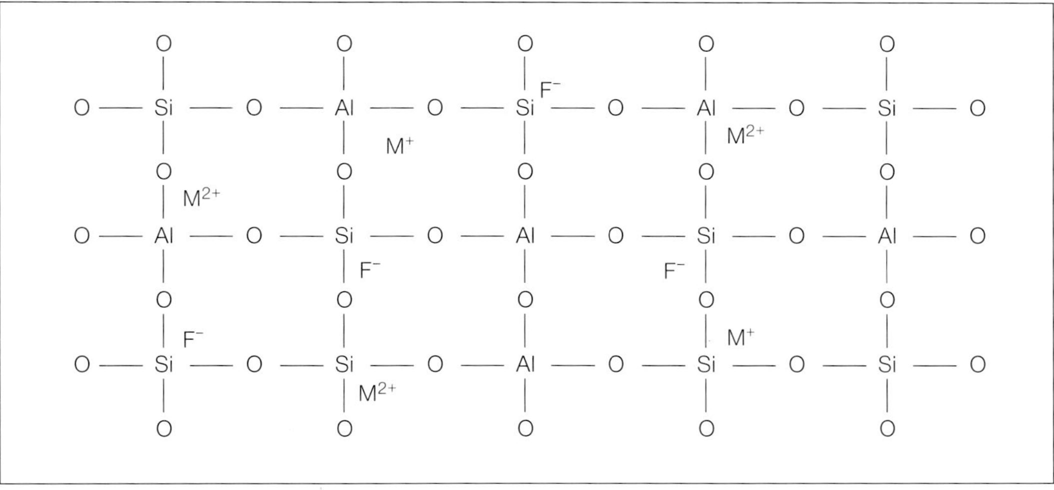

Fig 1-1 Skeletal structure of fluoroaluminosilicate glass (a tetrahedron). Si is in the center and O is at the vertex. Al can replace the Si site, is attacked by the H^+ ion, and can react with anion. The modified ion M^{2+} (Ca^{2+}, Sr^{2+}, Na^+, K^+, etc) also is reactive. F^- is not in the tetrahedron so it can diffuse through the glass structure.

Because fluorine does not exist in the skeletal structure of the glass, fluorine in the glass core probably diffuses throughout the cement matrix and is then released slowly. The physical properties of glass-ionomer cement do not deteriorate even after fluorine release. Many studies have suggested the ability of glass-ionomer cement to recharge fluorine is a feature of the fluorine movement within the cement matrix.[14–17] In other words, when the level of fluorine ions increases in the proximity of the glass-ionomer cement restoration, fluorine diffuses into and is accumulated in the cement. When the level of fluorine ions in the environment decreases, the accumulated fluorine ions are released again. This feature tries to maintain constant levels of fluorine in the oral environment. Figure 1-2 shows the levels of fluorine ions released from Fuji IX and Fuji III which are usable for fissure protection sealant as measured with fluorine electrodes. These results show the ability of a glass-ionomer cement to release small amounts of fluorine over an extended period.

Composition and structure of matrix-forming polyacid

The polyacid that reacts with the fluoroaluminosilicate glass in the glass-ionomer system is usually a polycarboxylic acid. Recently polyvinyl phosphonic acid also has been introduced to this system.[18] The acids that may be included in the glass-ionomer cement (Fig 1-3) are known as polyacrylic acid, polymaleic acid, acrylic acid–itaconic acid copolymer, acrylic acid–maleic acid copolymer, acrylic acid–2 butene dicarboxylic acid copolymer, and polyvinyl phosphonic acid. The reactivity of the poly-acid depends on the

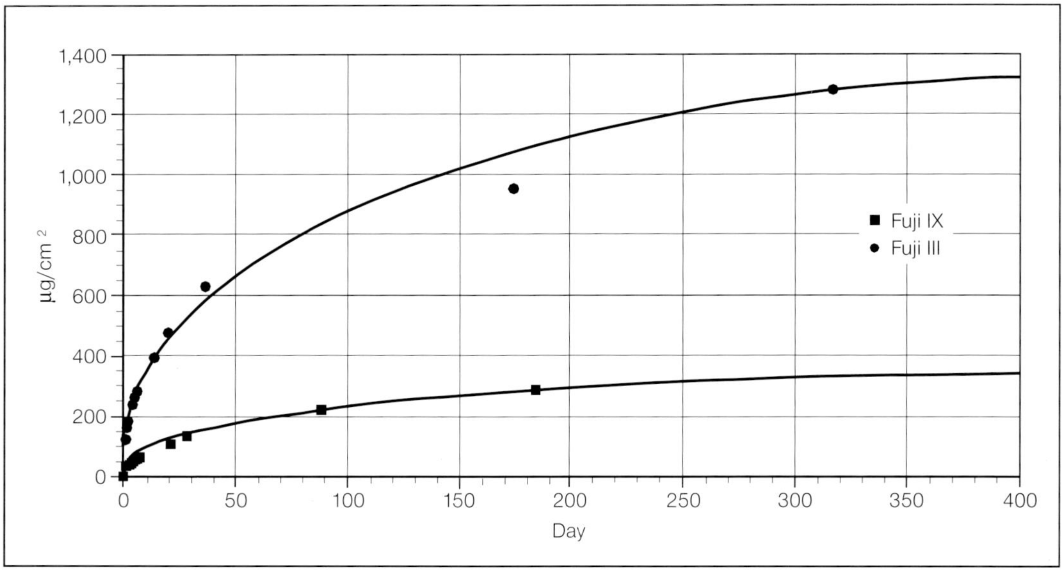

Fig 1-2 Mean cumulative fluoride release from fissure protection materials.

ingredients of the copolymer, as well as its molecular weight and concentration. By adding maleic or itaconic acid to the acrylic acid, the number of carboxylic groups based on the total molecular weight and reactivity are increased.

The polyacid either is part of the liquid as an aqueous solution or is incorporated into the cement powder as a freeze-dried powder. In the latter case, the liquid is simply water in which the freeze-dried polyacid dissolves on mixing.

Thanks to the presence of these particular acids, the glass-ionomer cement has the ability to adhere to tooth structures or metals without the additional step of a special substrate treatment. Although the mechanism of adhesion to the tooth structure and metal has not been elucidated completely, it is supposed that the primary source of this ability is the ionic reaction of the carboxyl group in the polymer acid with metal ions. It is also possibile that a chelating linkage exists, because glass-ionomer cements can adhere to metal. Measurements of the adhesion of glass-ionomer cements to metal using X-ray photoelectron spectroscopy (ESCA) suggest that the interaction occurrs between the carboxylic acid in the cement and metal ions.19 The mechanism of adhesion and bonding is discussed in detail in other chapters of this book.

Because glass-ionomer cement contains polyacrylic acid in its liquid component, its low pH can influence living tissues. The unset cement mixture exhibits an acidity which can adversely affect exposed pulp. On the other hand, the fully set cement has no acidic effect on the environmental fluid.[20] The biocompatibility of glass-ionomer cements is addressed elsewhere in this book.

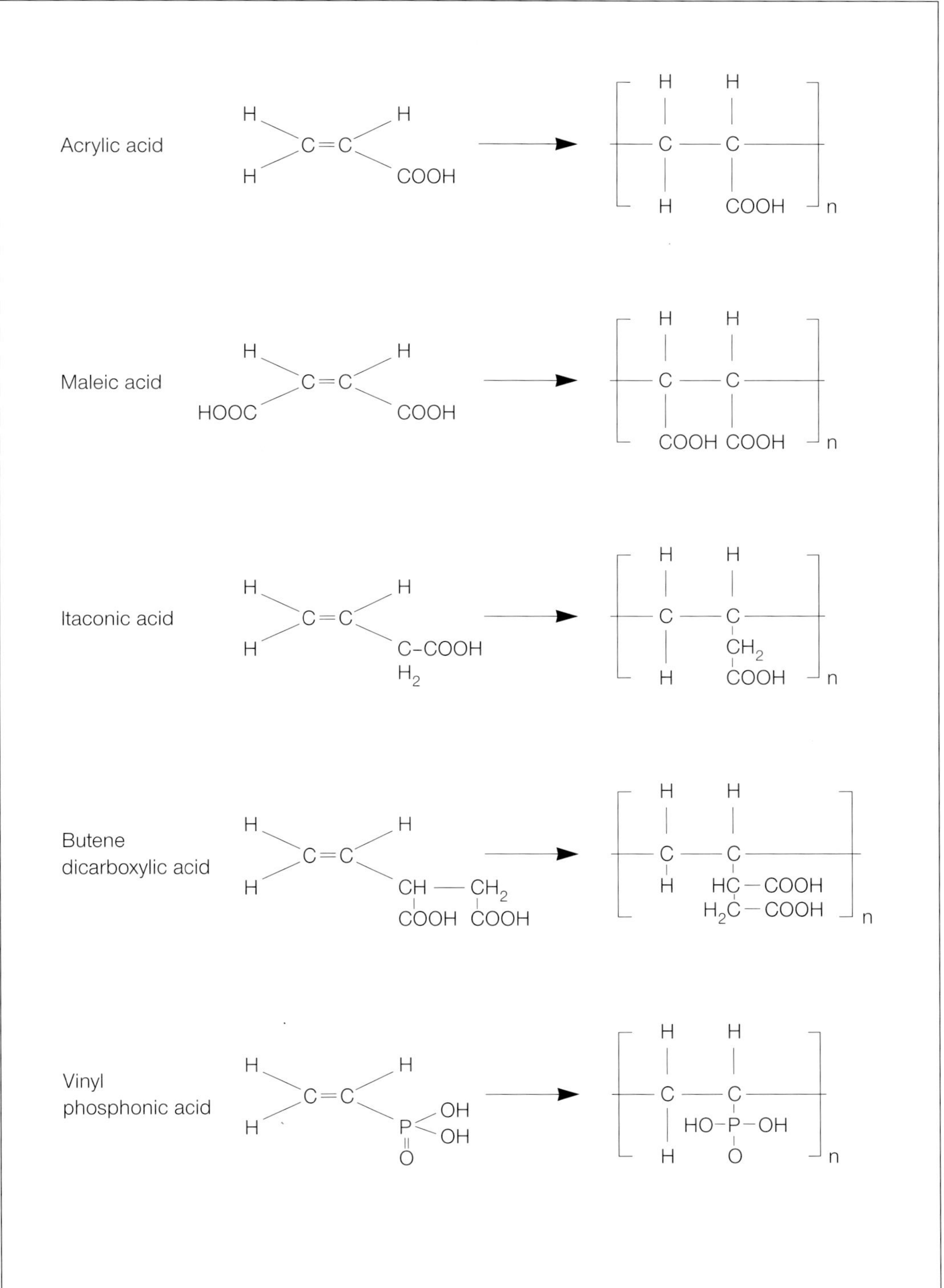

Fig 1-3 Acids that may form the polyacid component of glass-ionomer cements.

Fig 1-4 Setting reaction of glass-ionomer cement. Glass powder and polyacrylic acid are mixed, and the H^+ ion released from the polyacrylic acid attacks the glass surface. The metal ion is released from the glass following the H^+ ion attack. The metal reacts with the polyacrylic acid, and the surface of the glass particle forms a silica gel layer.

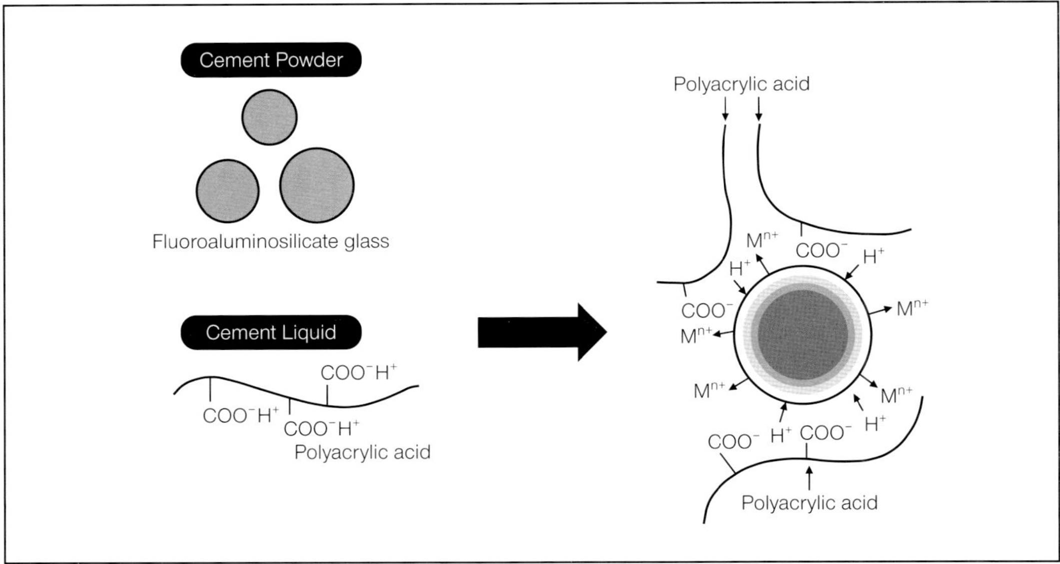

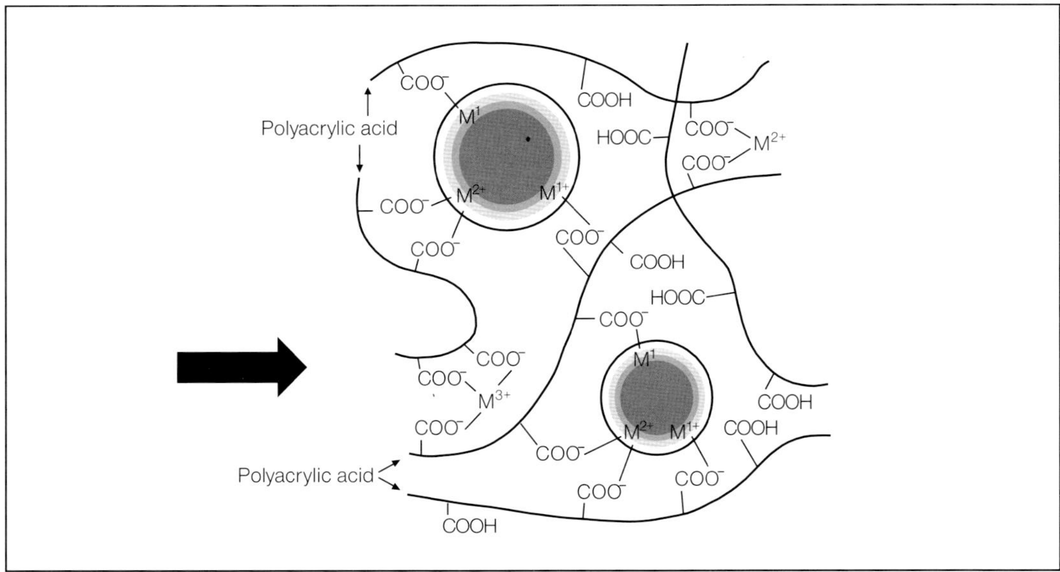

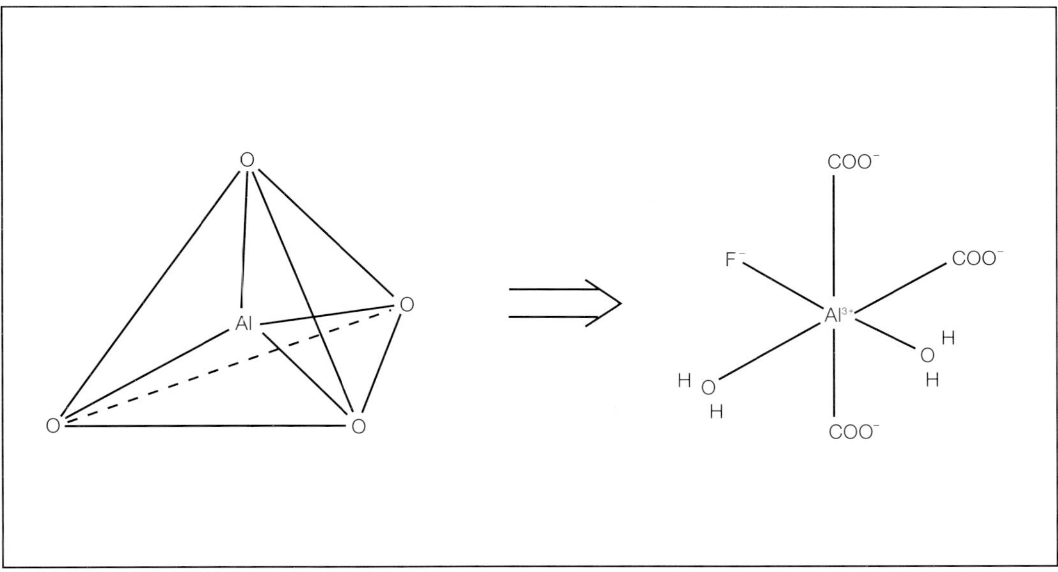

Fig 1-5 Ligand of aluminum ion in the hardened matrix. Al^{3+} ion is surrounded by four oxygen atoms in the glass and by six atoms in the set cement matrix. The six atoms should comprise the selected atoms the carboxylic acid group, water, the fluoride ion, and other anionic ions.

Setting reaction

The setting reaction of conventional glass-ionomer cements starts when the fluoroaluminosilicate glass powder and the aqueous solution of polyacrylic acid are combined, producing an acid-base reaction with the powdered fluoroaluminosilicate glass as the base:

Fluoroaluminosilicate glass (base) + Polyacid (acid) → Polyacid matrix (salts)

The hydrogen ions of the acid attack the glass particles in the presence of water, releasing calcium, strontium, and aluminum ions. The metal ions combine with the carboxylic acid groups of the polyacid to form the polyacid salts matrix, and the glass surface is changed to a silica hydrogel (Fig 1-4). Although the aluminum ion in the aluminum oxide does not react with acid, it does react when present in the silicate glass. It has been reported that the coordination state of the aluminum ion changes with the setting reaction.[21] The aluminum ion, which is initially surrounded by four oxygen atoms in the glass, is surrounded by six atoms in the set cement matrix.[22] The Al^{3+} ion in the set cement should be coordinated to six atoms selected from the carboxylic acid groups, water, fluoride ions, and other anionic ions (Fig 1-5).

The surface layer of the glass powder

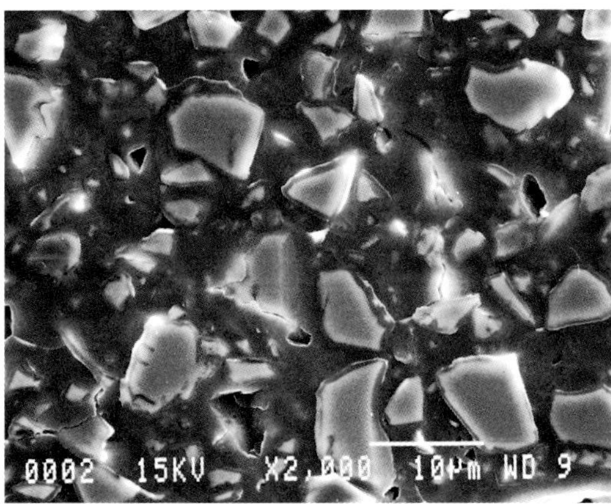

Fig 1-6a Scanning electron micrograph of hardened Fuji I glass-ionomer cement for luting. (Original magnification ×2,000.)

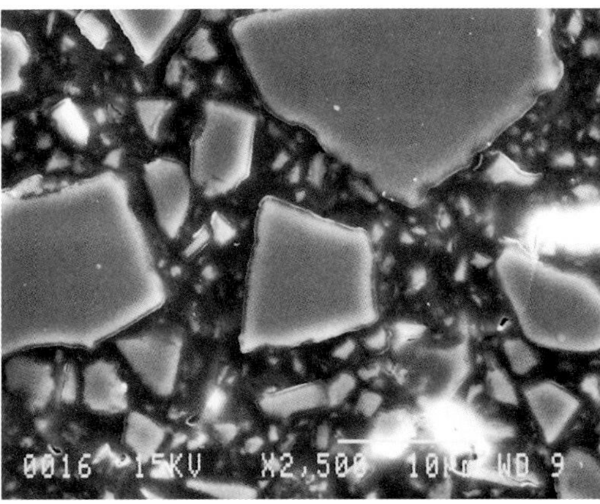

Fig 1-6b Scanning electron micrograph of hardened Fuji IX glass-ionomer cement for restorative filling. (Original magnification ×2,000.)

reacts with acid, whereas the glass core remains intact. The glass core exists as filler in the cement matrix. The reactivity of the glass surface controls the nature of the set cement. The surface layer of the glass powder becomes a silicon-rich layer. A silica gel layer is then formed at the interface between the cement matrix and the glass particles. This layer has not been analyzed, however, the concentration gradient of the elements should exist in this silica gel. The constitutional metal elements decrease from the inner core to the outer surface with a small gradient of silicon ions. The intersurface of a glass-ionomer cement is different from the intersurface of fillers in a resin composite. The filler and matrix in a resin composite only bind by way of a silane-coupling agent.

There is no concentration gradient in the interface of the filler particles and the hardened matrix for resin composite.

Scanning electron microscopy (SEM) of hardened Fuji I luting cement and Fuji IX restorative filling (Fig 1-6) shows there is a thicker silica gel layer in Fuji I. This layer needs a period of weeks or even months to harden fully. At any time during the reaction and the setting process, all these materials are sensitive to dehydration. The compressive strength of a glass-ionomer cement increases over 1 year (Fig 1-7).[23] Some studies have reported that the cement requires several months to become stable.

Types of conventional glass-ionomer cements

As shown in Table 1-1, glass-ionomers are currently used for various clinical applications. A large number of products are available, each with a more or less different formulation to fulfill the required characteristics for a specific field of application.

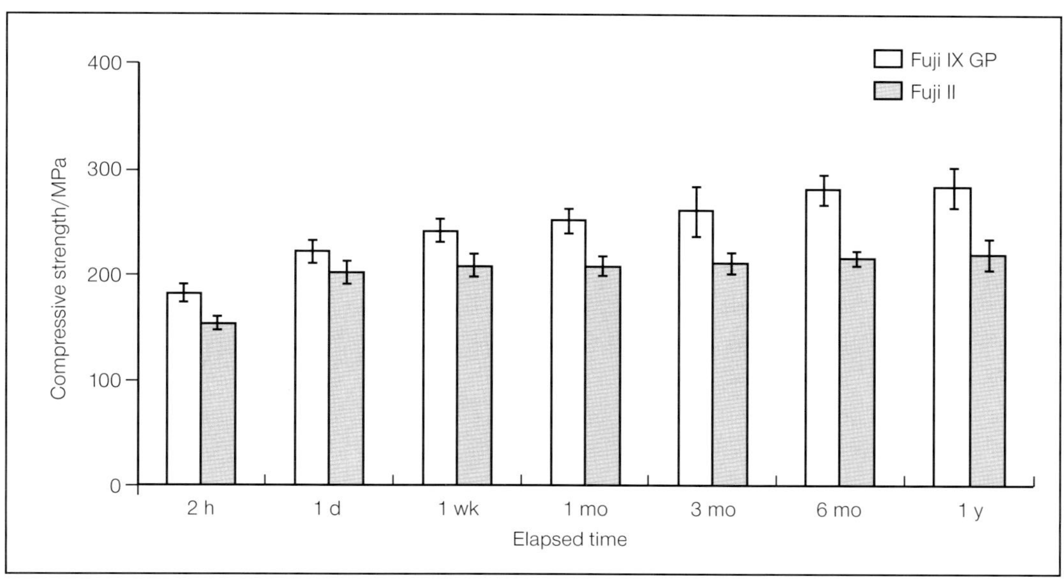

Fig 1-7 Long-term increase of compressive strength in glass-ionomer cements.

Glass-ionomers for direct restoration

The first glass-ionomer cement developed for filling was called Alumino Silicate Poly-Acrylate (ASPA; Dentsply). Currently, many glass-ionomer products are available for restorative purposes. Although resin based composites possess superior mechanical properties and better esthetics than glass-ionomer cements, composite resins require bonding agents because they are usually hydrophobic and thus do not adhere well to teeth. Glass-ionomer cements bond directly to tooth structures, offer easy handling, possess a coefficient of thermal expansion similar to that of the tooth,[24] and have a potential effect of remineralization. Glass-ionomers are widely used for pedodontic applications and for the restoration of Class III and Class V cavities (Figs 1-8a to 1-8d). They are not recommended for permanent filling of occlusal surfaces in adults where there is excessive load because of insufficient resistance to abrasion.

Metal-reinforced glass ionomers

In the interest of reinforcing glass-ionomer cements, the addition of metals to the filler component has been proposed.[25,26] The powder contains fluoroaluminosilicate glass and a silver alloy[25] or the glass is sintered with silver.[26] The latter product is called a *cermet* (*cer*amic, or glass, and *met*al). Due to the admixing of metals, these materials are no more tooth colored than other glass-ionomer cements. They have appropriate strength, are easy to manipulate, and are sufficiently radiopaque. These properties, added to their adhesive ability to the tooth structure make cermet cements appropriate for core buildup. Clinicians may like the

Fig 1-8 Long-term clinical case using a conventional glass-ionomer restoration in a cervical defect.

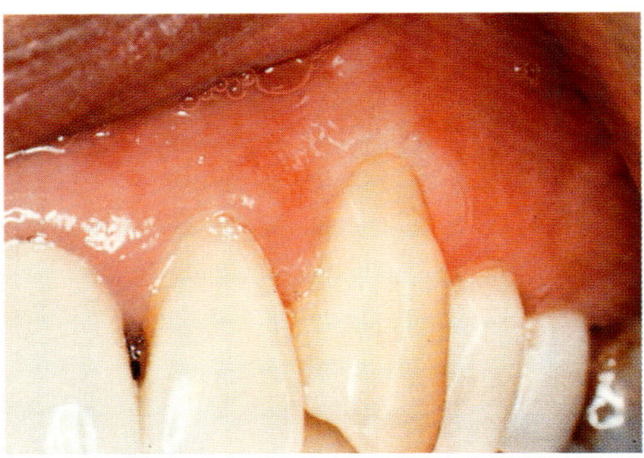

Fig 1-8a Prior to restoration.

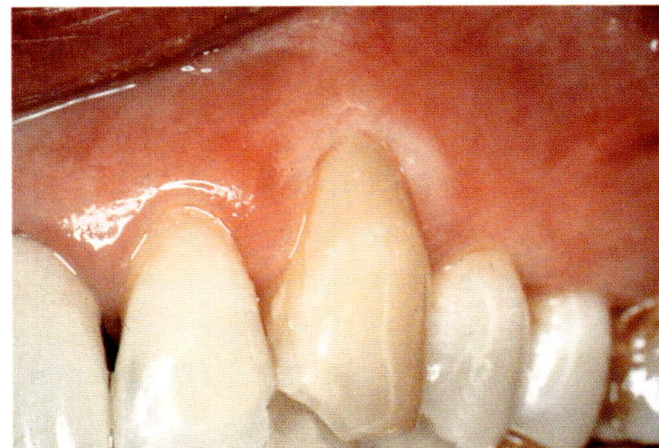

Fig 1-8b Immediately following restoration.

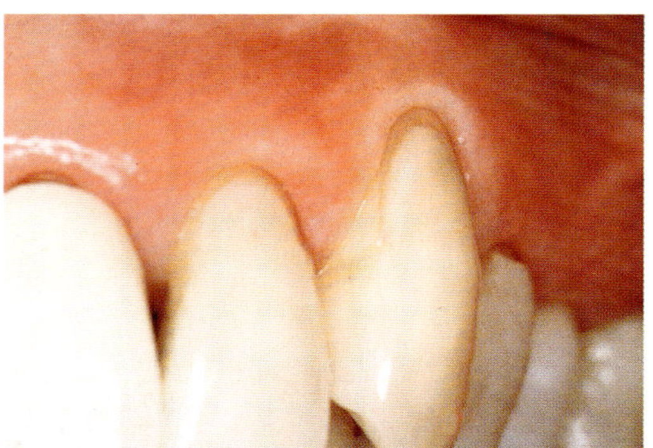

Fig 1-8c Eight years after restoration. Some wear can be seen, but there is no marginal discoloration.

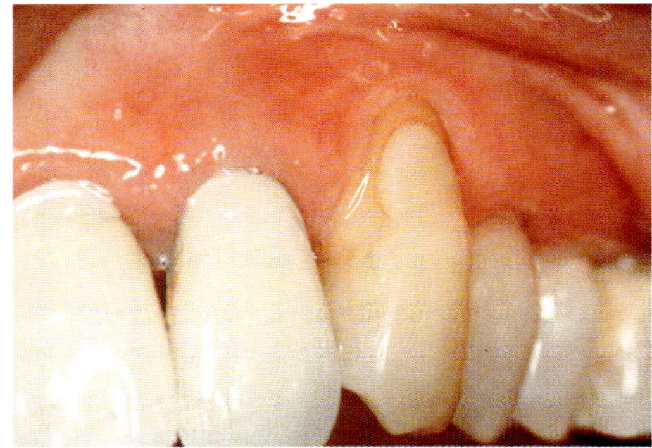

Fig 1-8d Fourteen years after restoration. The diagnosis is still good.

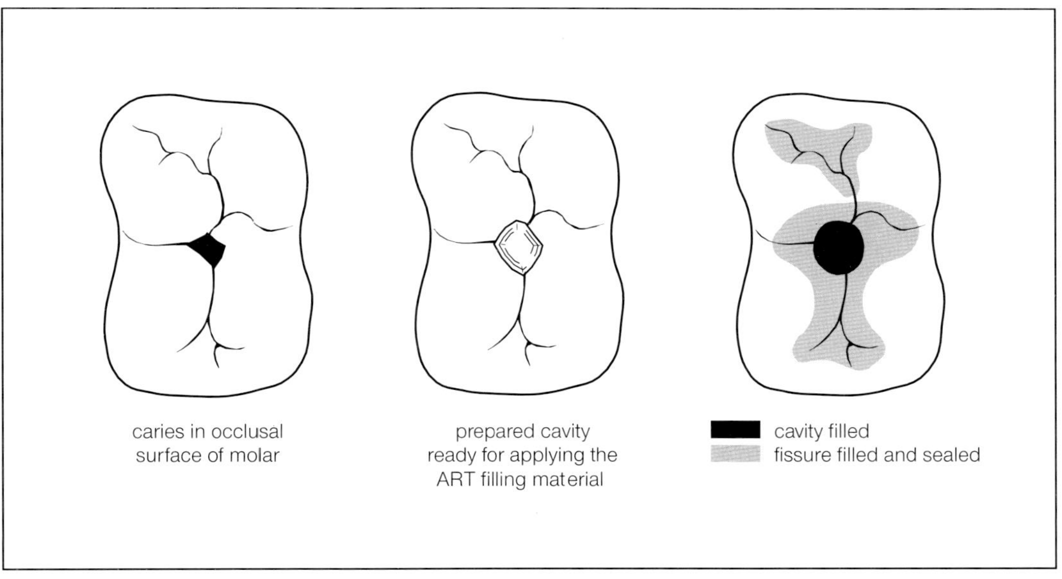

Fig 1-9 Atraumatic restorative treatment (ART) process. *(left)* Caries are identified in the occlusal surface of a molar. *(center)* The cavity is prepared for the highly viscous glass-ionomer filling material. *(right)* The cavity is filled and fissures are filled and sealed. Reprinted from World Health Organization. Manual of Atraumatic Restorative Technique, 1994.

difference between the surface hardness of the cement and the tooth structure, and the distinguished color may be helpful when preparing the tooth using burs. Metal-reinforced glass-ionomers also have been proposed as a temporary posterior restorative material.

Highly viscous glass-ionomers

The highly viscous glass-ionomer cements were designed as an alternative to amalgam for posterior preventive restorations. These glass-ionomers are particularly useful for the atraumatic restorative treatment (ART) technique. This is a procedure based on excavating carious dentin in teeth using hand instruments only and restoring the tooth with adhesive filling materials (Fig 1-9).[27] Examples of highly viscous glass-ionomer cements are Fuji IX and Ketac Molar. Such glass-ionomers are expected to be particularly effective in the ART technique when they are applied in the early stages of caries development.[28]

Due to their manipulative and mechanical characteristics, highly viscous glass-ionomers can be used for intermediate restorations, replacing amalgam, and for core buildup procedures. They are applied as glass-ionomer preventive restorations to fill cavities and to seal around them.

Low-viscosity glass ionomers

The low-viscosity glass-ionomers have been developed as liners, fissure protection materials, sealing materials for hypersensitive cervical areas,[29] and endodontic materials.[30] Such materials are designed with low powder–liquid ratios and are highly flowable.

The fluoride released from glass-ionomers strengthens the tooth structure. The low powder:liquid ratio material is expected to cause gradual dissolution from the occlusal surface when they are applied as fissure protection materials. Low-viscosity glass-ionomer cements should be suitable as fissure protection materials during the eruption period of the teeth.

Base and liner

Some glass-ionomers have been developed for base and lining applications. These materials are used for the "sandwich" technique in which they are applied as a dentin substitute and composite resin is applied as an enamel substitute.[31] Thus the advantages of both glass-ionomers and resin composite may be combined. The composite resin shows superior physical and esthetic properties, making it suitable for surface application. The glass-ionomers show a coefficient of thermal expansion similar to that of the tooth structure, good bonding to dentin, and good biocompatibility, making them suitable for application as a dentin substitute. Some studies also have reported the antibacterial effect of these materials.[32]

Luting

The glass-ionomer cements for luting are widely used for cementing metal inlays, crowns, and bridges. They are considered the most suitable luting cements, because of their ease of manipulation, bonding ability, fluoride release, and low solubility in the oral environment.[33,34] Their physical properties are well balanced compared to those of zinc phosphate cement, polycarboxylate cement, and resin cement. These cements have gone through many steps in their development.[35] Because the system is complicated, many problems had to be overcome. For example, when comparing the first version of Fuji I for luting and the current product, the physical properties have been improved significantly. As a result, the reliability and durability also have increased. Table 1-2 summarizes the long-term development of Fuji I physical properties.

Resin-Modified Glass-Ionomer Cement

Definition

Disadvantages of conventional glass-ionomer cements compared to a composite resin are inferior mechanical properties, namely bending strength, tensile strength, and fracture toughness. These properties need to be improved in order to widen the range of clinical applications.

For traditional glass-ionomer cements, some sort of hybridization at the interaction with the dentin surface has been demonstrated, as is the case with resin bonding and cements,[36] but this form of stable adhesion could be improved for the glass-ionomer cements. Resin modification of glass-ionomer cement was designed to produce favorable physical properties similar to

Table 1-2 Improvement of physical properties on Fuji I

	Fuji I (old)	Fuji I (conventional)	Fuji I (new)
Year of Development	1977	1986	1993
Powder:liquid ratio (g:g)	1.4:1.0	1.8:1.0	1.8:1.0
Working time	1 min, 00 s	1 min, 45 s	2 min, 00 s
Setting time	5 min, 30 s	5 min, 30 s	4 min, 30 s
Film thickness (μm)	25	18	15
Consistency (mm)	29	31	34
Compressive strength, 1 day (MPa)	139 (11)	177 (7)	207 (8)
Diametral tensile strength, 1 day (MPa)	8.0 (1.9)	12.0 (1.4)	12.4 (2.2)
Bond strength			
1 day, bovine enamel (MPa)	4.7 (1.2)	5.0 (1.4)	5.1 (1.3)
1 day, bovine dentin (MPa)	3.5 (0.9)	3.6 (1.2)	4.6 (1.0)
Solubility (%)			
Water	0.6	0.08	0.06
0.001M lactic acid	1.53	0.41	0.37
Radiopacity	–	+	+

Numbers in parentheses indicate standard deviations.

those of resin composites and resin cements while retaining the basic features of the conventional glass-ionomer cement.[37] This goal was achieved by incorporating water-soluble resin monomers into an aqueous solution of polyacrylic acid. In this way the system undergoes polymerization of the resin monomer while the acid-base reaction continues simultaneously. The resulting resin-modified glass-ionomer cements exhibit many advantages of both resin cements and glass-ionomer cements.

The resin-modified glass-ionomer cement is defined as a material that undergoes both polymerization reaction and acid-base reaction. The basic composition of the cement liquid is polycarboxylic acid, water, and 2-hydroxyethylmethacrylate (HEMA). It may also contain a small amount of cross-linking material. Some products, such as Vitremer, are said to contain a polycarboxylic acid modified with pendant methacrylate groups. The composition and structure of the fluoroaluminosilicate glass for resin-modified glass-ionomer cements are basically similar to those of conventional glass-ionomer cements.

Fig 1-10 Setting reaction of resin-modified glass-ionomer cement. The glass powder and cement liquid are mixed, and the H^+ ion in the liquid attacks the glass surface. The metal ion released from the glass particle reacts with polyacrylic acid while HEMA cures concurrently. The surface layer of the glass particle forms a silica gel layer.

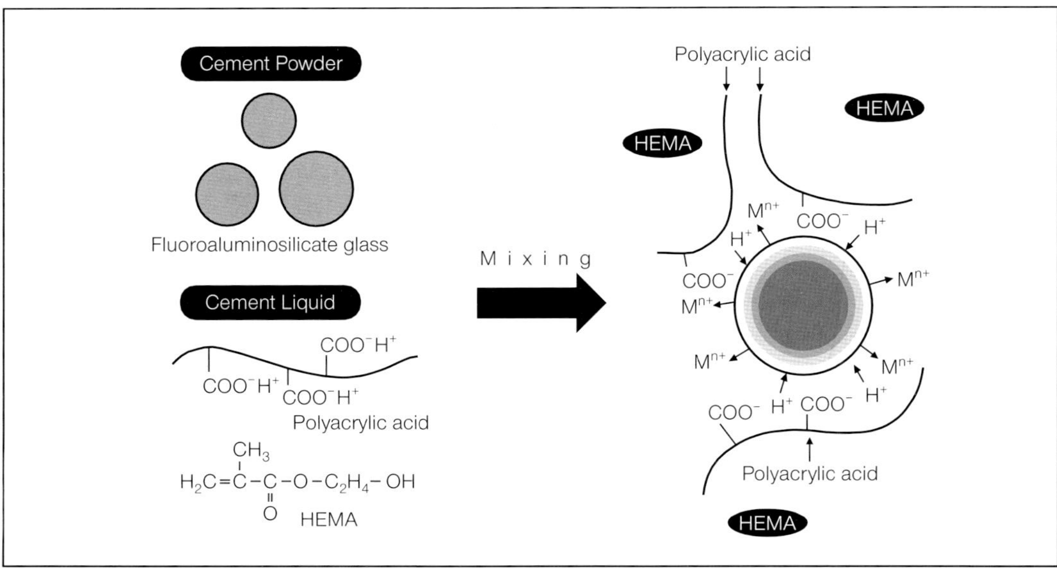

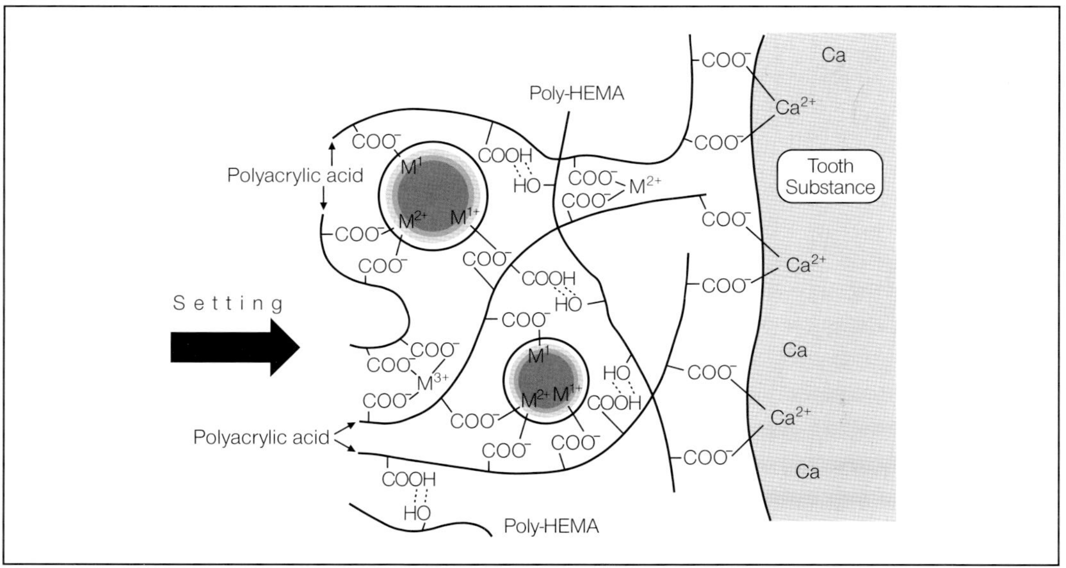

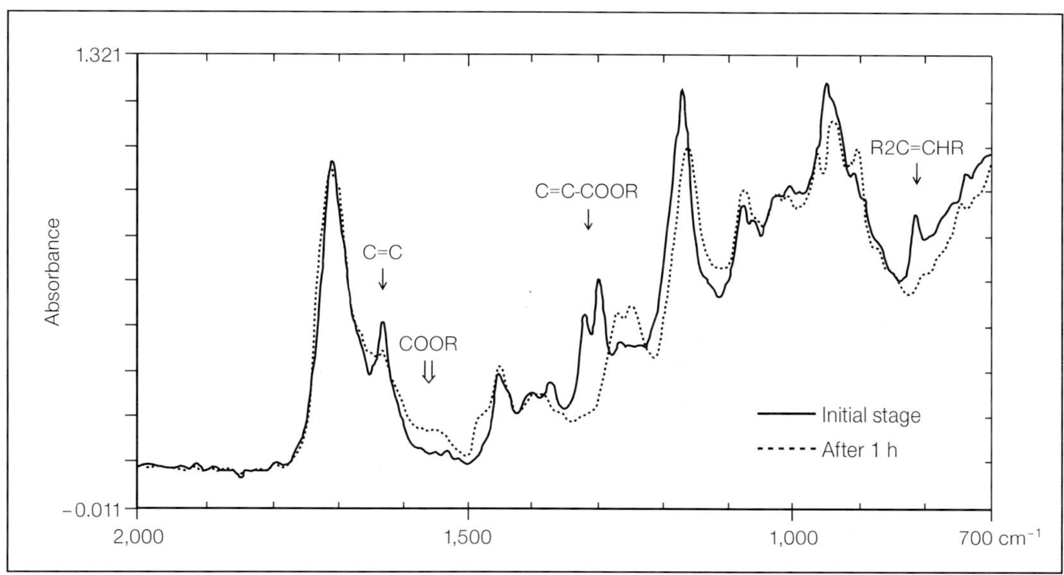

Fig 1-11 Infrared spectrum of Fuji Plus.

Setting reaction

The essential acid-base reaction between the fluoroaluminosilicate glass and the polycarboxylic acid is initiated by mixing the powder and liquid. At the same time, the polymerization of HEMA and cross-linking material is started by an oxidation-reduction or a photopolymerizing catalyst. This forms a hardened mixture in which HEMA polymer and polycarboxylic acid are supposed to be linked by hydrogen bonding (Fig 1-10). The acid with polymerizable double bonds that is included in some products is formed with a monomer. Figure 1-11 shows an infrared spectrum illustrating this mechanism in which the resin-modified glass-ionomer cement hardens. The double bonds of the polymerizable monomer included in the liquid disappear after hardening, and the number of carboxyl groups in the polyacrylic acid decreases as the acid-base reaction advances.[38,39]

One of the main disadvantages of conventional glass-ionomer cement is that when it comes in contact with water during the early stage of setting, the setting reaction is inhibited, damaging the surface of the cement. Water sensitivity could be reduced by incorporating photopolymerization, which promotes faster setting, into the setting reaction.

Rapid setting is also an advantage for color stability. Unlike conventional glass-ionomer cements, after the completion of photo-polymerization hardened resin-modified glass-ionomer cement shows the same shade as a specimen that has been immersed in water for 60 minutes

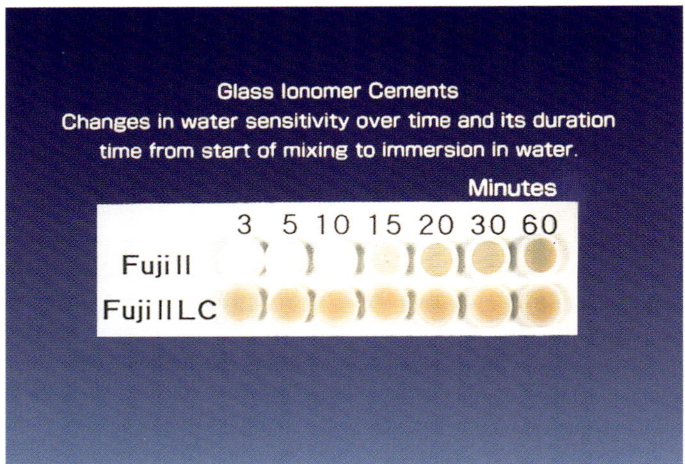

Fig 1-12 The effects of exposure to water after mixing of conventional (Fuji II) and photo polymerized (Fuji LC) glass-ionomer cements.

(Fig 1-12). In other words, water no longer inhibits the setting reaction by the time photo polymerization is completed. The color of the specimen immersed in water soon after photo polymerization is slightly lighter than the control because the resin-modified glass-ionomer cement undergoes both photo and chemical curing, (dual-cured or tricured systems). The chemical setting reaction continues even though the setting reaction initiated by light has been completed. The proportion of chemical setting in the entire process is only about 15%, but this reaction is affected by water. Although the application of varnish is much less effective for reducing water sensitivity in light-cured glass-ionomer cement than in conventional glass-ionomer cement (Figs 1-13a to 1-13d), it is beneficial to prevent contamination from water in resin-modified glass-ionomer cement.

The translucency of resin-modified glass-ionomer cements declines slightly with the lapse of time. The shade of the final restoration is slightly darker than the initial shade which should be taken into account during shade selection.

During the setting process, the pH of the liquid of resin-modified glass-ionomer cement is about 1.5 because it contains polycarboxylic acid. The pH increases as the acid-base reaction advances. This stage proceeds relatively quickly, probably because the polymerization heat of the monomer promotes the acid-base reaction. Figure 1-14 illustrates the method used to measure the pH of glass-ionomer cements; Fig 1-15 shows the results of surface pH measurements of four commercial products.

Fig 1-13 The effect of varnish application over glass-ionomer restorations.

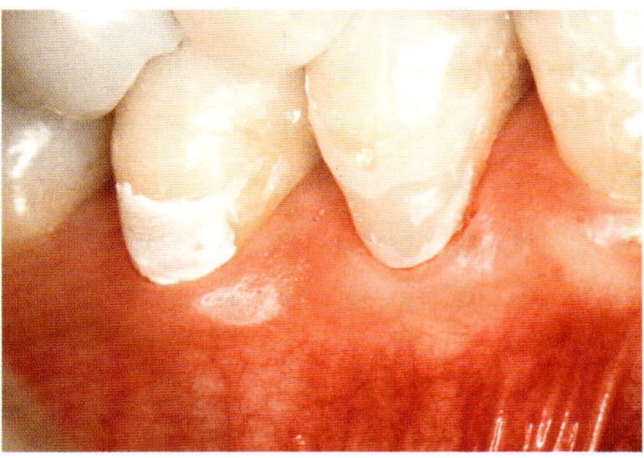

Fig 1-13a Teeth 44 and 45 were restored with conventional glass-ionomer. Varnish was applied on tooth 44 only.

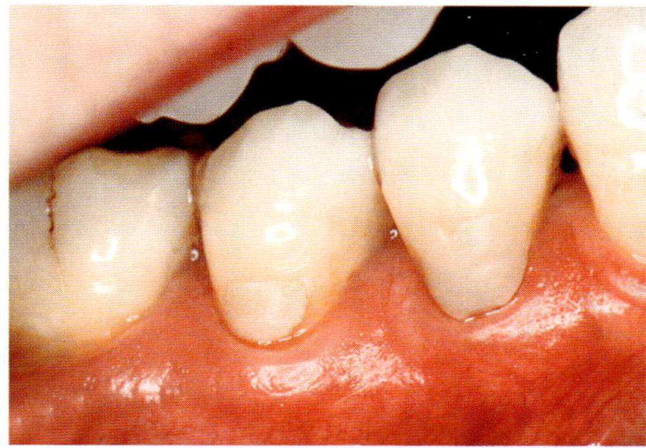

Fig 1-13b After 3 years, the effect of early water exposure on the restoration in tooth 45 can be observed as wear at the periphery of the filling.

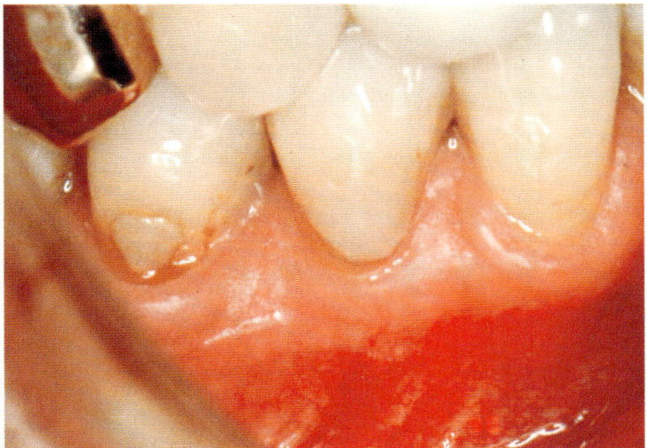

Fig 1-13c After 8 years, the condition of the restoration in tooth 45 is bad.

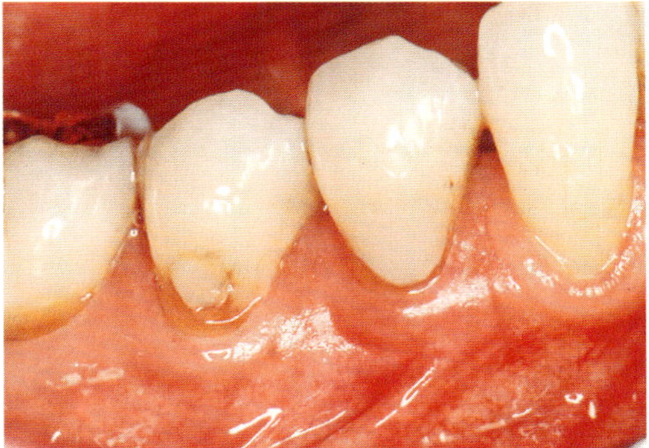

Fig 1-13d After 12 years, the restoration in tooth 45 looks worse, while that in tooth 44 is still in good condition.

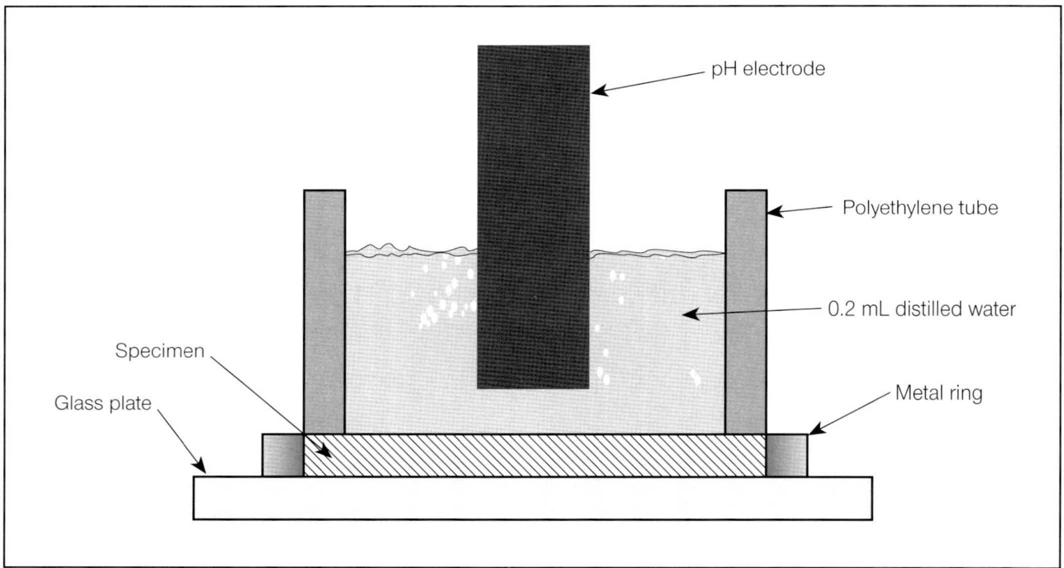

Fig 1-14 Surface pH measurement of glass-ionomer cement.

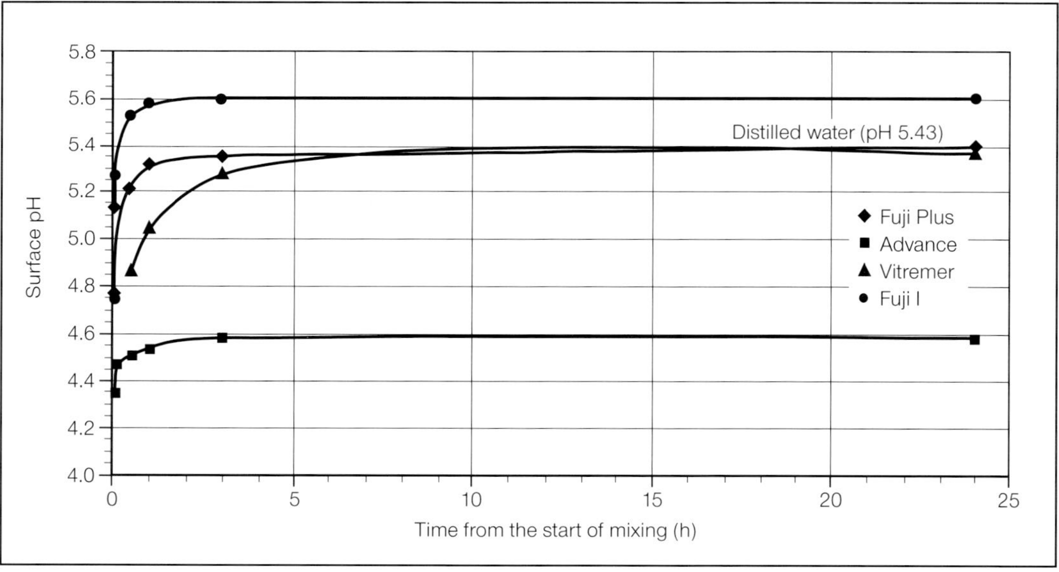

Fig 1-15 Changes in surface pH for four glass-ionomer luting cements.

Adhesion to tooth structures

It is presumed that the ionic reactivity of a resin-modified glass-ionomer cement to the tooth surface is lower than that of a conventional glass-ionomer cement. However, it can be markedly increased by treating the tooth surface with an acid conditioner. Preparation of the dentin surface with a strong acid such as phosphoric acid weakens the surface's adhesiveness, therefore polyacrylic acid or citric acid are usually used for this purpose. Ferric chloride and aluminum chloride are occasionally used in combination with these acids. It is supposed that these agents stimulate the astringent action of collagen at the interface between the tooth surface and the glass-ionomer cement.[40] Figures 1-16a and 1-16b illustrate the effects of treating the tooth surface with two different acid liquids.

The most notable determinant for how the tooth surface is treated is the use of resin-modified or conventional glass-ionomer cement.[41, 42] Scanning electron micrographs (Figs 1-17a and 1-17b) of the cement-enamel and cement-dentin interfaces with both resin-modified and conventional glass-ionomer cements show that, with conditioning, the resin-modified material apparently forms a hybrid layer whereas the conventional material does not. Treating the enamel surface with phosphoric acid does not decrease the bond of either type of cement, and the bond is stabilized. An aqueous solution of citric acid–ferric chloride or of polyacrylic acid–aluminum chloride also is effective in increasing either cement's adhesiveness. It is probably best to use conditioning materials that exhibit acidity at the same level as that of an aqueous solution of polyacrylic acid and aluminum chloride when both enamel and dentin are treated simultaneously. The bond strength of a resin-modified glass-ionomer cement increases because its tensile strength improves with the treatment. Figure 1-18 shows the bonding strength of a resin-modified glass-ionomer cement compared with that of a conventional glass-ionomer cement in bovine enamel and dentin. Bond strength was particularly stable after thermal cycling (Fig 1-19), suggesting the effectiveness of the surface conditioning. Further details related to the mechanism of adhesion to tooth structure are discussed elsewhere in this book. Figures 1-20a to 1-20d illustrate a clinical situation in which restoration with materials other than a resin-modified glass-ionomer cement as bonding agent would be difficult.

Types of resin-modified glass-ionomer cements

Restorative materials

One of the main disadvantages of conventional glass-ionomer cement as a direct restorative material is the need to avoid polishing immediately after placement. This clinical caution is required to prevent deterioration of the material's physical properties caused by water sensitivity during the initial stage of the setting process. The introduction of photo curing to the resin-modified glass-ionomer cement has made the material significantly less sensitive to water. The popular products in this category are Fuji II LC,

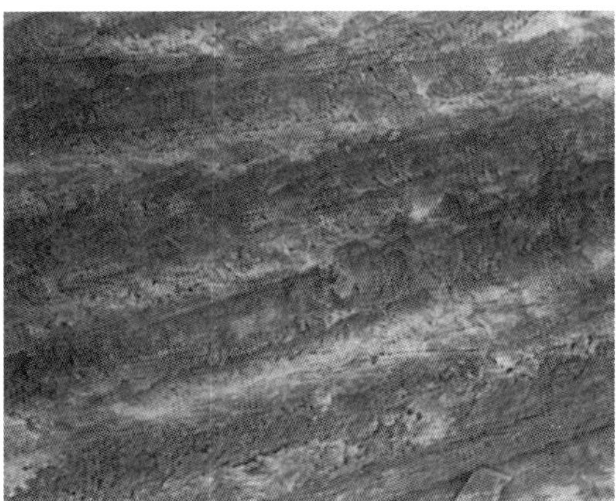
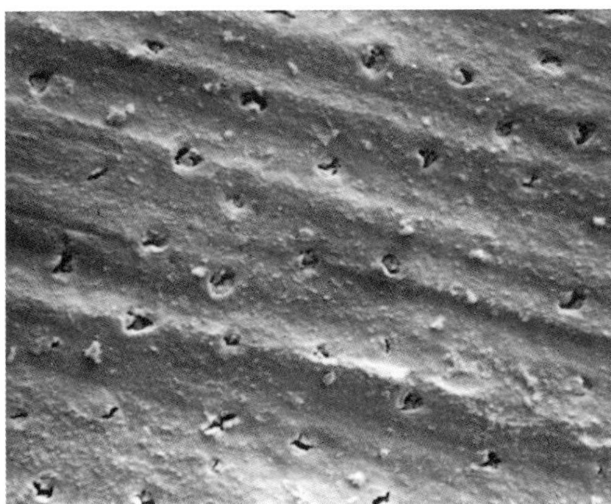

Fig 1-16a Scanning electron micrograph of human enamel and dentin treated GC Cavity Conditioner, with 20% polyacrylic acid + 3% aluminum chloride. (Original magnification ×2,000.)

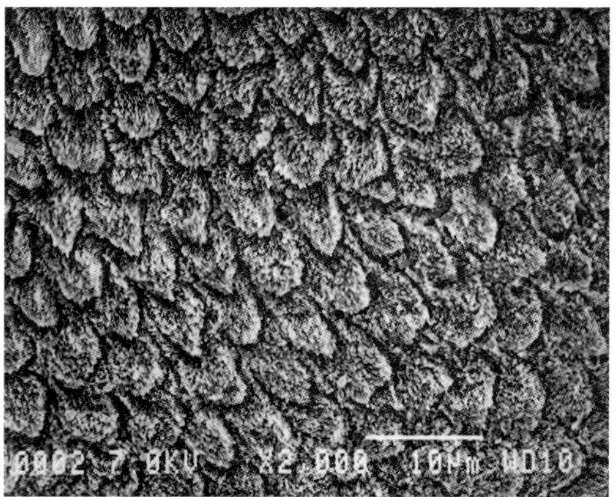

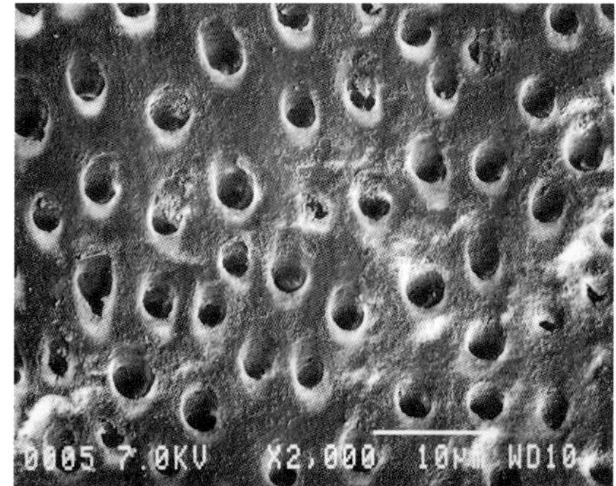

Fig 1-16b Scanning electron micrograph of human enamel and dentin treated with phosphoric acid. (Original magnification ×2,000.)

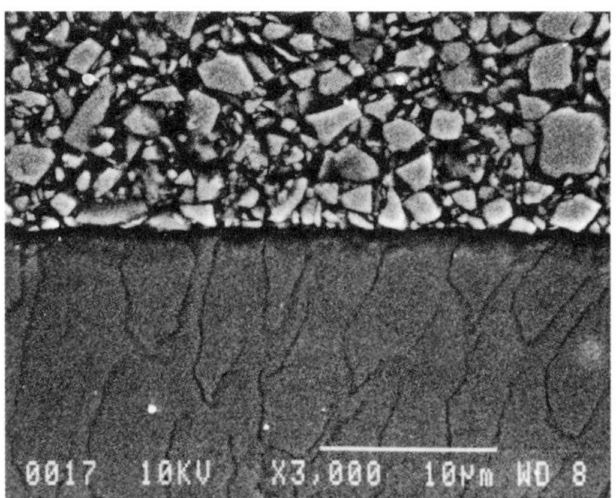

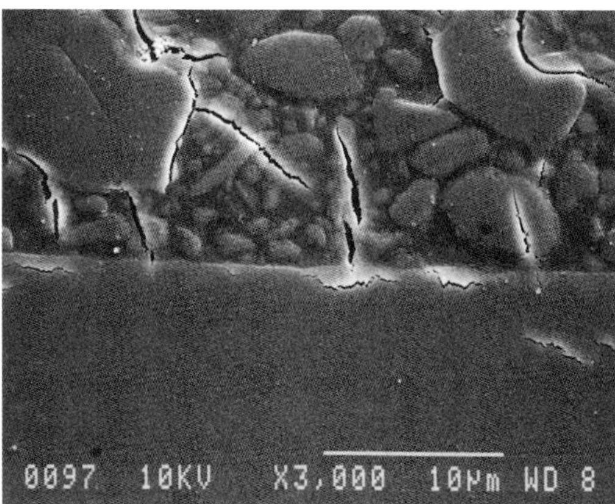

Fig 1-17a Scanning electron micrographs of the interface between glass-ionomer cements and human enamel. *(left)* Fuji II LC Improved, a resin-modified glass-ionomer. (Original magnification ×3,000.) *(right)* Fuji IX, a conventional glass-ionomer. (Original magnification ×3,000.)

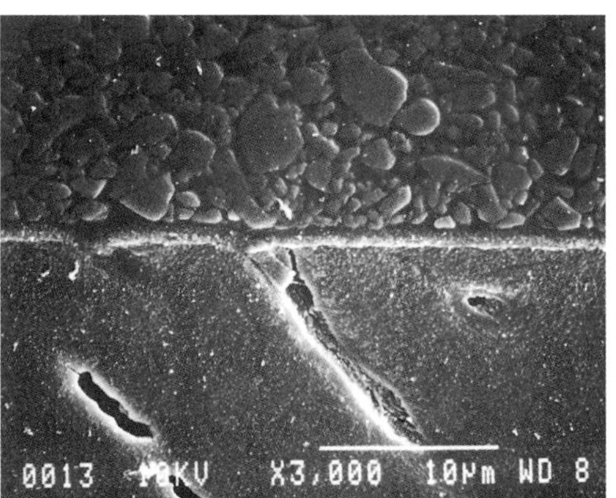

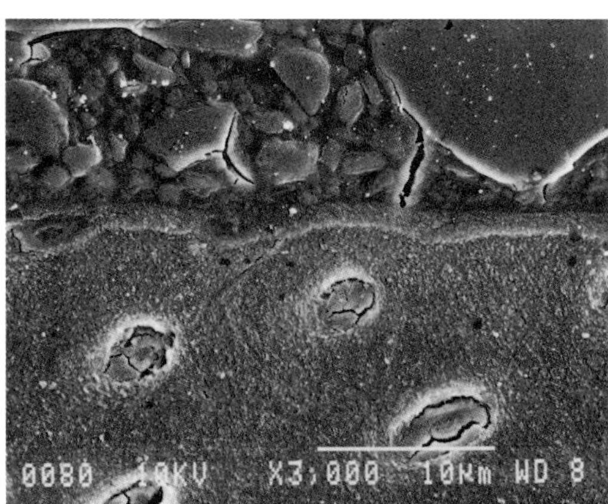

Fig 1-17b Scanning electron micrographs of the interface between glass-ionomer cements and human dentin. *(left)* Fuji II LC Improved, a resin-modified glass-ionomer. (Original magnification ×3,000.) *(right)* Fuji IX, a conventional glass-ionomer. (Original magnification ×3,000.)

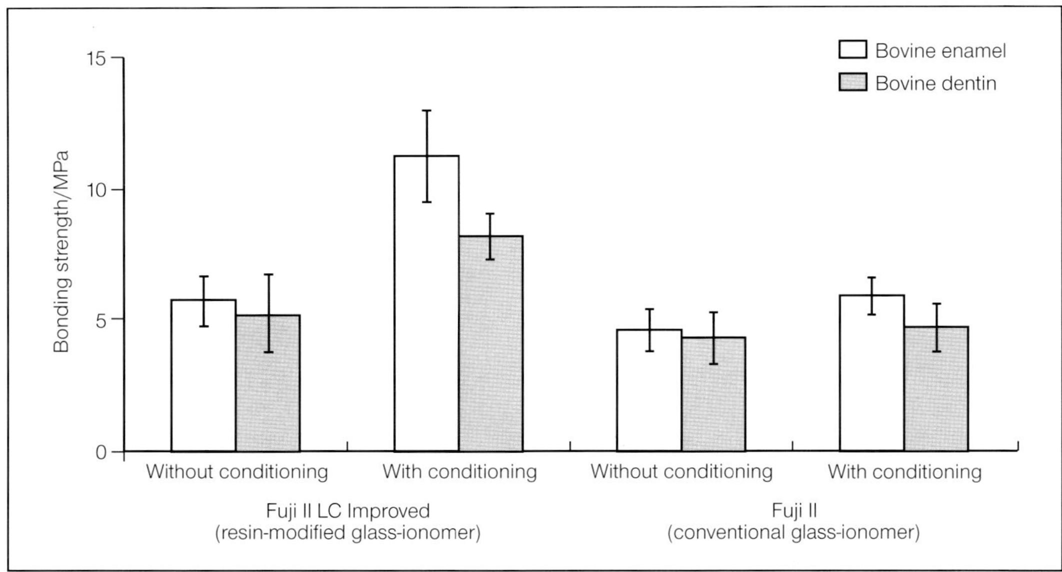

Fig 1-18 Bond strength of two glass-ionomer restorative materials in bovine enamel and dentin.

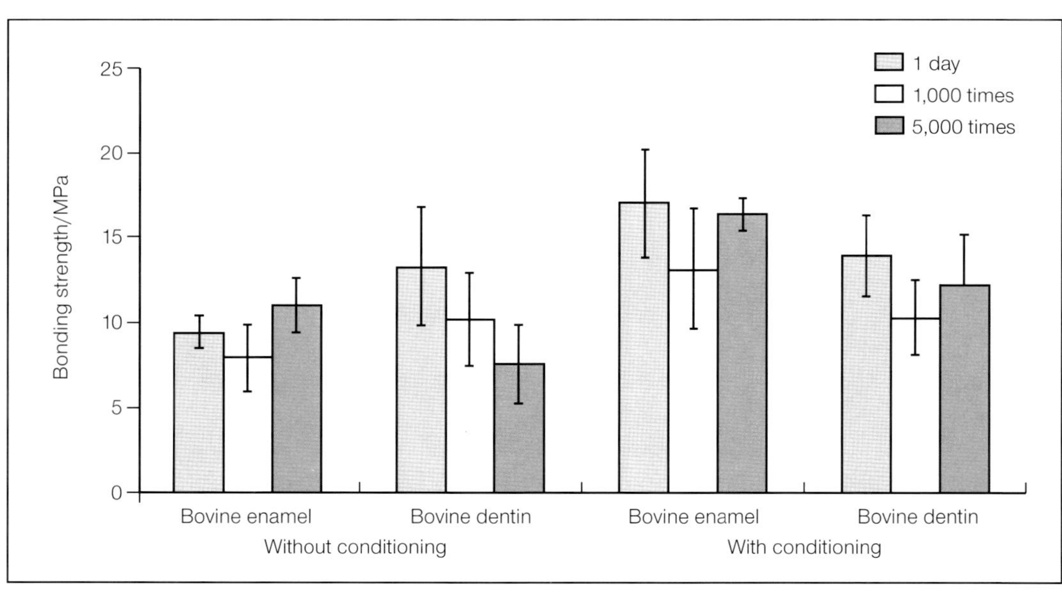

Fig 1-19 The effect of conditioning on the bonding strength of Fuji Plus following thermal cycling 4°C, 30s - 55°C, 30s.

Fig 1-20 A clinical case involving a composite resin restoration with resin-modified glass-ionomer used as a bonding material.

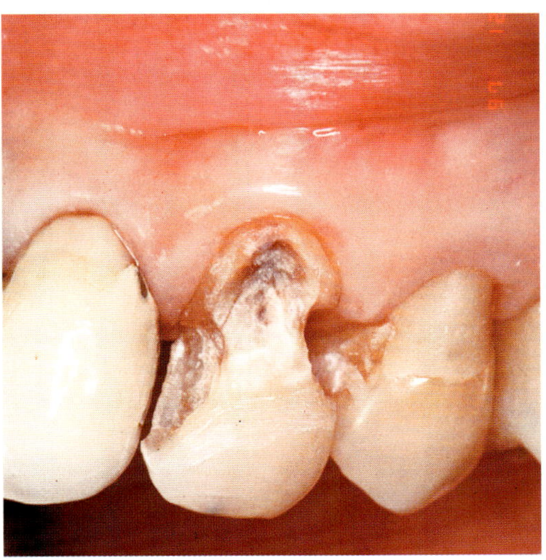

Fig 1-20a After preparation, discolored hard dentin is left.

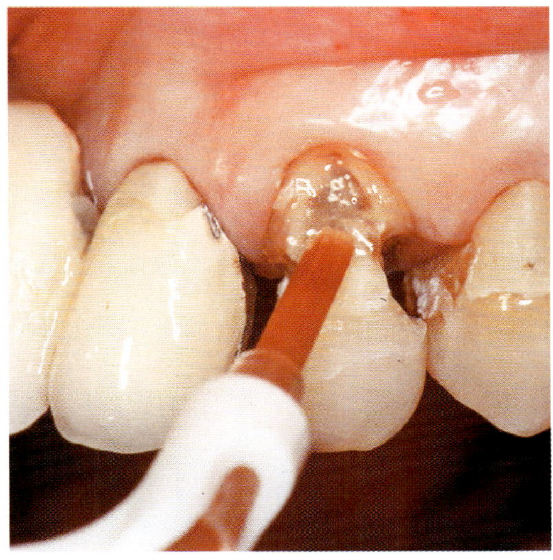

Fig 1-20b Application of Fuji Bond LC.

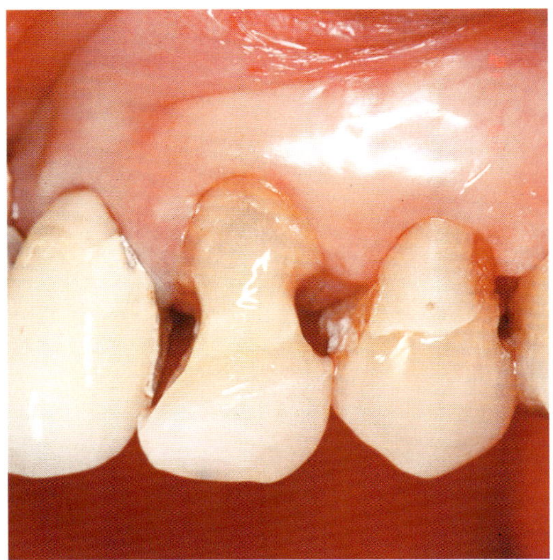

Fig 1-20c The bonding material concealing the discolored dentin.

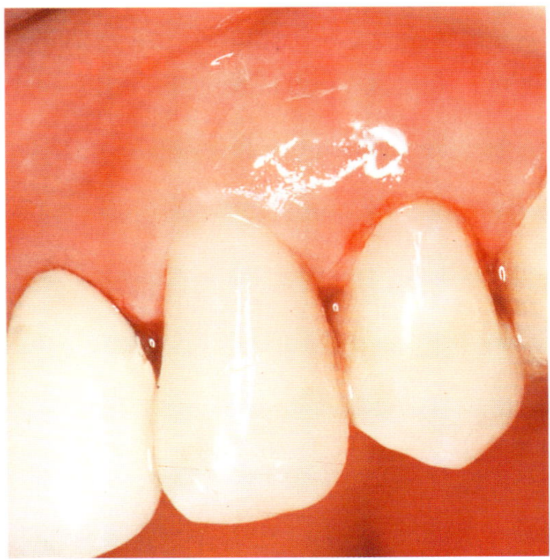

Fig 1-20d Good esthetics after restoration with a composite resin.

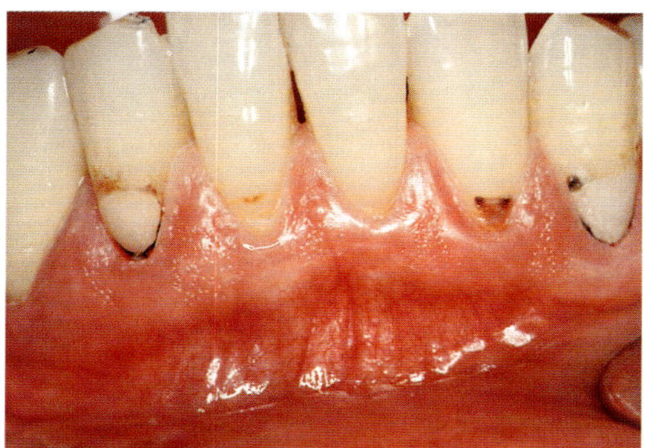

Fig 1-21a Prior to restoration.

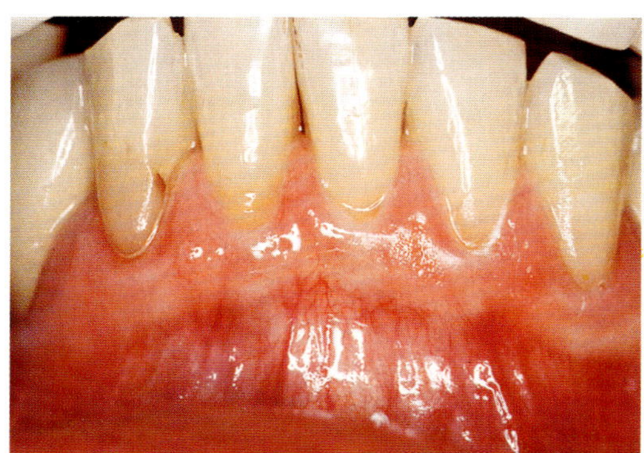

Fig 1-21b Restoration after 5 years. Fuji II LC resin-modified glass-ionomer restorations in teeth 41, 31, 32, and 33. Resin composite restoration for comparison in tooth 42.

Vitremer, and Photac Fil, although their composition and setting mechanisms differ.

There have been four major improvements in the resin-modified glass-ionomer cement for filling: decreased water sensitivity and improved mechanical properties, manipulability, and translucency. The incorporation of monomers and photo polymerization make the material less water-sensitive, while giving it greater mechanical strength and ease of manipulation.[43,44] It also makes the material more translucent than conventional cements by better matching the refractive indexes of the liquid and the filler.[45] The incorporation of monomers to the cement liquid increases the refractive index of the liquid. In the case of the conventional glass-ionomer Fuji II with a refractive index of 1.42, the liquid of Fuji II LC has a refractive index of 1.44, that brings it nearer to that of the applied glass powder which has a refractive index of 1.50 (Figs 1-21a and 1-21b).

Base and liner

The first clinical application of resin-modified glass-ionomer cement was as a base and liner. Conventional glass-ionomer products also have been successfully used for these purposes. However, the base and liner applications are usually followed by restorative or temporary filling procedures. Thus, the quick set with photo polymerization of the resin-modified glass-ionomer cement, as opposed to the relatively slow setting of conventional glass-ionomer products, exactly meets the requirements for these applications.

Vitrebond and Fuji Lining LC, products with base and liner applications, opened a new era of resin-modified glass-ionomer cements. This type of cement is applied as a liner prior to placement of a composite resin restoration. Fuji Bond LC is a further modification to the lining materials.[46,47] It was designed to be applied after surface treatment with GC Cavity Conditioner, an aqueous solution of 20% polyacrylic acid with 3% aluminum chloride. The smear layer, which is formed on the cut surface, is removed by a 10-second treatment with the cavity conditioner. The aluminum chloride conditions the dentin surface to enable formation of a hybrid layer with the cement. The powder and liquid of Fuji Bond LC is then thinly mixed with a disposable brush and applied directly to the cavity surface. A thin layer (approximately 10 to 40 μm thick) should be used, allowing the cement to work as both a bonding and a lining material. The monomers penetrate into the demineralized dentin, forming a hybrid layer which is expected to contribute to long-term stable adhesion of the cement to the tooth. The lining layer of Fuji Bond LC has a low modulus of elasticity and works as a stress relaxation layer, compensating for the stresses developed by the polymerization shrinkage of the composite resin during light curing.[48] Fuji Bond LC also has shown remineralization effects on demineralized cavity walls due to fluoride release.[41]

Resin-modified glass-ionomer cements used as bonding agents prior to placement of composite resins are remarkably different from resin bonding agents. Further development of the former materials are anticipated.

Fissure protection

Conventional glass-ionomer cements for pit and fissure protection offer several advantages. Their ability for long-term fluoride release is beneficial. In addition, glass-ionomers adhere to the tooth structure without acid etching, allowing their use on partially erupted teeth with difficult access for rubber dam isolation. However, although the merits of glass-ionomers used as protection material were accepted in some countries, they were not recognized worldwide. Their retention rate was not as high as that of a resin sealant, and they require prevention of moisture contamination in the early stages of setting. Fuji III LC, a resin-modified glass-ionomer fissure protection material, comprises improved mechanical and handling properties. This material shows a high fluidity and ability to penetrate into fissures.[49] Because the caries morbidity rate is comparatively high for teeth during the eruption period, it is thought that the resin-modified glass-ionomer cement could be an efficient fissure protector. Although this material is retained in the fissure for a required period of time, it does not have to be retained as long as a resin sealant material. Presently, the glass-ionomer cement is the only material that increases the acid resistance of the tooth.

Luting

The bond strength of conventional glass-ionomer cement for luting is not as high as that of resin cement. Failure often occurs as cohesive fractures within the cement.[50] There are many resin-modified

Table 1-3 Comparison of mechanical and bonding properties of luting materials

	Conventional Glass-Ionomer Cement	Resin-modified Glass-Ionomer Cement	Resin Cement
Product	Fuji I	Fuji Plus	Panavia 21
Manufacturer	GC	GC	Kuraray
Compressive strength, 1 day (MPa)	207 (8)	155 (7)	252 (11)
Diametral tensile strength, 1 day (MPa)	12 (2)	24 (2)	—
Flexural strength, 1 day (MPa)	18 (4)	27 (3)	105 (6)
Bond strength to bovine dentin, 1 day (MPa)			
Polished and without surface treatment and/or bonding material	4.6 (1.0)	13.4 (3.5)	Does not bond
With surface treatment and/or bonding material as recommended by manufacturer	No treatment recommended	14.1 (2.4)	15.1 (3.7)

Numbers in parentheses indicate standard deviations.

glass-ionomers available that contain a monomer component in the liquid to strengthen the matrix of the cured material. Also, the bond strength of the material to the tooth structure has been improved with the incorporation of monomers.[51] Fuji Plus and Vitremer luting cement are popular products in this category. They have significantly higher bonding strengths, which has to be attributed to their improved mechanical properties (Table 1-3). They undergo the setting reaction of polymerization by the oxidation-reduction catalyst and conventional acid-base reaction simultaneously. These materials show a sharp setting characteristic in the oral environment, because the polymerization reaction is strongly influenced by environmental temperature, making the material less sensitive to saliva (Figs 1-22a and 1-22b).

A major feature of all types of resin-modified glass-ionomer cements is the early development of mechanical strength. Figure 1-23 shows how the mechanical strength of the resin-modified

Fig 1-22 Cementation with a resin-modified glass-ionomer (Fuji Plus).

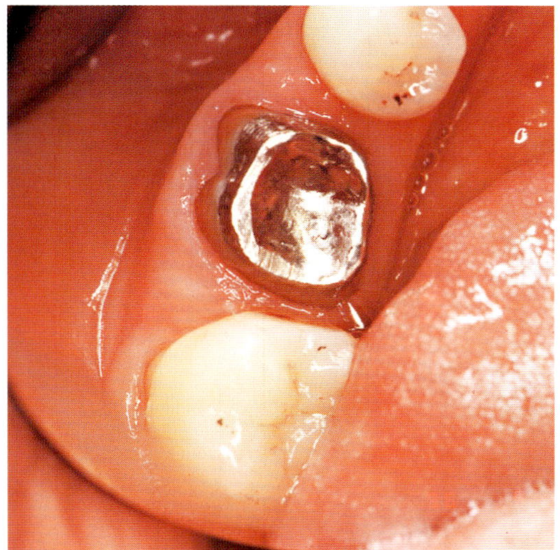

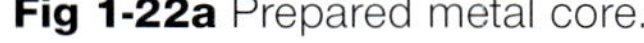

Fig 1-22a Prepared metal core.

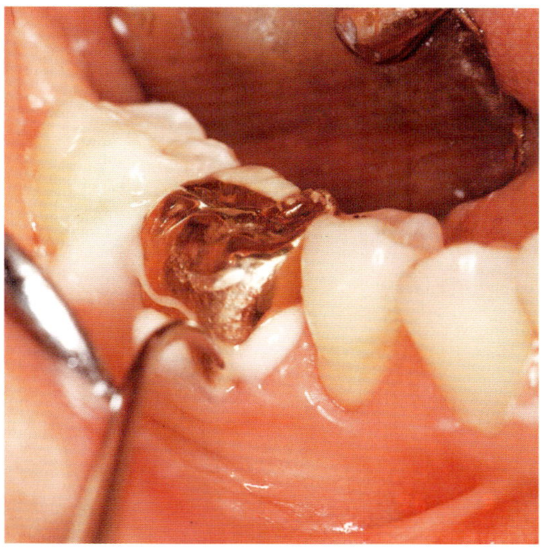

Fig 1-22b Removal of the excess cement.

glass-ionomer cement (Fuji II LC) developed significantly earlier (at 10 minutes after the start of mixing) than that of the two conventional glass-ionomer cements. This early development contributes to the reliability of the resin-modified material in the clinical application.

Orthodontic cementing material

Significant improvements in its adhesion have made resin-modified glass-ionomer cement applicable as an orthodontic cementing material.[52–55] Fuji Ortho LC, Fuji Ortho, and Unitek Multi-Cure Glass Ionomer Orthodontic Band Cement have been developed specifically for orthodontic applications. Fuji Ortho is chemically cured and Fuji Ortho LC and Multi-Cure are cured both chemically and by photo polymerization. Although resin cements are the more popular materials for bonding orthodontic brackets because of their reliable bonding strength to both enamel and brackets, they have a major disadvantage. They require acid etching of the substrate prior to bonding procedures. Moreover, the debonding procedure may damage the enamel surface; it has even been reported that the enamel surface of a bonded area was torn off with the bracket during debonding. The treatment of the enamel surface required for bonding with Fuji Ortho LC and Fuji Ortho is conditioning with GC Ortho Conditioner, a 10% aqueous solution of polyacrylic acid. It does not dramatically change the enamel surface like phosphoric acid etching does, but it cleans the surface and promotes a suitable bonding substrate for application of the cement.[56] During orthodontic treatment, the cement releases

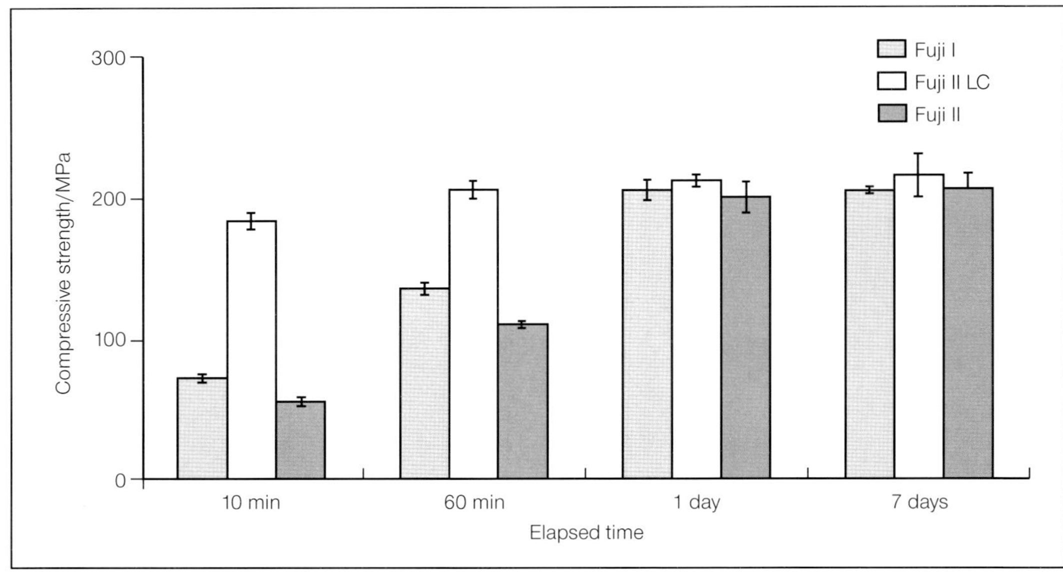

Fig 1-23 Development of the compressive strength of resin-modified glass-ionomer cements over time.

fluoride and prevents demineralization of the enamel around the brackets. The debonding of the brackets is easy and the bonded material can be removed easily with scalers and brush cones. The Unitek Multi-Cure Glass-Ionomer Orthodontic Band Cement is specially designed to bond the orthodontic bands. This material sets chemically and also snap-sets with photo polymerization.

Polyacid-Modified Resin Composites

In the search for a new restoration material, an attempt was made to polymerize an acid monomer in the presence of fluoroaluminosilicate glass. This attempt led to the development of a compound that releases fluoride slowly in the oral environment; it is called a *compomer*. The compomer shows physical properties quite similar to those of a composite resin. At the same time, the acid monomer which has been polymerized exhibits acidity when in contact with water from the saliva and reacts with the basic glass which contains fluoride.

Definition

Two types of material exist between the extremes represented by composite resins and conventional glass-ionomer cements: resin-modified glass-ionomer cements and compomers. The nature and physical properties of these materials can be modified consecutively between the two extremes. Therefore, several products claim to have the nature of both conventional glass-ionomer cements and composite resin, making the classification of such materials complicated. The compomer is one of the materials in this category. It basically has a similar nature and similar physical properties to resin composites. According to the manufacturers, it also has the ability to release fluoride and undergoes an acid-base reaction between the acidic monomer and basic glass filler in the presence of water in the saliva. However, the compomer does not contain water and does not self-adhere to the tooth structure, which distinguishes it from a resin-modified glass-ionomer material. The compomer is mainly a resin composite with fluoride-releasing potential.

Basic composition

The compomer is a one-paste material consisting of fillers and a matrix that is similar to that of composite resin. Each compomer product has a different composition of fillers and matrix, depending on the manufacturer's technology. The material usually contains fluoroaluminosilicate glass powder as filler to release fluoride. Metal fluoride also is included in some materials for the same purpose. The fluoroaluminosilicate glass contains strontium or some other metal to make the material radiopaque. The compomer's original composition contained the acidic monomer in its matrix, although the other part of the matrix is similar to that of composite resin.

Setting reaction

The polymerization reaction of the monomer components, initiated by photo polymerization rules the setting reaction of the compomer. The acidic monomer is polymerized with other monomer components of the matrix to the acidic polymer, or the polymer with acidic group, in the initial setting reaction. The acid-base reaction is inhibited until the material hardens and absorbs water. The material is said to have its acid-base reaction between the acid group in the polymer and the basic glass filler in the presence of water from the saliva.

Clinical application of compomers

Some of the compomers available are Dyract AP, Compoglass F, F2000, and Ionosit Fil. These products are light-cured, one-paste materials that are capable of fluoride release. The main clinical application for compomers is restorative filling, because they are not adhesive and require a separate bonding agent. Compomers possess better mechanical properties and manipulability than glass-ionomer filling materials, and their flowability in the cavity is better than that of resin composite. However, the need for application of a bonding agent prior to filling is a disadvantage, and the mechanical properties of compomers are inferior to those of resin composites. Presently, the compomer can be classified as an intermediate material between the glass ionomer for filling and the resin composite. Long-term clinical

Table 1-4 Physical properties of restorative filling materials

	Conventional Glass-Ionomer Cement	Resin-modified Glass-Ionomer Cement	Compomer	Resin Composite
Compressive strength, 1 day (MPa)	160 ~ 240	180 ~ 240	220 ~ 340	240 ~ 340
Flexural strength, 1 day (Mpa)	10 ~ 20	40 ~ 70	120 ~ 160	120 ~ 200
Fluoride release	+ +	+ +	+	–
Translucency	Poor	Good	Good	Good
Surface smoothness	–	– ~ ±	± ~ +	± ~ +
Radiopacity	+	+	+	+
Bond strength to bovine dentin, 1 day (MPa)				
To polished dentin	3 ~ 6	4 ~ 10	Does not bond	Does not bond
With treatment and/or bonding material	3 ~ 6	6 ~ 20	3 ~ 15	10 ~ 20

studies with the compomers are expected, in which the clinical benefits to patients will be identified clearly (Table 1-4).

Summary and Future Perspectives

For the purposes of this book, restoration materials are classified into four major categories: glass-ionomer cements, resin-modified glass-ionomer cements, compomers, and resin composites. The glass-ionomer cement category includes both conventional and resin-modified materials. The basic composition, setting chemical reactions, and structures of the set materials are compared in Table 1-5.

Conventional and resin-modified glass-ionomer cements have been widely applied in clinical procedures. They originally possess the basic features required for dental materials, such as slow release of fluoride, the ability to adhere to the tooth structure, and biocompatibility. Because of these features, glass-ionomer materials could be the mainstream of the restorative materials used in a dental practice where cariology is emphasized. Glass-ionomer materials have a great potential for widely continued use, and the further advancement of glass-ionomer technology is expected.

Table 1-5 Classification of glass-ionomer cement, compomer, and resin composite

Material	Basic Composition	Setting Reaction	Structure of Set Material
Glass-ionomer cement	Powder: Fluoroalumino-silicate glass Liquid: Polyacrylic acid Polybasic carboxylic acid Water	Acid-base reaction	Filler: Fluoroaluminosilicate glass powder Matrix: Polyacid salt
Resin-modified glass-ionomer cement	Powder: Fluoroaluminosilicate glass Liquid: Polyacrylic acid Water-soluble methacrylate monomer (HEMA, etc) Catalyst	Acid-base reaction Polymerization	Filler: Fluoroaluminosilicate glass powder Matrix: Polymer acid salt Methacrylate polymer
Compomer	Paste: Filler (containing fluorine, etc) Methacrylate monomer Acidic monomer Catalyst	Polymerization	Filler: Filler containing fluorine Matrix: Methacrylate polymer Acidic polymer
Resin composite	Paste: Filler (oxide filler, etc) Methacrylate monomer Catalyst	Polymerization	Filler: Oxide filler Matrix: Methacrylate polymer

References

1. Olea N, Pulgar R, Perez P, et al. Estrogenicity of resin-based composites and sealants used in dentistry. Environ Health Perspect 1996; 104(3):298–305.

2. Komatsu M, Ikeda T, Ohshima K, et al. Enamel fluoride uptake from glass-ionomer cement designed for use as a fissure sealant. J Conserv Dent 1989;32(3):688–695.

3. Swift EJ Jr. Effect of glass-ionomers on recurrent caries. Oper Dent 1989;14:40–43.

4. Tyas MJ. Cariostatic effect of glass-ionomer cement: A five-year clinical study. Aust Dent J 1991;36(3):236–239.

5. Ten Cate JM, Van Duinen RNB. Hyper-mineralization of dentinal lesions adjacent to glass-ionomer cement restoration. J Dent Res 1995;74:1266–1271.

6. Park S-H, Kim K-Y. The anticariogenic effect of fluoride in primer, bonding agent, and composite resin in the cavosurface enamel area. Oper Dent 1997;22:115–120.

7. Nagamine M, Itota T, Torii Y, Irie M, Staninec M, Inoue K. Effect of resin-modified glass-ionomer cements on secondary caries. Am J Dent 1997;10(4):173–178.

8. Perreira PNR, Inokoshi S, Tagami J. In vitro secondary caries inhibition around fluoride releasing materials. J Dent (in press).

9. Dental water-based cements. ISO 9917:1991(E).

10. Wilson AD, Kent BE. The glass-ionomer cement: A new translucent dental filling material. J Appl Chem Biotechnol 1971;21:313.

11. Wilson AD, Kent BE. A new translucent cement for dentistry. The glass ionomer cement. Br Dent J 1972;132(2):133–135.

12. Wilson AD. Dental cements based on ion-reachable glasses. In: von Fraunhofer JA (ed). Dental Materials. London: Butterworths, 1975.

13. Takigawa T. Study on glass-ionomer cement, influence of powder. J Conserv Dent 1982; 25(3):812–813.

14. Forsten L. Fluoride release and uptake by glass-ionomers. Scand J Dent Res 1991;99:241–245.

15. Takahashi K, Emilson CG, Birkhed D. Fluoride release in vitro from various glass-ionomer cements and resin composites after exposure to NaF solutions. Dent Mater 1993;9:350–354.

16. Diaz-Arnold AM, Holmes DC, Wistrom DW, Swift EJ. Short-term fluoride release/uptake of glass ionomer restoratives. Dent Mater 1995; 11:96–101.

17. Hirasawa M, Tosaki S, Hirota K. Fluoride release and uptake of glass-ionomer cement. Presented at the 3rd International Congress on Dental Materials, 1997.

18. Anstice HM, Nicholson JW. Investigation of the post-hardening reaction in glass-ionomer cements based on poly(vinyl phosphonic acid). J Mater Sci Mater Med 1995;6:420–425.

19. Nasu T. Polyacrylic acid-metal adhesive bond joint characterization by x-ray photoelectron spectroscopy. J Biomed Mater Res 1986; 20:347–362.

20. Kawahara H, Imanishi Y, Oshima H. Biological evaluation on glass-ionomer cements. J Dent Res 1979;58:1080–1086.

21. Maeda T, Matsuya S, Ohta M. Application of solid-state NMR to the study on setting mechanism of glass-ionomer cements. Dent Jpn (Tokyo) 1993;30:106–109.

22. Matsuya S, Maeda T, Ohota M IR and NMR analyses of hardening and maturation of glass-ionomer cement. J Dent Res 1996;75(12): 1920–1927.

23. Suzuki Y, Tosaki S, Hirota K. Physical properties of glass-ionomer for restorative filling. [abstract 1282] J Dent Res 1995;74:561.

24. Hirota K, Akahane S, Tosaki S, Tamiya Y, Tomioka K. Thermal expansion coefficient of glass-ionomer cements. [abstract 225A] J Dent Res 1988;67:141.

25. Simmons J. The miracle mixture glass-ionomer and alloy powder. Tex Dent J 1983;100:6–12.

26. McLean JW, Gasser O. Glass-cermet cements. Quintessence Int 1985;5:333–343.

27. Frencken J, Phantumvanit P, Pilot T. Manual Atraumatic Restorative Treatment Technique of Dental Caries. 2d ed. Groningen: WHO Collaborating Centre for Oral Health Services Research University of Groningen, 1994.

28. Frencken J, Pilot T, Songpaisan Y, Phantumvanit P. Atraumatic restorative treatment (ATR): Rationale, technique, and development. J Public Health Dent 1996;56(3):135–140.

29. Tosaki S, Sato H, Akahane S, Hirota K, Tomioka K. Thickness of glass-ionomer cement applied for sealing hypersensitive sites. [abstract 1621] J Dent Res 1990;69:311.

30. Ray H, Seltzer S. A new glass-ionomer root canal sealer. J Endod 1991;17(12):598–603.

31. McLean JW, Prosser HJ, Wilson AD. The use of glass-ionomer cements in bonding composite resins to dentine. Br Dent J 1985;158:410–414.

32. McComb D, Ericson D. Antimicrobial action of new proprietary lining cements. J Dent Res 1987;66(5):1025–1028.

33. Mitchem JC, Gronas DG. Continued evaluation of the clinical solubility of luting cements. J Prosthet Dent 1981;45(3):289–291.

34. Pluim LJ, Arends J. The relation between salivary properties and in vitro solubility of dental cements. Dent Mater 1987;3:13–18.

35. Van Zeghbroeck LM, Davidson CL. Evolution in physical properties of glass-ionomer luting cements. [abstract 2423] Presented at the 75th General Session IADR, 1997.

36. Ferrari M, Davidson CL. Interdiffusion of a traditional glass-ionomer cement into conditioned dentin. Am J Dent 1997;10:295–297.

37. Yoshii E, Kanaoka T, Hirota K. Biological evaluation of a new light cured glass-ionomer cement for restorative filling. p.53, Fourth World Biomaterials Congress, 1992.

38. Yoshikawa T, Hirasawa M, Tosaki S, Hirota K. Concentration of HEMA eluted from light-cured glass-ionomers. [abstract 254] J Dent Res 1994;73:133.

39. Hirasawa M, Yoshikawa T, Tosaki S, Hirota K. Setting characteristics of resin-modified glass ionomer for luting. [abstract 0698] J Dent Res 1995;74:488.

40. Kato S, Tosaki S, Hirota K. Effect of tooth surface conditioning materials on glass-ionomer bonding. [abstract 759] J Dent Res 1995;74:106.

41. Kato S, Tosaki S, Hirota K. Fluoride release of resin reinforced glass ionomer bonding agent. Presented at the 3rd International Congress on Dental Materials, 1997.

42. Nakaseko H, Kato S, Tosaki S, Hirota K. Effect of tooth treatment on bonding strength of a resin-modified GI. [abstract 2395] J Dent Res 1997;76:313.

43. Ishihara Y, Tosaki S. Comparison of physical properties between conventional type and light-cured type glass-ionomer cement. Presented at the 2nd International Congress on Dental Materials, 1993.

44. Todo A, Hirasawa M, Tosaki S, Hirota K. The surface roughness of glass-ionomer cement. [abstract 415] J Dent Res 1996;75:69.

45. Fusejima F, Sato H, Tosaki S, Hirota K. Comparison of transmittance between two types of glass ionomer cement. [abstract 936] J Dent Res 1992;71:632.

46. Knight GM. The co-cured, light-activated glass-ionomer cement composite resin restoration. Quintessence Int 1994;25:97–100.

47. Yamada T, Kanemaru N, Inokoshi N, Tagami J, Kato S. Tensile bond strength and interfacial ultrastructure of a new resin bonding system based on a glass-polyalkenoate cement. [abstract 1920] J Dent Res 1996;75:257.

48. Davidson CL. Glass-ionomer bases under posterior composites. J Esthet Dent 1991; 6:223–226.

49. Yoshii E, Kanaoka T, Katoh S. Physical and biological evaluation of a new light-cured sealant. [abstract 0261] J Dent Res 1994;73:134.

50. Davidson CL, Van Zeghbroeck L, Feilzer AJ. Destructive stresses in adhesive luting cements. J Dent Res 1991;70:880–882.

51. Yoshikawa T, Tosaki S, Hirota K. Effect of tooth treatment for bonding strength of resin-modified

glass-ionomer. [abstract 222] J Dent Res 1995;74:428.

52. Fricker JP. A 12-month clinical evaluation of a light-activated glass-polyalkenoate (ionomer) cement for the direct bonding of orthodontic brackets. Am J Orthod Dentofac Orthop 1994;105: 502–505.

53. Fricker JP. A 12-month clinical comparison of resin-modified light-activated adhesives for the cementation of orthodontic molar bands. Am J Orthod Dentofac Orthop 1997;112:239–243.

54. Silverman E, Cohen M, Demke RS, Silverman M. A new light-cured glass-ionomer cement that bonds brackets to teeth without etching in the presence of saliva. Am J Orthod Dentofac Orthop 1995;108:231–236.

55. Komori A, Ishikawa H. Evaluation of a resin-reinforced glass-ionomer cement for use as an orthodontic bonding agent. Angle Orthod 1997; 67(3):189–196.

56. Todo A, Tosaki S, Hirota K. The bonding strength of light-cured glass-ionomer cement for orthodontics. Presented at the 3rd International Congress on Dental Materials, 1997.

Chapter 2

Physical Properties of Glass-Ionomer Cements: Setting Shrinkage and Wear

Anton J. de Gee

In resin composite research, a great deal of attention has focused on setting shrinkage because of its importance for sealing composite restorations. Although composites form an acceptable alternative to amalgam for an increasing number of indications, the polymerization shrinkage is still a major problem. As a result of contraction during the setting stage, loss of adhesion to the cavity walls may occur where the tensile shrinkage stresses on the adhesive bonds reach levels that surpass the bond strength.

Setting shrinkage of glass ionomers is equally important, because these materials may be used as an alternative to composites. The first half of this chapter examines this issue, notably the setting shrinkage stresses resulting from shrinkage in bonded situations and the ability to relieve these stresses by water sorption.

While a property such as setting shrinkage is mainly concerned with the clinical success of a restoration in terms of retention and sealing, the longevity of the surface contour is determined by the restorative material's resistance to wear. The second half of this chapter addresses the durability of glass-ionomer cements.

Setting Shrinkage of Glass-Ionomers

To facilitate the discussion, the setting processes for the different types of glass-ionomers are summarized first.

Setting of conventional glass-ionomers

The setting of conventional glass-ionomer cements starts when the liquid and powder are brought into contact with each other. This produces an acid-base reaction in which the acid is a polyalkenoic (eg, polyacrylic or polymaleic) acid, and the base is a finely powdered glass consisting of fluoroaluminosilicates. The polyacid is either part of the liquid as an aqueous solution or incorporated into the powder in a freeze-dried state. In the latter case, the liquid is simply water in which the freeze-dried polyacid dissolves on mixing.

The hydrogen ions of the acid penetrate the glass particles and release calcium, strontium, and aluminum ions, which combine with the polyalkenoic

Table 2-1 Setting shrinkage at 23°C after 24 hours of conventional, metal-modified, and resin-modified glass-ionomers

Material	Type	Manufacturer	Setting Shrinkage (vol%)
Ketac-Fil Aplicap	Conventional	Espe	3.4
Ketac-Molar	Conventional	Espe	4.4
Fuji II Capsule	Conventional	GC	3.6
Fuji IX Capsule	Conventional	GC	3.6
Chem-Fil Superior	Conventional	DeTrey/Dentsply	4.1
Shofu Hi-Dense	Metal-modified	Shofu	2.6
Miracle Mix	Metal-modified	GC	3.5
Ketac-Silver	Metal-modified	Espe	3.1
Photac-Fil Aplicap	Resin-modified	Espe	3.8
Fuji II LC Capsule	Resin-modified	GC	4.8
Vitremer	Resin-modified	3M	4.3

chains of the acid to form an initial rubbery hydrogel structure. In the following phase of the setting reaction, the metal ions form cross-links between the polyalkenoic chains, creating a highly rigid material. This portion of the reaction may continue over a period of weeks or even months.[1–4] During all stages of the reaction and also in the set state, all these materials are sensitive to dehydration. Table 2-1 lists several examples of conventional and modified glass-ionomer cements.

Setting of resin-modified glass-ionomers

The slow rate of setting[4–6] and the sensitivity to dehydration of conventional glass-ionomer cements are unfavorable properties in comparison with resin composites. In an attempt to overcome these disadvantages, hybrid materials were developed that combine resin composite and conventional glass-ionomer technologies. These resin-modified glass-ionomers are light curable and less sensitive to dehydration,[7] while retaining most of the advantages of conventional glass-ionomers.[8] Some of these materials

Table 2-2 Reactions that take place in resin-modified glass-ionomer cements

Reacting Components	Reaction Type
Polyacid + fluoroaluminosilicate glass particles	Acid-base
Monomer + photoinitiator + light	Polymerization (light-initiated)
Monomer + initiator + catalyst	Polymerization (chemical-initiated)

are now widely used in such products as Fuji II LC, Photac-Fil, and Vitremer (see Table 2-1). They are derived from conventional glass-ionomer cements, in which part of the water content is replaced by the water-soluble and photopolymerizable 2-hydroxyethylmethacrylate (HEMA) monomer.

The setting of resin-modified glass-ionomers involves the polymerization of the HEMA monomer by light activation and the classic acid-base reaction between a polyacid and the basic glass particles. However, in many cases the monomer will polymerize even without light because the manufacturer has added a catalyst to the composition. Table 2-2 provides an overview of the three reactions which can occur in resin-modified glass-ionomer cements.

The rubbery hydrogel phase seen with conventional glass ionomers is not expressed after light curing. This is because the polymerization reaction of the monomer rapidly lends the material considerable strength. The acid-base reaction proceeds within the polymer network that has been formed, and the two reactions ultimately result in the formation of two interpenetrating matrices.

Setting shrinkage

Using measuring devices which make it possible to determine the dimensional changes which take place during the setting of restorative materials (such as the mercury dilatometer),[9] it has been demonstrated that both types of glass-ionomer cements undergo considerable setting shrinkage (see Table 2-1). In the case of resin-modified glass-ionomers, shrinkage occurs for both the polymerization reaction of the monomers and the acid-base reaction, depending on the moment of light activation. For example, when light activation is started within 2 minutes after mixing, shrinkage occurs only for the polymerization reaction. No shrinkage of the acid-base reaction can take place, because it is completely blocked by the polymer network. However, when light activation is omitted or delayed for a time, the shrinkage of the acid-base reaction can be expressed during this period. If the manufacturer has included a catalyst in the composition for the polymerization of the monomer (see Table 2-2), there is a contributory shrinkage effect as a result of the chemically initiated polymerization

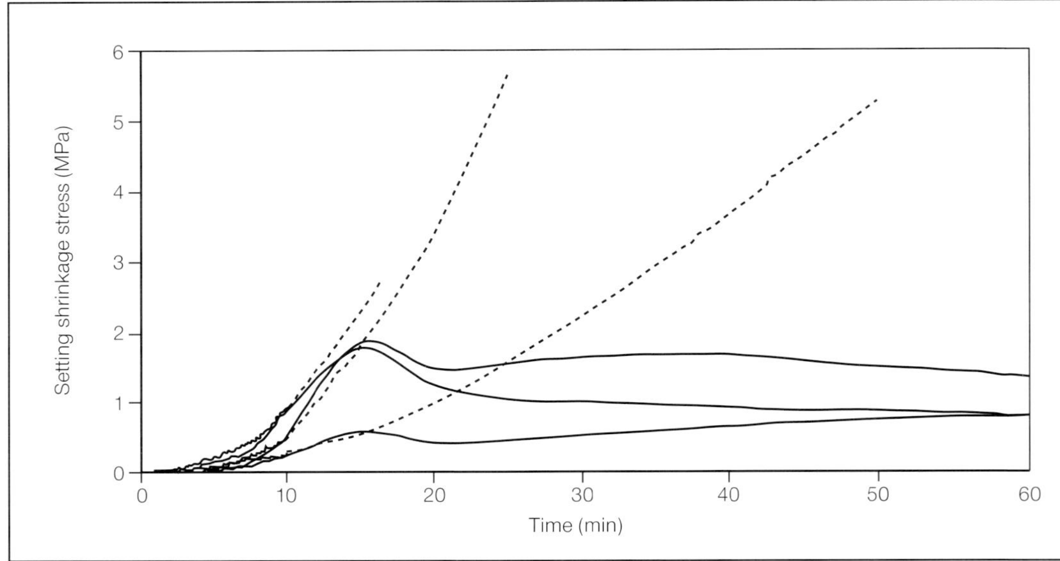

Fig 2-1 Setting shrinkage stress development in conventional glass-ionomers simulated for a shallow Class V cavity. (·····) The recording of these curves was interrupted as a result of premature cohesive or adhesive failure of the sample from dehydration in the test setup. From top to bottom at 10 minutes: Ketac-Fil, Fuji II, and Chem-Fil Superior. (——) Contact of the samples with water at 15 minutes after mixing results in a considerable reduction of shrinkage stress and preservation of cohesive and adhesive integrity. From top to bottom at 10 minutes: Ketac-Fil, Fuji II, and Chem-Fil Superior. For self-curing composites (not shown in this figure), the shrinkage stress reaches values of approximately 15 Mpa.[11]

reaction. The extent of the ultimate shrinkage when light activation is delayed or omitted is different for each resin-modified material. Although further examination of this phenomenon is beyond the scope of this chapter, it is important to note that resin-modified glass-ionomers also cure in the absence of light activation. This is known as the *dark curing* of resin-modified glass-ionomers. The process generally proceeds slowly, but if a situation occurs that prevents the light from the light source reaching deep parts of a restoration, curing ultimately takes place.

Shrinkage stress in bonded restorations

In a restoration that is adhesively bonded to the cavity walls, the material exerts a tensile stress on the walls during setting. The ultimate extent of the shrinkage stress in a cavity determines whether bonding to the cavity wall is retained.

One of the most important factors influencing the degree of stress is the shape of the cavity. The larger the surface of the cavity walls to which the restoration bonds, the greater the stress. Conversely, a fairly large unbonded surface keeps the shrinkage stress low, because a relatively large amount of material from the free

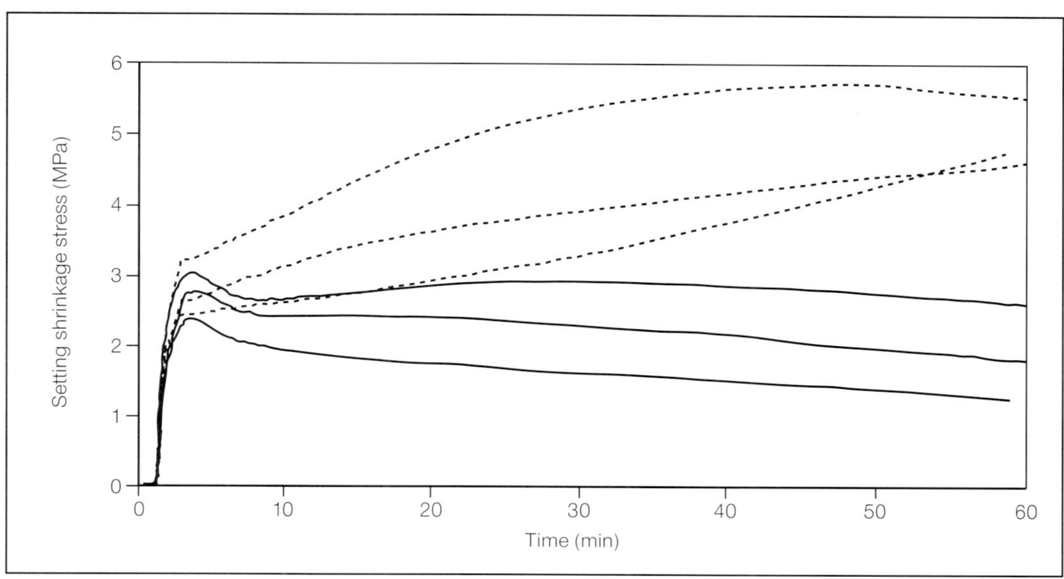

Fig 2-2 Setting shrinkage stress development in resin-modified glass-ionomers simulated for a shallow Class V cavity. (·····) The shrinkage stress gradually increases when the samples are not in contact with water, but cohesive and adhesive integrity is maintained. From top to bottom at 15 minutes: Photac-Fil, Fuji II LC, and Vitremer. (——) Contact of the samples with water directly after light curing results in a considerable reduction of shrinkage stress. From top to bottom at 15 minutes: Photac-Fil, Fuji II LC, and Vitremer. For light-curing composites (not shown in this figure), the shrinkage stress reaches values of approximately 18 Mpa.[11]

surface is able to flow to the stress area. Thus, the final shrinkage stress depends on the geometry of the cavity preparation.

With the aid of a simulation model, the details of which are not presented here, it is possible to study the development of shrinkage stress during setting for any cavity geometry.[10] Experiments with this model show that the shrinkage stress developed by glass-ionomer cements is considerably lower than that of resin composites, despite the fact that glass-ionomer cements display a much higher setting shrinkage (see Table 2-1) than do composites (2.0 to 3.0 vol%). In the case of a simulated shallow Class V restoration, the stresses in composites can reach values of 15–18 MPa, whereas those for conventional and resin-modified glass-ionomers do not exceed 2 to 3 MPa (Figs 2-1 and 2-2). Thus, there is a strong possibility that a Class V composite restoration will detach from the cavity wall during setting, because the shrinkage stresses may exceed the bond strength.

The low shrinkage stress of conventional glass-ionomer cements is due largely to the rubbery stage these cements pass through during the setting process. Besides flow, elastic yielding also relieves the shrinkage stress. When both factors are favorable, there is a strong possibility that the bonding to the cavity walls, which is approximately 6 MPa

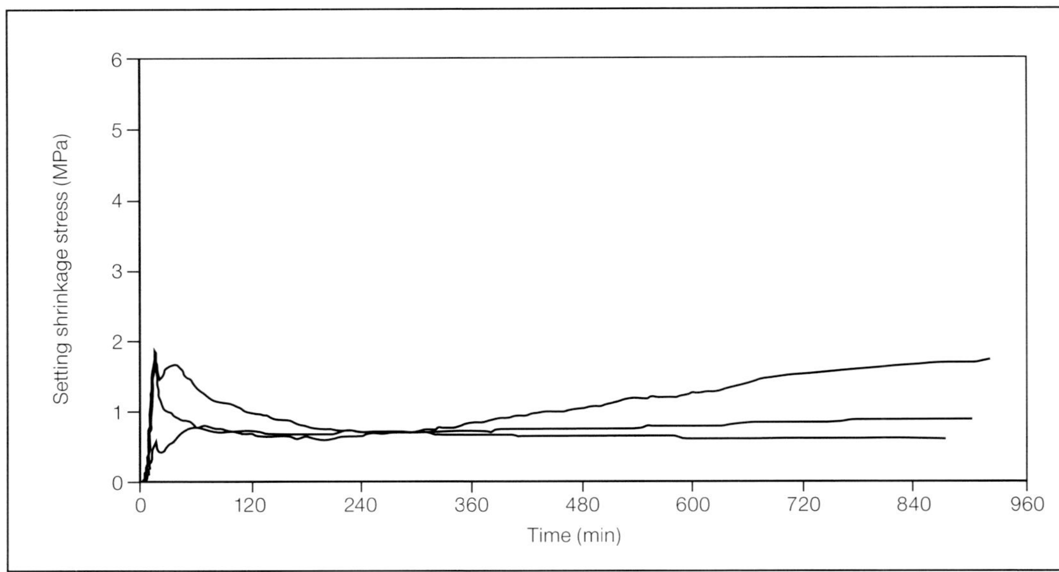

Fig 2-3 Setting shrinkage stress development measured over a period of 14 hours in conventional glass ionomers simulated for a shallow Class V cavity. The samples were immersed in water 6 minutes after the start of mixing. No continuous reduction of stress occurred within the test period. From top to bottom at approximately 30 minutes: Fuji II, Ketac-Fil, and Chem-Fil Superior.

for enamel and 3 MPa for dentin, will be retained during setting. However, when the material is subject to dehydration, adhesive or cohesive failure may occur (see Fig 2-1).

The shrinkage stresses recorded for resin-modified glass-ionomers are somewhat higher than those of the conventional materials (see Fig 2-2). This is due to the fact that the shrinkage is totally dominated by the light-initiated polymerization reaction. No rubbery phase can be distinguished, as in the case of the acid-base reaction. Therefore, the shrinkage stresses do not experience elastic relaxation. In most materials the degree of shrinkage stress following light activation is approximately 3 MPa. It is not surprising that the stresses are again lower than the 18 MPa recorded for light-curing composites, because the amount of monomer in resin-modified glass-ionomers is only 6% as opposed to 30% to 50% in composites. As yet, little is known about the effect of shrinkage stress on the bonding of the restoration to the cavity wall, but leakage tests have shown that resin-modified materials are comparable to conventional cements in this respect.[12]

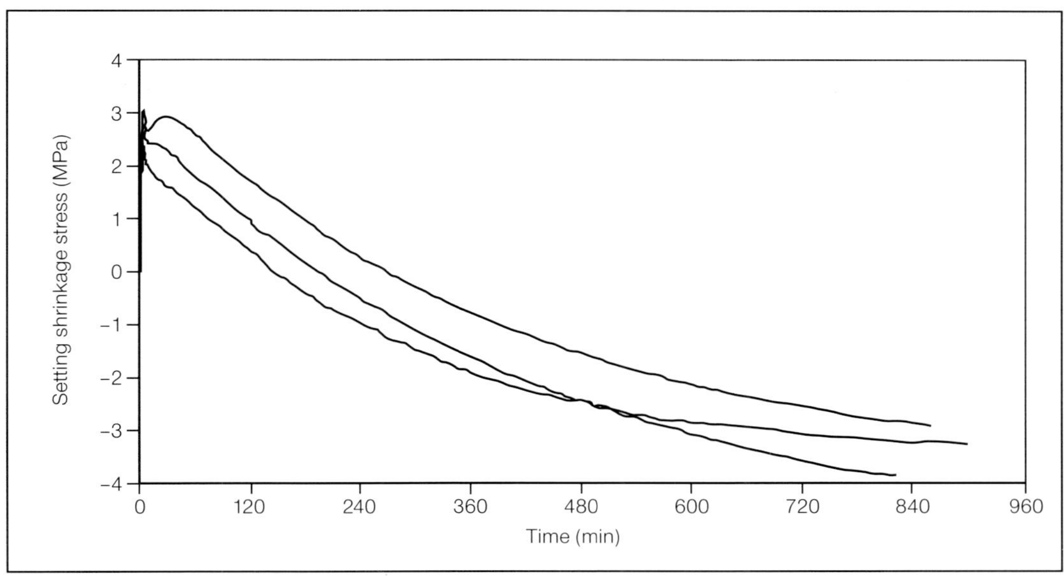

Fig 2-4 Setting shrinkage stress development measured over a period of 14 hours in resin-modified glass ionomers simulated for a shallow Class V cavity. The samples were immersed in water directly after light curing. Within the test period, tensile stresses converted to compression stresses due to water sorption. From top to bottom at approximately 30 minutes: Photac-Fil, Fuji II LC, and Vitremer.

Water sorption and relaxation of setting stresses

It is generally assumed that shrinkage stress can be wholly or partially counteracted by hygroscopic expansion as a result of water sorption. The solid curves in Fig 2-1 show what happens when contact with water occurs after 15 minutes. The stress decreases almost immediately, but then increases again. The decrease shows that glass-ionomer cements are capable of absorbing water and that this occurs quite rapidly. The stress then increases, due to the advanced stage of the reaction, so the development of shrinkage stresses again predominates. From this moment, however, hygroscopic expansion actively opposes shrinkage stress. This is particularly evident in the upper curves in Fig 2-1, where it continues to rise because the materials have not been brought into contact with water. It may be concluded from this experiment that as soon as wet finishing in the mouth begins, the development of shrinkage stress is slowed by water sorption.

An unexpected result is that total relaxation is not attained within a period of 14 hours. A downward trend is visible (Fig 2-3), and it is possible that this process lasts for several days.

In the case of resin-modified glass-ionomers, hygroscopic expansion also occurs following exposure to water. Total relaxation is attained within 5 hours and from that point the reverse process takes place, building up expansion forces (Fig 2-4). Nevertheless, any marginal crevice that may appear as a result of shrinkage stress does not achieve a perfect attachment, because the planes of fracture will never fit together as perfectly as before.

After 14 hours the expansion has still not come to an end and may continue for a long time. Obviously, the ultimate compressive stress must not be too high, because this can lead to cracks in the tooth material.

In contrast to conventional cements, the omission of water contact does not necessarily lead to cohesive or adhesive failure in resin-modified materials, but shrinkage stresses continue to increase (see Fig 2-2). In the clinical situation, contact with water almost always takes place directly after setting by light activation, which occurs within 5 minutes.

Wear of Glass-Ionomers

Although the loss of substance displayed by restorations in the occlusal area is caused by a number of wear mechanisms, occlusal wear is thought to be primarily three-body in nature.[13,14] This type of wear results from the abrasive activity of solid particles in a food bolus when it is pressed onto and sheared across the occlusal surfaces of opposing teeth during mastication. Lutz et al[15] have described this as wear in the occlusal contact-free areas (CFA). The wear resulting from direct contact is defined as wear in the occlusal contact area (OCA), which involves such mechanisms as two-body abrasive wear, adhesive wear, and surface fatigue.[15–17] Another type of wear is corrosive in nature, where chemical factors soften or degrade the surface of the restoration.[18–20]

Although it is only in the mouth that the wear mechanisms described come into play simultaneously and thus interact with each other, some of the wear components can be imitated simultaneously or separately using the ACTA wear machine.[14] Research has demonstrated that this machine not only makes possible a good simulation of clinical CFA,[21] but also provides an impression of the wear caused by surface fatigue in the OCA.[22] The role of chemical components, such as acids, also can be studied.

Characteristics of wear

Due to their limited mechanical strength, brittleness, and high degree of wear, applications of glass-ionomer cements have thus far been limited to erosion and abrasion lesions, or Class III and Class V cavities. Metal-modified cements, including cermets, have been employed occlusally in primary molars with varying degrees of success[23,24] and in permanent teeth where chewing stresses are low.[25–27]

The limited wear resistance of glass-ionomer cements on chewing surfaces is thought to be due to insufficient strength directly after placement. It is only after the cements have had time to build up a greater degree of strength that wear resistance reaches an acceptable level. This increase in mechanical properties may take weeks or even months.

Another factor that may influence wear resistance is the sensitivity to acids.[28] This is liable to be a problem in those areas where mechanical forces and acids are active at the same time, such as on occlusal surfaces during mastication of acidic food substances.

Despite the general view that glass-ionomers are not yet suitable for occlusal applications, the temptation to use them has often been too great to resist. With the advent of resin-modified glass-ionomer cements, which appear to set fully after light activation, an occlusal filling is often considered an attractive option.

The rest of this section examines the wear performance of conventional, metal-modified, and resin-modified glass-ionomers in contact-free and occlusal contact areas during the early stages after placement and in the long-term, as well as the susceptibility of these materials to acids as studied using the ACTA wear machine.

Early and long-term wear of glass-ionomer cements

Unlike composite resins, in which the polymerization reaction ceases within a week after initiation,[29] the setting process for all types of glass-ionomers continues over a period of several months.[2,3,30] This is reflected in the high early wear rates determined directly after preparation of the samples, and the declining wear over time (Table 2-3). Even between 4 months and 1 year there is evidence of a reduction in wear.[6] The continuing improvement in mechanical properties is probably the result of the slow displacement of calcium ions by aluminum ions, which further enhances the cohesion of the matrix.

The wear of resin-modified glass-ionomers appears to be significantly higher than that of the conventional materials (see Table 2-3), probably due to differences in matrix formation. The matrix of a conventional glass-ionomer consists of an ionically cross-linked polyalkenoate network resulting from an acid-base reaction. The set cements of resin-modified Photac-Fil and Fuji II LC have similar cross-linked polyalkenoate networks, but these are entangled with HEMA polymer chains. In the case of Vitremer, the polyalkenoate network and polymer chains are connected through pendant methacrylate groups on the polyalkenoate chains. The greater wear displayed by resin-modified materials may indicate that the coherence of filler particles embedded in the interpenetrating matrices of polyalkenoate and polymer is inferior to that of the particles in the conventional matrix. This may be due to the partial replacement of the rigid polyalkenoate network by the flexible polymer chains. The increased deformation of the surface caused by the load of mastication, as simulated in the wear machine, can lead to the formation of subsurface microcracks in the ionic cross-linked polyalkenoate matrix with a subsequent loss of coherence.

In fact, this type of wear is related to subsurface fatigue, which takes on dramatic proportions under the conditions prevailing at occlusal contact areas (Fig 2-5). While Photac-Fil and Fuji II LC show an approximate increase in wear of 200% from CFA to OCA, the increase is limited to 50% in the case of Vitremer. The superior performance of Vitremer indi-

Table 2-3 Contact-free area wear of glass-ionomers directly after preparation and finishing and in the long term as determined with the ACTA wear machine

			Wear (μm)		
Material	Type	Manufacturer	1 day	4 months	1 year
Ketac-Fil Aplicap	Conventional	Espe	116	35	30
Ketac-Molar	Conventional	Espe	88	42	36
Fuji II Capsule	Conventional	GC	167	65	57
Fuji IX Capsule	Conventional	GC	119	57	51
Chem-Fil Superior	Conventional	DeTrey/Dentsply	128	58	53
Shofu Hi-Dense	Metal-modified	Shofu	116	32	27
Miracle Mix	Metal-modified	GC	154	65	48
Ketac-Silver	Metal-modified	Espe	95	64	52
Photac-Fil Aplicap	Resin-modified	Espe	522	172	152
Fuji II LC Capsule	Resin-modified	GC	308	155	138
Vitremer	Resin-modified	3M	211	90	82

cates that the chemical integration of its two matrices leads to a higher stability than a coherence based on entanglement. Also, the conventional glass-ionomers, with the exception of Ketac-Silver, are more sensitive at occlusal contacts as simulated in the wear machine, but the wear on these materials increases by only about 30% (Fig 2-6).

It is noteworthy that the metal-modified Ketac-Silver cermet, which is indicated for use on occlusal surfaces in primary molars, does not perform any better with respect to long-term CFA wear than Ketac-Fil (see Table 2-3). Thus, the superior clinical performance of Ketac-Silver must be due to its more favorable early CFA wear and its higher resistance to OCA wear (Fig 2-6). In this respect, the highly viscous Ketac-Molar and Fuji IX also show better performance than their predecessors, Ketac-Fil and Fuji II.

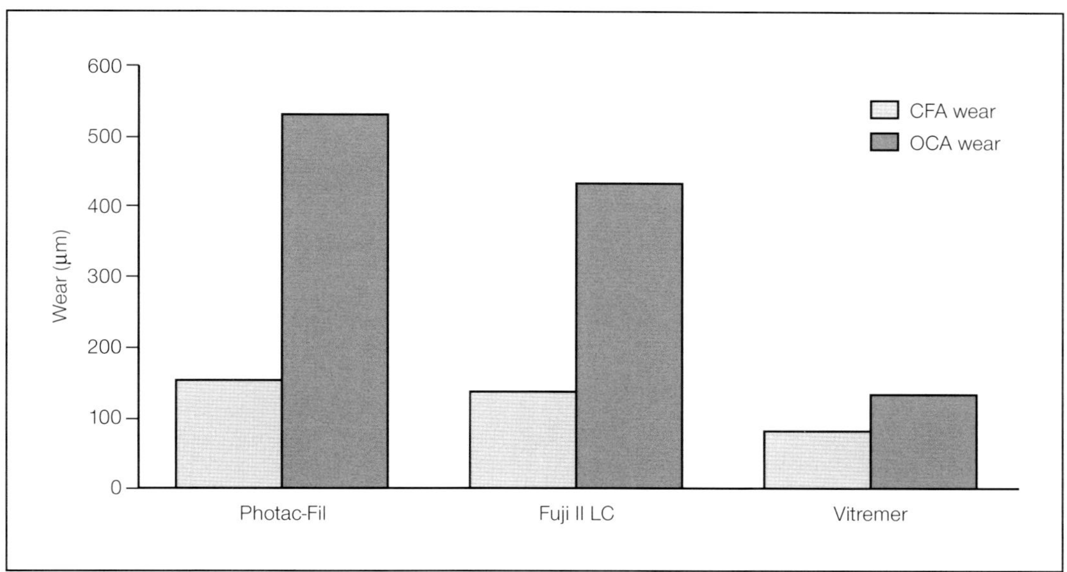

Fig 2-5 Comparison of CFA and OCA wear of fully matured resin-modified glass-ionomers as determined with the ACTA wear machine. Note that the height of the vertical axis is four times of that in Fig 2-6.

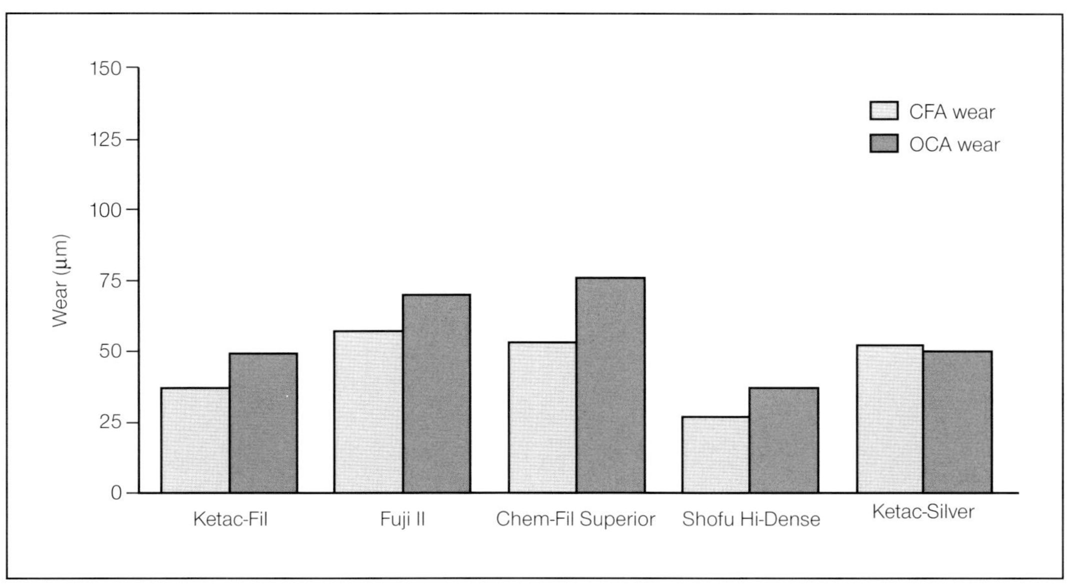

Fig 2-6 Comparison of CFA and OCA wear of fully matured conventional and metal-modified glass-ionomers as determined with the ACTA wear machine.

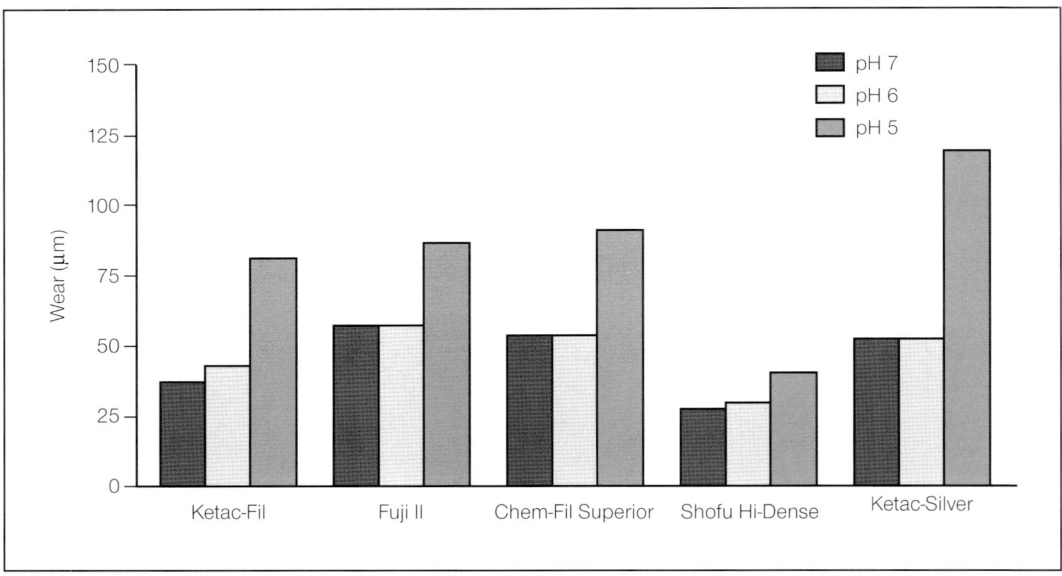

Fig 2-7 Comparison of CFA wear at different pHs of fully matured conventional and metal-modified glass-ionomers as determined with the ACTA wear machine.

Wear under acidic conditions

Acids directly attack the surface of glass ionomers, causing the dissolution of the cement. The extent to which this occurs depends on the degree of acidity. When acids and wear mechanisms operate simultaneously, as on occlusal areas during mastication of acidic food substances or directly after consumption of acidic drinks, their influence is noticeable at a pH as low as 5. Figure 2-7 shows that the CFA wear of conventional and metal-modified glass ionomers at pH 6 differs only marginally from that at pH 7, but a considerable degree of wear is evident at pH 5. The material's degree of sensitivity to acid is considered important, because it may be one of the factors contributing to clinical durability. A test that is commonly used to determine the acid sensitivity of cements is the lactic acid jet test.[28] Cement surfaces are exposed to a powerful jet comprising a solution of lactic acid in water which has a pH of 4. The classification of conventional and metal-modified glass-ionomer cements with respect to acid sensitivity as determined by this test corresponds to the increase in wear under acid conditions in the ACTA wear machine (see Fig 2-7): Fuji II = Shofu Hi-Dense < Chem-Fil Superior < Ketac-Fil < Ketac-Silver.

Tests for the stability of resin-modified glass-ionomers under acidic conditions (Fig 2-8) resulted in interesting findings which have not yet been explained. It would appear that the presence of the

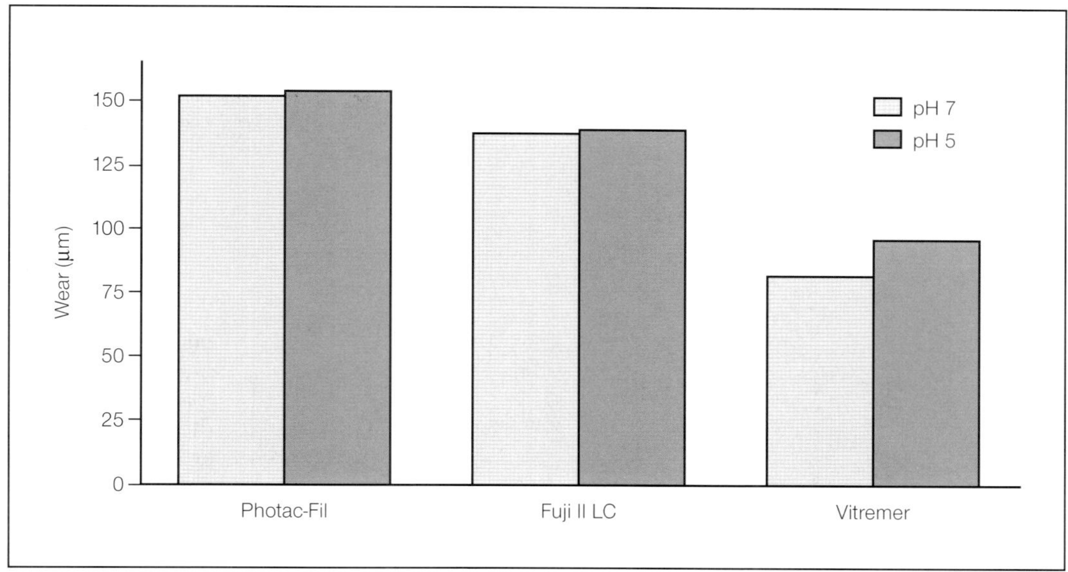

Fig 2-8 Comparison of CFA wear at different pHs of fully matured resin-modified glass-ionomers as determined with the ACTA wear machine.

resin is sufficient to provide a certain degree of protection against acid. It is possible that in the early stages after setting this category of materials is sensitive to pH values of 5 or lower, as has been demonstrated for comparable cements such as Vitrebond and XR-ionomer at pH 4 using the lactic acid jet test.[31]

It is clear from the marked degree of early CFA wear (> 100 μm) compared to that of resin composites (30 to 60 μm) that resin-modified materials are not yet suitable for occlusal restorations. However, some glass-ionomers, such as conventional Ketac-Fil and metal-modified Shofu Hi-Dense, may be able to compete with composites as their long-term wear falls in the 20- to 50-μm range (see Table 2-3). Moreover, because of the high intraoral temperature, setting in the mouth is expected to proceed more rapidly, so that under clinical conditions a higher wear resistance will be attained sooner.

References

1. Pearson GJ, Atkinson AS. Long-term flexural strength of glass-ionomer cements. Biomaterials 1991;12:658–660.

2. Williams JA, Billington RW, Pearson GJ. Increase in compressive strength of glass-ionomer restorative materials with respect to time: A guide to their suitability for use in posterior primary dentition. J Oral Rehabil 1989;16:475–479.

3. Williams JA, Billington RW. Changes in compressive strength of glass-ionomer restorative materials with respect to time periods of 24 h to 4 months. J Oral Rehabil 1991;18:163–168.

4. Williams JA, Billington RW, Pearson GJ. The effect of maturation on in vitro erosion of glass-ionomer and other dental cements. Br Dent J 1992;173:340–342.

5. Cattani-Lorente MA, Godin C, Meyer JM. Mechanical behavior of glass-ionomer cements affected by long-term storage in water. Dent Mater 1994;10:37–44.

6. De Gee AJ, Van Duinen RNB, Werner A, Davidson CL. Early and long-term wear of conventional and resin-modified glass-ionomers. J Dent Res 1996;75:1613–1619.

7. Cho E, Kopel H, White SN. Moisture susceptibility of resin-modified glass-ionomer materials. Quintessence Int 1995;26:351–358.

8. Sidhu SK, Watson TF. Resin-modified glass-ionomer materials. A status report for the American Journal of Dentistry. Am J Dent 1995;8:59–67.

9. Feilzer AJ, De Gee AJ, Davidson CL. Curing contraction of composites and glass-ionomer cements. J Prosthet Dent 1988;59:297–300.

10. Feilzer AJ, Kakaboura AI, De Gee AJ, Davidson CL. The influence of water sorption on the developments of setting shrinkage stress in traditional and light curing glass-ionomer cements. Dent Mater 1995;11:186–190.

11. Feilzer AJ, De Gee AJ, Davidson CL. Setting stresses in composites for two different curing modes. Dent Mater 1993;9:2–5.

12. Hallett KB, Garcia-Godoy F. Microleakage of resin modified glass-ionomer cement restorations: An in vitro study. Dent Mater 1993;9:306–311.

13. Mair LH. The measurement and analysis of clinical abrasion—a modified approach. Dent Mater 1990;6:271–275.

14. De Gee AJ, Pallav P. Occlusal wear simulation with the ACTA wear machine. J Dent 1994; 22(suppl 1):21–27.

15. Lutz F, Phillips RW, Roulet JF, Setcos JC. In vivo and in vitro wear of potential posterior composites. J Dent Res 1984;63:914–920.

16. Roulet J-F. Mechanisms of degradation. In: Degradation of Dental Polymers. New York: Karger, 1987:60–63.

17. Mair LH. Wear in dentistry. Current terminology. J Dent 1992;20:140–144.

18. Wu W, McKinney JE. Influence of chemicals on wear of dental materials. J Dent Res 1982;61:1180–1183.

19. McKinney JE. Environmental damage and wear of dental composite restoratives In: Vanherle G, Smith DC (eds). International Symposium on Posterior Composite Resin Dental Restorative Materials. The Netherlands: Peter Szulc, 1982.

20. Mair LH. Effect of surface conditioning on the abrasion rate of dental composites. J Dent 1991;19:100–106.

21. Pallav P, Davidson CL, De Gee AJ. Wear rates of composites, an amalgam and enamel under stress-bearing conditions. J Prosthet Dent 1988;59:426–429.

22. Pallav P, De Gee AJ, Werner A, Davidson CL. Influence of shearing action of food on contact stress and subsequent wear of stress-bearing composites. J Dent Res 1993;72:56–61.

23. Forsten I, Karjalainen S. Glass-ionomers in proximal cavities of primary molars. Scand J Dent Res 1990;98:70–73.

24. Mjör IA, Jokstad A. Five-year study of class II restorations in permanent teeth using amalgam, glass-polyalkenoate (ionomer) cermet and resin-based composite materials. J Dent 1993; 21:338–343.

25. Hickel R, Petchelt A, Maier J, Voss A, Sauter M. Nachuntersuchung von Fullungen mit Cermet-Zement (Ketac-Silver). Dtsch Zahnarztl Z 1988;43:851-853.

26. Smales RJ, Gerke DC, White IL. Clinical evaluation of occlusal glass-ionomer, resin, and amalgam restorations. J Dent 1990;18:243-249.

27. Croll TP, Killian CM. Glass-ionomer-silver-cermet interim Class I restorations for permanent teeth. Quintessence Int 1992;23:731-733.

28. Billington RW, Williams JA, Pearson GJ. In vitro erosion of 20 commercial glass-ionomer cements measured using the lactic acid jet test. Biomaterials 1992;13:543-547.

29. Watts DC. Kinetic mechanisms of visible-light-cured resins and resin composites. In: Watts DC (ed). Proceedings of a Symposium on Setting Mechanisms of Dental Materials, June 30, 1992. Scotland:1992.

30. Soltész U, Leupolz M. Hârte- und Festigkeitsverhalten von Glasionomerzementen. Dtsch Zahnarztl Z 1993;48:237-241.

31. Hegarty AM, Pearson GJ. Erosion and compressive strength of hybrid glass-ionomer cements when light activated or chemically set. Biomaterials 1993;14:349-352.

Chapter 3

Physical Properties of Glass-Ionomer Cements: Fatigue and Elasticity

Marc J. A. Braem

The clinical application of restorative materials has always been preceded by extensive laboratory research into their physical and mechanical properties. As evidenced by the material in this book, the same is true for glass-ionomer cements. This chapter first examines research that has been done pertaining to the fatigue behavior of these materials. The second half of the chapter addresses the property of elasticity and how it affects the usability of glass-ionomers in clinical applications.

Elements of Fatigue Behavior

Stiffness and wear resistance

Stiffness has long been one of the primary focuses in dental material research. The advantage of studying this property is that a quick, straightforward methodology can easily be used to study the influence of a variety of test and environmental variables. Whereas studies of stiffness initially were used mainly in a purely quantitative way, this property has gradually evolved into a verification instrument for qualitative information such as elasticity gradients in hybrid layers.[1]

Such an approach can only be used if one accepts that it is impossible to use a single parameter, or even a combination of parameters, quantitatively to predict more complex processes, such as wear.[2] As a consequence, research has been initiated to study complex processes as quasi-solitary phenomena, mainly by trying to imitate and simulate the clinical environment, which restorative materials need to function properly. Gradually, the influence of diverse individual factors such as chewing force and the composition of the saliva can be sorted out, while the simulator is normalized using the results of clinical studies.[3] In this way, researchers can gain insight into the different types of wear occurring under simulated clinical conditions. In dentistry, the loss of material due to nonantagonistic contacts has been defined as occlusal contact-free area (CFA) wear. Occlusal contact area (OCA) wear has been designated as material loss caused by direct interaction of an antagonist with the restorative material. For one major group of restoratives, resin composites, CFA wear is no longer considered a problem. Also, most of these materials have highly improved OCA wear, with some showing wear resistance equal to that of amalgam. However, in spite of excellent wear resistance, some restorations fail all of a sudden.[4] Therefore, something else must come into play: fatigue.

Fatigue

As with wear, *fatigue* is only a nonspecific descriptive term that stands for several different expressions of damage accumulation inside a material caused by static fatigue conditions, dynamic and/or cyclic fatigue. They all have one basic feature in common: crack growth.

Studying wear phenomena occurring under OCA conditions emphasizes the presence of cracks in both the wear facet itself and its immediate vicinity. This lends credence to the hypothesis that there is something like fatigue wear, which causes delamination of wear particles following subsurface crack growth in situations where there is cyclic sliding of a plunger on a test surface (eg, an antagonistic cusp on the surface of a filling). Such subsurface cracks have been identified both in vitro[5] and in vivo.[6]

Given that wear and fatigue seem to be related, at least by the basic underlying damage mechanism, it becomes of primary importance to study a cement's crack sensitivity or its reciprocal, crack resistance, together with the influences on the clinical environment on this property. It must be realized that the corrosive action of oral fluids, certainly in cements and even in polymers, may contribute significantly to the crack growth sensitivity of a material.[7]

However, even for traditional engineering materials such as metals, for which fatigue has been a recognized problem for decades, the fundamental causes of failure are not yet completely understood. Therefore, one can readily accept that for materials such as dental resin composites and cements, the era of fatigue studies has just started and that fatigue data are only sparsely available. Although current knowledge on the fatigue behavior of materials, such as fiber-reinforced composites, is growing rapidly, it is highly unlikely that the same effort will be directed toward the relatively small market of dental restoratives.

Furthermore, despite the volume of work undertaken to discover the fatigue properties of plastics, very little effort is being made to design standardized test methods. As a consequence, standards developed in fatigue testing of metals have been adapted for use with plastics, although extreme care must be exercised because metals behave differently than do viscoelastic plastics. Furthermore, the fatigue properties of plastics are often influenced to a large extent by the environment in which they are used and/or tested.[8] This certainly holds true for dental restorative materials.

The present situation points to the necessity of establishing standardized testing and gathering fatigue data for dental restorative materials, thereby allowing a better understanding of the major failure processes of wear and fatigue. However, strength also is a factor in failures of restorations and should be integrated with wear and fatigue as a subject of study.

Strength

Two types of loading conditions cause a material to lose strength over time. The first is static loading in the presence of a chemical agent, and the second is cyclic loading. It is obvious that both conditions occur simultaneously in the mouth, and that one can speak about cyclic loading in a chemically active environment.

Under cyclic stress (eg, in extension), a material may fail at stresses well below its known ultimate stress limit. Often tens of thousands of cycles will elapse without incident, followed by a rapid and sudden catastrophic failure, as has been described in the literature for microfilled composites.[4] In general, the higher the stress, the shorter the life of the restoration. Furthermore, composition and chemical structure, as well as environmental conditions, exert profound influence on mechanically induced crack propagation.

Fatigue failure involves two mechanisms: weakening due to energy-dissipating modes of relaxation, and mechanical initiation and propagation of a crack. The latter mechanism is especially dominant at low frequencies, as in the mouth where generally a chewing frequency of 1 to 2 Hz is present. A simple fatigue scenario would then be a progressive loss of strength due to the gradual spread of one or more cracks. Fatigue is the growth of these cracks under cyclic loading conditions.[9] Thus, it is necessary to find out why cracks develop and grow.

In most if not all materials, the onset of crack growth initiates from a preexisting flaw or defect. In dental ceramics, intrinsic defects may arise from microstructural features, whereas extrinsic defects may be introduced by grinding during occlusal adjustment. One must also take into consideration that crack growth may be complicated by crack healing or blunting of the crack tip during prolonged nonstressed periods.[10]

In composite materials, frictional sliding or debonding between the reinforced phase and the matrix also may occur.[8] In the latter case, the effect of an aqueous environment on subcritical crack growth and mechanical degradation will be profound: silicate glasses are among the most (corrosive) fatigue-susceptible of all ceramics.[7,11] Furthermore, although voids can be helpful in the reduction of curing stresses, they are also structural imperfections that encourage crack growth.

Evaluation of Glass-Ionomers for Fatigue

Glass-ionomer cements are considered particle-reinforced materials.[12] The generally low strength of conventional glass ionomers can be explained by a mismatch in the mechanical properties of the glass-ionomer matrix and the glass-particles, causing large stresses to accumulate at the interface.[13] Numerous voids can be detected in these materials. The voids vary substantially in size and diameter, depending on the processing method followed. In metal-reinforced glass-ionomers, the well-bonded, high-strength discrete metal particles may act as pinning sites of the crack front, thus retarding crack growth, perhaps altogether.[13] It is not yet known what the effect of the added resinous components in resin-modified glass-ionomers may be in terms of fatigue behavior. There also is little to nothing known about the fatigue behavior of polyacid-modified composites, also called *compomers*.

The rest of this section discusses how to test for fatigue behavior. The focus is on one particular study involving resin composites and glass-ionomer cements. In the following sections, resin composites will be denoted only by *composites*.

Testing techniques

One way of studying crack growth is by creating test samples that contain an artificially induced crack of known length. This can be achieved rather easily through polymerization of a material against a sharp raiser knife or by indentation. The disadvantage of this technique is that an artificial crack cannot truly mimic naturally occurring defects that are caused by processing, occlusal adjustment, or occlusal forces. Furthermore, although the artificial crack tends to grow in a constant direction, real fatigue cracks can deviate significantly from their normal and expected growth plane due to interactions of the crack tip with microstructural inhomogeneities, environmental elements, and other factors. Fracture toughness tests, which have been carried out on many composite restorative materials, use this methodology.[14]

Indents can be produced with hardness indenters, and this type of experiment has been used to study composites[15] and porcelains.[16] Results with polymeric materials all indicate that the presence of an aqueous environment yields to plasticizing of the matrix phase, thereby lowering most mechanical properties.[7] When indenters that mimic the tips of natural tooth cusps are used,[15] it is found that the matrix phase can undergo considerable plastic deformation without failure. It also has been shown that cracks can be formed at loads of about 50 N, which are easily achieved during mastication.

Unfortunately, all these tests lack the effect of cyclic loading. It might be expected that cyclic loading is less harmful to a material than steady loading, because the average deflection over the cyclic period is less than the steady deflection. However, it is the cyclically loaded material that breaks and the statically loaded one that survives. So, in spite of the important knowledge that can be gathered from static and dynamic fatigue tests, they must be combined with data obtained from cyclic fatigue tests. A common way to establish the fatigue behavior of materials is by studying the number of cycles survived at different stresses, the Wohler curve.

Fracture is the final fatigue criterion that needs to be included in testing. However, this is not possible for the study of cyclic fatigue in particulate-reinforced materials which have widely varying compositions, resulting generally in anisotropic behavior. Furthermore, the establishment of a fatigue criterion becomes complicated, due to the several modes of damage and damage accumulation. Therefore, most fatigue criteria for such materials are dictated by the application area of the structure or the specific properties of the material itself; for example, the percentage of stiffness loss at an established point of fiber and matrix decomposition can be used. Models for the mathematical approach of measuring fatigue in composites are not readily available. Often, the analytical approach is based on linear fracture mechanics, which may or may not apply to glass-ionomer cements. Because many dental materials are heterogeneous in structure and are likely to contain faults or imperfections such as porosity in varying amounts and sizes, the time taken for crack propagation and fracture or material loss by wear is expected to vary considerably. However, at this time, more appropriate equations have not been reported.[15–17]

One could conclude that each group of materials seems to fail by mechanisms specific to that group, and generalizations are hard to make.[9] Rather than looking for the absolute answer in terms of fatigue behavior, a more interesting approach may be to study different dental restoratives under identical testing conditions, which ideally should resemble the clinical service environment. Experimentally, there are several valid approaches.

First, a series of tests can be performed at various levels of stress, and the number of cycles survived can be observed. This Wohler-type of experiment requires many samples and a lot of time. Another approach is to compare the relative levels of stress at which different materials can survive for a pre-set number of stress cycles. This approach is often referred to as a *staircase method.* Tests are conducted sequentially with the maximum applied stress in each test being increased or decreased by a fixed increment, according to whether the previous test resulted in failure or nonfailure.[18]

A comparable method is the *boundary method*, which has some advantages over the staircase method. It is less time-consuming if more than one testing machine is available. Once suitable load levels have been selected, it also allows for simultaneous testing, unlike the staircase method, in which the outcome of any one test must be known before the next can be started.[19]

Materials and methods

Based on the preceding review, a fatigue test was developed[20,21] using a staircase methodology, with the pre-set number of cycles at 10,000. Samples were tested in a stress-controlled mode at a test frequency of 2 Hz. Dynamic creep was compensated for by clamping of the samples. Prior to fatigue testing, the clamped fracture strength was determined (n = 6), and the amount of increase or decrease of fatigue stress following nonfailure or failure, respectively, was arbitrarily set at 4% of this strength. Tests were performed at 35°C.

After preparation, samples were stored for 1 month, either dry (n = 12) or in distilled water (n = 12), at 35°C. In an additional test, freshly prepared samples (n = 12) for selected products were subjected to the fatigue regimen under wet testing conditions, and the fatigue limit was immediately determined. The samples that did not fail were tested again after 1 month of wet storage.

Representative composites, conventional glass-ionomers, resin-modified glass ionomers, and polyacid-modified composites were evaluated (Table 3-1).

Table 3-1 Products and batches used for testing

Brand Name	Type	Curing	Shade	Batch	Manufacturer
Silux Plus	Microfilled composite	L	U	0AM2 92LO8A	3M
Z100	Hybrid composite	L	A2	Lot 92D14A	3M
P50-APC	Hybrid composite	L	U	Lot E8JD03	3M
Charisma	Microfilled composite	L	OA22	22	Kulzer
Artglass	Hybrid composite	L	U	CH121	Kulzer
Herculite XRV	Hybrid composite	L	U	1-2193	Kerr
HiFi Master Palette	Glass-ionomer cement	AB	A3.5	P:BN069428-4 L:BN039430-1	Shofu
Shofu Type II	Glass-ionomer cement	AB		9401	Shofu
Shofu FX	Glass-ionomer cement	AB		9702	Shofu
Ketac-Fil	Glass-ionomer cement	AB	U	044/18 X 204	Espe
Vitremer	Resin-modified glass-ionomer	L, AB, S	A4	P: 199-30-405 L: 199-31-218	3M
Fuji II LC Capsules	Resin-modified glass-ionomer	L, AB, S	B3	Lot 121-045 Lot 021-231	GC
Fuji II LC Powder/Liquid	Resin-modified glass-ionomer	L, AB, S	B3	P: lot 160-931 L: lot 240-831	GC
Fuji IX GP Capsules	Glass-ionomer cement	AB	A2	020967	GC
Dyract	Polyacid-modified composite	L, (AB)	A2	Lot 94-05-20-Z	DeTrey/ Dentsply

AB = acid-based reaction; S = self-curing; L = light-curing; ( ) = hypothetical.
Data reported previously.[9,10,12]

Results

The results are summarized in Table 3-2. In general, for all composite materials tested, the flexural fatigue limit (FFL) after water sorption was significantly lower. This was also the case for the glass-ionomer HiFi Master Palette. It was not true for Shofu FX, the resin-modified glass ionomers, or the polyacid-modified composite.

The results for the immediate fatigue test reveal that all materials tested showed a significant decrease in FFL at 5 minutes compared to the dry FFL. When examining the wet FFL, all materials but the composites had a significantly decreased FFL, with the resin-modified glass

Table 3-2 Results for flexural fatigue limits (MPa)

Product	Postcure FFL		Immediate FFL	
	Dry (SD)	Wet (SD)	5 min (SD)	1 mo (SD)
Silux Plus	72.5* ± 3.4	54.6* ± 3.4	54.6 ± 2.1	58.2 ± 2.3
Charisma	91.4* ± 4.4	60.1* ± 3.0		
Artglass	108.1 ± 2.8	77.8 ± 2.7		
P50-APC	103.7* ± 11.9	74.9* ± 3.6		
Z100	126.3* ± 3.1	94.5* ± 3.7	83.6 ± 8.7	68.5 ± 6.5
Herculite XRV	128.4* ± 6.4	112.0* ± 15.9		
HiFi Master Palette	58.5 ± 4.2	35.2 ± 3.0		
Shofu Type II	44.3 ± 1.8	26.9 ± 1.6		
Shofu FX	31.6 ± 2.4	28.8 ± 4.6		
Vitremer	53.0 ± 10.2	53.2 ± 2.0	24.6 ± 3.4	51.6 ± 2.3
Fuji II LC Capsules	51.3* ± 7.9	51.0* ± 3.5	27.1 ± 1.6	47.8 ± 1.7
Fuji II LC Powder/Liquid	48.8* ± 5.1	51.1* ± 8.2		
Fuji IX Capsules	40.5 ± 3.5	27.3 ± 2.4		
Dyract	72.9* ± 14.7	67.2* ± 5.1	45.4 ± 3.5	56.8 ± 5.0

SD = standard deviation.

*Data reported previously.[20,21]

ionomers scoring only about 50%. One month later, however, only Z100 had a significantly lower FFL than the wet samples.

The investigation into fractured surfaces revealed several common fracture characteristics. Regardless of the type of material tested, most often the fracture was initiated at an inclusion or imperfection: a void (Fig 3-1), a filler particle (Fig 3-2), and so on. In the microfilled materials, markings of the cyclic nature of the crack growth could be identified clearly at both the filler particles and the matrix phase (Fig 3-3). The crack retardation effect of optimal particle size distribution on crack growth also could be seen (Fig 3-4).

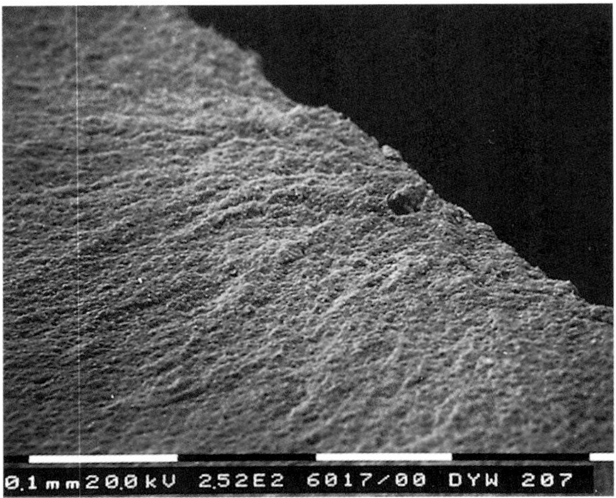

Fig 3-1 Failure initiated by the presence of a void. The surface texture shows diverging patterns originating at the defect. (Dyract, wet storage and testing.)

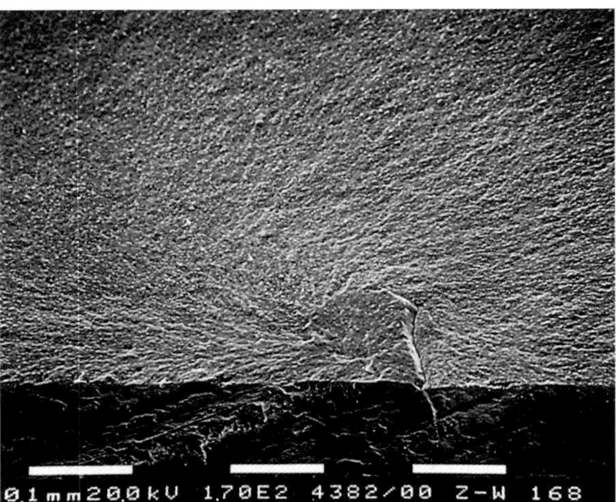

Fig 3-2 Failure probably initiated by a defect created during finishing procedures. The crack started at the edge of the sample. Again, the surface texture reveals a specific pattern. (Z100, wet storage and testing.)

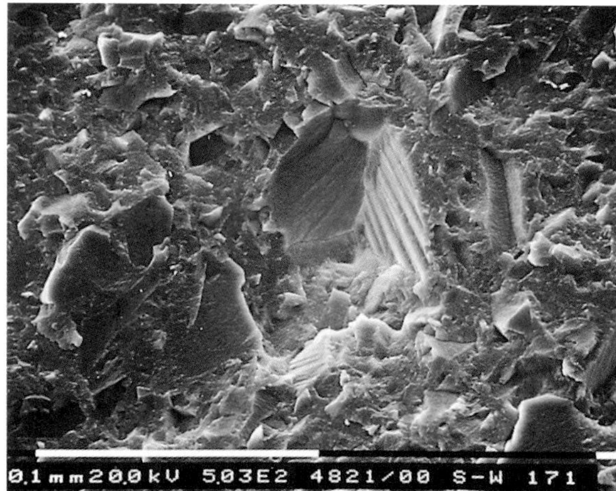

Fig 3-3a Stress striae observed at the particle–matrix interphase. (Silux Plus, wet storage and testing.)

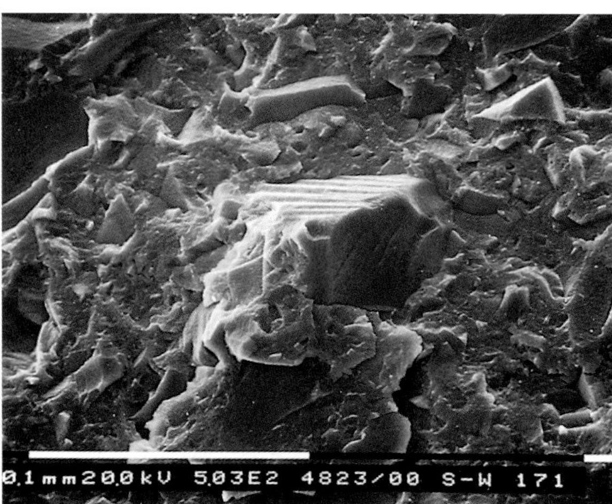

Fig 3-3b The opposite surface where the particle is still present, showing identical marks.

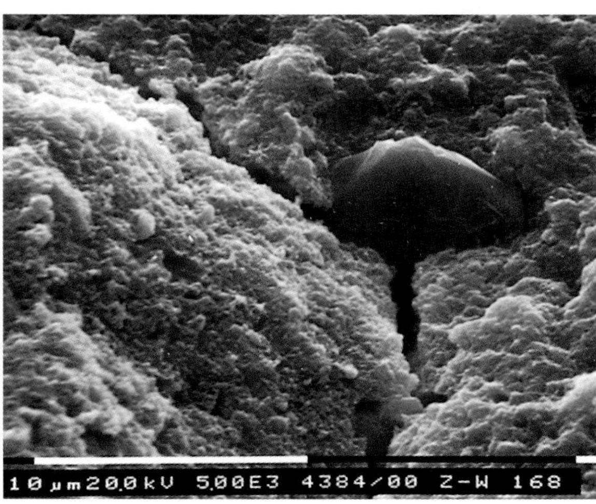

Fig 3-4 The obvious effect of optimal particle size distribution on crack pinning.

Discussion

Water plays a major role in filler-matrix bond failures in resin-based matrices. It leaches out filler elements; it induces filler failures and filler-matrix debonding, thereby reducing the strength of the matrix material because debonded fillers may act as stress concentrators and significantly multiply the number of potential crack growth sites;[22] and it has a plasticizing effect on the matrix. Therefore, it is extremely important that fatigue tests are run in a humid environment, in which composites are immersed in water for at least 30 days.[23] The present results show that water decreases the flexural fatigue limits of the tested composite materials.

The hydrophilic 2-hydroxyethylmethacrylate (HEMA) is used in most resin-modified glass-ionomers,[24] at a concentration of about 5% in the final set material.[25] Neither version of Fuji II LC or of Vitremer deteriorated after water sorption, thus supporting the hypothesis that "self-healing" or "repair" could be possible in glass-ionomer cements.[26] However, this healing may be a retardation in crack growth or a crack growth toughening mechanism, possibly due to the plasticizing effect of the resinous component.

The results for conventional glass-ionomers add to the controversy about the influence of time and water on their properties. A decline following exposure to an aqueous environment is attributed to the plasticizing and erosive effect of water on the cement, as reviewed by Gladys.[27] A healing mechanism is apparently not present in HiFi Master Palette because its fatigue resistance decreased 13.5% after water uptake. It is suggested that extrinsic water inhibits the matrix-forming process of a conventional glass-ionomer, leading to a strength reduction.[28]

In Dyract, the acidic polymerizable monomer (tetracarboxylbutane) has two methacrylate groups, as well as two carboxyl groups, and accounts for about 28% of the composition (technical information from DeTrey/Dentsply). This monomer not only can cross-link when initiated through radical polymerization, but also undergoes an acid-base reaction with the reactive glass particles if water is absorbed from the tooth and the oral environment. This is reflected in the results where Dyract performs better than the other composites tested. In the dry-storage samples, the postpolymerization predominated over the acid-base reaction, and was even reinforced by storage in the oven at 35°C. Once placed in a wet environment, the active carboxylic groups undergo the acid-base reaction.[29] This delayed reaction may compensate for the plasticizing effect of water on the resin component.

The fatigue results of the freshly prepared samples show that the composites tested already have a flexural fatigue limit after about 5 minutes, comparable to that after 1 month of undisturbed postcuring in wet storage conditions. After 1 month, however, there are significant differences among the products tested.

The microfilled composite has not suffered from the stress applied during the initial formation of the cross-linked polymer network. The hybrid composite, however, clearly shows evidence of loss in fatigue resistance, probably due to damage encountered during the first fatigue test at 5 minutes, which then created opportunities for water to further attack the weakened material. Because the hybrid composite is highly filled, at some spots the matrix remaining between the filler particles became too vulnerable with regard to fatigue stresses.

The resin-modified glass-ionomers showed a remarkable increase in fatigue resistance 1 month after the immediate fatigue test, resulting in a fatigue resistance that was no different from that obtained under unstressed storage conditions. Thus, the acid-base reaction continued following water uptake.[30]

The polyacid-modified material also did not suffer from the imposed fatigue regimen immediately after curing. It is not clear whether this can be attributed strictly to postcuring of the resinous matrix or the continued acid-base reaction, or to a combination of both factors.

Most fatigue tests apply a given load at a given stress rate without taking into account the stress state of the tested surface. Only a few studies have determined the actual fatigue stress.[20,31] Indeed, a load of 100 N may result in a stress of 10 MPa with a surface contact of 10 mm^2 versus 1 MPa for a contact surface of 100 mm^2. Thus, it is important to know the stress limits to which fillings will be subjected during clinical service.

The maximum biting force varies between 108 and 608 N for natural teeth, with the greatest forces exhibited by the molars.[32] The forces used during mastication show peak values of 32 to 374 N, with an average of about 20 N.[33] These values may differ substantially during the chewing cycle and the progressive reduction in the size of food particles. Generally, the load remains smaller during 95% of the chewing cycle. When the load rises, the functional maximal values are about 71 N.[33] The force exerted on the teeth during swallowing is, on average, twice the force exerted during mastication. These values are, of course, force values and should be considered as forces exerted on a surface. To be able to calculate the stress at the occlusal contact area, one must consider the surface area of an antagonistic cusp, which can be estimated at about 1 mm^2. The average stress state of a restorative under antagonistic load can be estimated at between 10 to 20 MPa, with short peaks of about 70 MPa during chewing. Consequently, the stress increases from 40 MPa up to 160 MPa during swallowing.

It is interesting to note that some work[34] using finite element analysis with an applied load of 100 N at 90 degrees to the internal inclined plane of the buccal cusp, reports tensile stresses in the filling of 12.4, 22.5, and 42.5 MPa, ranging up to 82.5 MPa.

After wet storage, conventional glass-ionomers score below the arbitrary 40 MPa criterion. Even more important is that resin-modified materials seem to be very vulnerable at the early stages of placement, with a fatigue resistance of about 25 MPa. Thus, it must be remembered that one of the primary characteristics of fatigue is that a material will fail at stresses below its static strength.

Conclusion

The fatigue resistance of resin-modified glass ionomers after water sorption is between that of microfilled composites and polyacid-modified composites. Resin-modified composites, however, seem to be vulnerable at the early stages after curing, although this is not reflected in the fatigue behavior at later stages. Fatigue resistance is still a matter of concern and stress-bearing restorations should, therefore, be avoided. Hybrid composites also can be vulnerable during early fatigue stresses, probably due to their high filler content.

Elasticity

As stated at the beginning of this chapter, it is important to have a good understanding of the underlying principles that rule the properties of restorative materials. One of these principles is that mechanical and physical properties originate from a material's internal structure, which involves atoms and the way these atoms are associated with their neighbors. This internal structure may be altered when the material is deformed.[35]

Under clinical circumstances, fillings are put under stress in a chemically active environment with superimposed thermal fluctuations. As a consequence, properties change. Some changes can be spotted easily, such as wear and failure which have already been discussed. These changes are symptoms, expressing that the internal structure has been modified due to applied stimuli. It is of interest, therefore, to study a property that is capable of reflecting the internal structure of materials and the changes this structure undergoes: elasticity.

The modulus of elasticity

One of the few principal properties capable of providing a basis for understanding the relationship between structure and properties, is Young's modulus, or the modulus of elasticity.[35] This property can be derived from the stress-strain characteristics of a given material.

Stress is the measure of force per unit area. Strain is the dimensional response to this stress. Plastic strain occurs when the stress exceeds a critical value that initiates a permanent displacement of atoms from their neighbors and, therefore, is irreversible. Elastic strain is reversible; when the stress is removed, the strain disappears. Elastic strain is commonly a linear function of stress. The modulus relating unidirectional elastic strain and stress is the modulus of elasticity (E).

The modulus of elasticity also reflects the strain capacity of a given material, acting more or less as the reciprocal of the modulus itself. The higher the modulus of elasticity, the lower the strain capacity within certain limits.

Clinical considerations

Many studies have shown that it is difficult to obtain a proper and lasting seal of the cervical border for a cavity filled with resin composite, especially when this border is situated in dentin. This is mainly due to the polymerization shrinkage of the composite toward the enamel, where a string bond can be obtained.[36] The direction of shrinkage, combined with the almost instantaneous polymerization reaction of the light-cured resin composite, increases the polymerization contraction stresses to a level that exceeds the weak and slowly developing dentin bond.[37]

This problem can be solved by taking advantage of the strain capacity of a given filling material: the results of tests for bonding strength indicate that materials with proper sealing ability do not necessarily show high bond strengths. They do, however, show an increased flexibility, or strain capacity, of the restorative system. Such a system can benefit from the application of an intermediate layer of a low-modulus material between tooth structures, corresponding with decreased marginal leakage scores.[38] The importance of creating such an elasticity gradient down to the dentin-resin interface scale has been substantiated by nano-indentation measurements.[1] Given these findings, glass-ionomer cements could be good materials to serve as such an intermediate layer, because they bond almost spontaneously to dentin, and on the condition that the strain capacity and modulus of elasticity would render them suitable for such a system.

Using the Modulus of Elasticity to Evaluate Restoration Materials

Materials and methods

Although simplified, the modulus of elasticity can be considered a parameter that describes a material's resistance against deformation. When applied to multiphase materials such as glass-ionomers and composites, both elastic and plastic effects may occur simultaneously under certain conditions: the deformation is said to be viscoelastic. Furthermore, most elastic and plastic deformation phenomena are influenced by environmental factors such as time and temperature. Although the modulus of elasticity might seem a straightforward property to determine, the experimental determination and the subsequent interpretation of data must be done with great care.

In dental research, most of the investigations of the modulus of elasticity rely on static or quasi-static tests, such as tensile or compressive testing methods. Such an approach has led to considerable difficulties in assessing and comparing the results for materials that show viscoelastic behavior.[39] Dynamic testing should take such phenomena into account, although the results obtained with such tests generally show higher values than those arising from static testing.[40]

One of the possible dynamic testing methods is based on the measurement of the duration of the fundamental period for the first harmonic of a freely oscillating sample.[41] The samples are set in transverse vibration with a single pulse excitation generated by means of a small hammer. While the sample is vibrating, a microphone located underneath the sample picks up the first harmonic, from which the fundamental frequency of the sample can be determined. The dynamic modulus of elasticity under flexure can than be calculated as a function of this frequency.

Table 3-3 Moduli of elasticity for static and dynamic testing, as a function of different storage conditions, after 1 month of storage

	Static Testing		Dynamic Testing
	Dry	Wet	Wet
Silux Plus	10.2 ± 0.5	7.7 ± 0.3	10.4 ± 0.1
Charisma	13.0 ± 0.5	11.5 ± 2.1	14.0 ± 0.6
P50-APC	23.2 ± 0.9	19.1 ± 1.3	25.0 ± 0.7
Z100	21.3 ± 0.8	16.7 ± 0.7	22.0 ± 0.1
Herculite XRV	17.1 ± 0.6	16.7 ± 0.1	—
HiFi Master Palette	—	—	18.1 ± 1.7
Ketac-Fil	—	—	26.5 ± 1.1
Vitremer	16.5 ± 0.5	10.2 ± 1.0	14.5 ± 1.5
Fuji II LC Capsules	15.0 ± 1.2	8.7 ± 0.5	18.9 ± 1.4
Fuji II LC Powder/Liquid	20.3 ± 2.6	8.6 ± 0.4	17.3 ± 1.0
Dyract	15.1 ± 0.5	11.6 ± 0.4	15.0 ± 0.6

Data previously reported.[20,21,42,44]

The static modulus of elasticity was measured prior to the fatigue limit tests described earlier.[21] The classic three-point flexural test setup was used to calculate the static modulus of elasticity.[20]

Several representative restorative materials were tested (see Table 3-1) under both static and dynamic testing conditions. Rectangular samples (length = 35 mm, width = 5 mm, height = 1.2 mm) were prepared for each type of test and were identical in geometry for both testing conditions. The samples were stored for 1 month in distilled water at 35°C prior to testing. For the static test, a separate group of samples was prepared and stored dry at 35°C prior to testing. Samples that were stored wet were tested under continuous water spray at 35°C, while samples stored dry were tested under dry conditions at 35°C.

Results

Table 3-3 shows the moduli of elasticity under dry and wet storage conditions for both test methods. The results confirm that the values from dynamic testing are higher than those obtained from static tests under wet conditions, as would be expected.[40] In general, the static test results allow for a more detailed ranking of the test materials according to their composition.

The results obtained from static testing emphasize the influence of water sorption on the elastic property of the test materials: generally, the modulus of elasticity decreases following water sorption. This decrease is most pronounced for the resin-modified glass-ionomer Fuji II LC.

For Ketac-Fil and HiFi Master Palette, both conventional-glass ionomers, the static modulus of elasticity could not be determined. These materials were so brittle that the extremely low deformation applied either caused failure of the samples before any valid reading could be made or yielded unrealistic values for the modulus of elasticity because the calculation was based on a nonlinear portion of the load-deflection curve.

Discussion

The finding that the ranking of the test materials is more pronounced for the static test results may be explained by the extremely low deformation that goes along with the dynamic test.[40] This test places less stress on the internal bonds that might be weakened by stress corrosion,[20] caused by the presence and action of water. Indeed, the difference between the two test methods is most pronounced for the wet storage samples, especially for Fuji II LC. The static test results show a drop of about 50% in the modulus of elasticity for resin-modified glass ionomers compared to the dry state. If the products are compared with the dynamic test results of Vitremer, it becomes clear that the low deformation test did not pick up the changes in the internal structure of the Fuji II LC materials, because they scored even higher than Vitremer.

The inability to determine the static modulus of elasticity for conventional glass ionomers emphasizes the brittle nature of these materials, which show virtually no strain capacity.

Resin-modified glass-ionomers, microfilled composites, and the polyacid-modified composite show comparable static moduli of elasticity after 1 month of water storage. Their collective results are about 40% lower than the results obtained for highly filled composites. These differences suggest that a favorable modulus of elasticity gradient may be needed to obtain proper bonding to dentin and preservation of the marginal integrity. However, before decisions can be made on a given material, more information is required about the internal structure and the corresponding strain capacity (eg, the properties of the matrix phase) of the materials.

The matrix phase in light-cured composites and light-cured polyacid-modified composites, which closely resemble composites, is formed by rapid cross-linking of the original low-molecular-weight molecules through high-energy covalent bonds. This results in an almost instantaneous, rigid, three-dimensional network with a considerable number of unreacted methacrylate groups. This is due to the fact that the probability of a given reactive group bonding covalently with a corresponding group on another molecule decreases as the molecule itself starts to grow. Furthermore, because covalent bonds are stable, the yielding capacity inherently present due to the unreacted groups is not likely to contribute to strain capacity. Finally, there is an absence of spontaneous bonding of composites to tooth structure. All these factors render the microfilled materials unsuitable as lining materials and elastic buffers.

Although the nature of the cohesive forces binding the matrix of glass ionomers together is still speculative, it is probable that a mixture of ionic cross-links, hydrogen bridges, and chain entanglements[42] may form both primary bonds that are not easily modified and secondary low-energy bonds that could reestablish broken bonds. The filler system can also provide better strain capacity because the filler particles are covered with a siliceous hydrogel or, in the case of smaller filler particles, are composed entirely of such a gel and link the filler core to the matrix phase.[43] In this way, the filler particles not only enhance the mechanical properties of the material, but participate in the setting reaction. This setting reaction is characterized by a gelation stage, also called the initial stage, which takes place during the initial set, thereby loosing its plastic behavior and becoming more rigid.[42] However, these conventional cements are very vulnerable to water sorption and generally show low mechanical properties, thereby limiting their application.

The results show that the addition of photocurable resins to conventional glass-ionomer cements has improved the mechanical properties, based on the modulus of elasticity. It is not yet completely understood how the leachable filler particles of the glass-ionomer could interact with the resin matrix. The results, however, do show that the resin component has modified the most brittle conventional glass-ionomer into a flexible material with strain capacity, that can cope with the sudden polymerization contraction stresses that arise from light curing a resin composite restorative on top of it. As a result, the adhesive bond remains intact, and marginal integrity can be preserved.[38,42]

Conclusions

The available resin-modified glass-ionomer cements open interesting perspectives with regard to marginal sealing and preservation of marginal integrity, due to their ability to bond to tooth structure combined with their strain capacity. Further research as to their long-term mechanical properties is required, especially in situations where the restorative system is stressed by both thermal and mechanical stimuli.

References

1. Van Meerbeek B, Willems G, Celis JP, Roos JR, Braem M, Lambrechts P, Vanherle G. Assessment by nano-indentation of the hardness and elasticity of the resin-dentin bonding area. J Dent Res 1993;72:1434–1442.

2. Harrison A, Draughn RA. Abrasive wear, tensile strength, and hardness of dental composite resins—Is there a relationship? J Prosthet Dent 1976;36:395–398.

3. Pallav P, Davidson CL, de Gee AJ. Wear rated of composites, an amalgam, and enamel under stress-bearing conditions. J Prosthet Dent 1988;59:426–429.

4. Lambrechts P, Braem M, Vanherle G. Evaluation of clinical performance for posterior composite resins and dentin adhesives. Oper Dent 1987;12:53–78.

5. Wu W, Cobb EN. A silver staining technique for investigation wear of restorative dental composites. J Biomed Mater Res 1981;15:343–348.

6. Mair LH. Staining of in vivo subsurface degradation in dental composites with silver nitrate. J Dent Res 1991;70:215–220.

7. Söderholm K. Degradation of glass-filler in experimental composites. J Dent Res 1981; 60:1867–1875.

8. Brown RP. Fatigue. In: Handbook of Plastic Test Methods. 2d ed. London: Longman, 1986:205–211.

9. Reid CN, Fisher J, Jacobsen PH. Fatigue and wear of dental materials. J Dent 1990;18:209–215.

10. Fairhurst CW, Lockwood PE, Ringle RD, Twiggs SW. Dynamic fatigue of feldspathic porcelain. Dent Mater 1993;9:269–273.

11. Morena R, Beaudreau GM, Lockwood PE, Evans AL, Fairhurst CW. Fatigue of dental ceramics in a simulated oral environment. J Dent Res 1986;65:993–997.

12. Wilson AD, McLean JW. The setting reaction and its clinical consequences. In: Glass-ionomer Cement. Chicago: Quintessence, 1988:43–56.

13. Nakajima H, Watkins JH, Arita K, Hanaoka K, Okabe T. Mechanical properties of glass-ionomers under static and dynamic loading. Dent Mater 1996;12:30–37.

14. Lloyd CH, Ianetta RV. The fracture toughness of dental composites. I. The development of strength and fracture toughness. J Oral Rehabil 1982;9:55–66.

15. Baran G, Shin W, Abbas A, Wunder S. Indentation cracking of composite matrix materials. J Dent Res 1994;73:1450–1456.

16. White SN. Mechanical fatigue of a feldspathic dental procelain. Dent Mater 1993;9:260–264.

17. Drummond JL. Cyclic fatigue of composite restorative materials. J Oral Rehabil 1989; 16:509–520.

18. Draughn RA. Compressive fatigue of composite restorative materials. J Dent Res 1979; 58:1093–1096.

19. Huysmans MC, van der Varst PGT, Schafer R, Peters MC, Plasschaert AJM, Soltesz U. Fatigue behavior of direct post-and-core-restored premolars. J Dent Res 1992;71:1145–1150.

20. Braem MJA, Davidson CL, Lambrechts P, Vanherle G. In vitro flexural fatigue limits of dental composites. J Biomed Mater Res 1994; 28:1397–1402.

21. Braem MJA, Lambrechts P, Gladys S, Vanherle G. In vitro fatigue behavior of restorative composites and glass-ionomers. Dent Mater 1995;11:137–141.

22. Sakaguchi RL, Cross M, Douglas WH. A simple model of crack propagation in dental restoartions. Dent Mater 1992;8:131–136.

23. Fan PL, Edahl A, Leung RL, Stanford JW. Alternative interpretations of water sorption values of composites resins. J Dent Res 1985;64:78–80.

24. Gasser O. Evolution of the glass systems. In: Hunt P (ed). Glass Ionomers: The Next Generation. Proceedings of the 2nd International Symposium on Glass-Ionomers, June 1994. Philadelphia: International Symposia in Dentistry, 1994:23–33.

25. Sidhu SK, Watson TF. Resin-modified glass-ionomer materials: A status report for the American Journal of Dentistry. Am J Dent 1995;8:59–67.

26. Davidson CL. Glass-ionomer bases under posterior composites. J Esthet Dent 1994; 6:223–226.

27. Gladys S. Mechanical and physical properties. In: In Vitro and In Vivo Characterization of Hybrid Restorative Materials. Belgium: Leuven University Press, 1997:12–13.

28. Shen C, Grimaudo N. Effect of hydration on the biaxial flexural strength of a glass-ionomer cement. Dent Mater 1994;10:190–195.

29. Hammesfahr PD. Developments in resionomer systems. In: Hunt P (ed). Glass-Ionomers: The Next Generation. Proceedings of the 2nd International Symposium on Glass-Ionomers, June 1994. Philadelphia: International Symposia in Denistry, 1994:47–55.

30. Jevnikar P, Jarh O, Sepe A, Pintar MM, Funduk N. Micro magnetic resonance imaging of water uptake by glass ionomer cements. Dent Mater 1997;13:20–23.

31. Sutow EJ, Jones DW, Hall GC, Milne EL. The response of dental amalgam to dynamic loading. J Dent Res 1984;64:62–66.

32. Hagberg C. Assessments of bite force: A review. J Craniomandib Disord 1987;1:162–169.

33. De Boever JA, McCall WD Jr, Holden S, Ash MM Jr. Functional occlusal forces: An investigation by telemetry. J Prosthet Dent 1978;40:326–333.

34. Van Noort R, Cardew GE, Howard IC. A study of the interfacial shear and tensile stresses in a restored molar tooth. J Dent 1988;16:286–293.

35. Van Vlack LH. Review of selected properties of materials. In: Elements of Materials Science and Engineering. 5th ed. Addison-Wesley, 1987:633.

36. Crim GA. Assessment of microleakage of 12 restorative systems. Quintessence Int 1987;17: 21–24.

37. Davidson CL, de Gee AJ, Feilzer AJ. The competition between the composite-dentin bond strength and the polymerization contraction stress. J Dent Res 1984;63:1396–1399.

38. Kemp-Scholte CM, Davidson CL. Complete marginal seal of Class V resin composite restorations effected by increased flexibility. J Dent Res 1990;59:1240–1243.

39. Nakayama WT, Hall DR, Grenoble DE, Katz JL. Elastic properties of dental resin restorative materials. J Dent Res 1974;53:1121–1126.

40. Braem M, Davidson CL, Vanherle G, Van Doren V, Lambrechts P. The relationship between test methodology and elastic behavior of composites. J Dent Res 1987;66:1036–1039.

41. Braem M, Lambrechts P, Van Doren VE, Vanherle G. The impact of composite structure on its elastic response. J Dent Res 1986;65:648–653.

42. Gladys S. In vitro and in vivo characterisation of new hybrid restorative materials. Doctoral thesis, 1997.

43. De Moor R. Composition and setting reaction of the glass-ionomer cements. In: De Moor R (ed). Evaluation of the Long-Term Fluoride Release of Self-Curing Glass-Ionomer Cements. Kortrijk: Acopy, 1995:7–29.

44. Willems G, Lambrechts P, Braem M, Celis JP, Vanherle G. A classification of dental composites according to their morphological and mechanical characteristics. Dent Mater 1992;8:310–319.

Chapter 4

Chemical and Biological Properties of Glass-Ionomer Cements

George Eliades

Glass-ionomer cements are considered the most durable dental cements currently available, even though in an aqueous environment they are susceptible to hydrolytic degradation through erosion, ion release, and water sorption.[1] Immediately after hardening, glass-ionomers are very sensitive to erosion because the matrix-forming ions are still soluble. When fully set, these cements release ions and absorb water in an aqueous environment. Conventional materials release sodium, fluoride, silica, and traces of calcium,[2] whereas admixed amalgam alloy and cermets release additional ionic silver.[3] The release of various ionic species from resin-modified glass-ionomers also has been confirmed.[4]

The water sorption phenomena from glass-ionomers have not been thoroughly investigated. From the early work of Wilson and Crisp[5] it is known that the labile, loosely bound fraction of water in glass-ionomers reaches up to 5% by weight of the set cement. This fraction varies depending on the environmental conditions and results either in hygroscopic expansion or in shrinking and material crazing. These structural changes do not allow for a reliable gravimetric determination of water sorption employing wet and dry weighing methods. Nevertheless, in one study 3.8% water sorption was measured for a conventional product[6] and considered as a clinical advantage because it exceeded the setting shrinkage of the material,[2] although no values were provided for the latter.

The introduction of visible light-cured resin-modified glass-ionomers was expected to provide protection against initial water sensitivity by the rapid formation of the polymer network,[7] which would set up a barrier to water diffusion. However, it has been shown that these materials also absorb water because of the hydrophilic nature of their polymer networks, which incorporate 2-hydroxyethylmethacrylate (HEMA) or poly-HEMA[1] and may adversely affect their properties.[8] It seems that the retardation observed in the acid-base reaction rate of these products after the rapid formation of the photo polymerizable network[9] minimizes the benefits of any short-term shielding effect of the polymer matrix as opposed to the slow-developing polysalt matrix.

The solubility of glass-ionomers—the outcome of ion release and water uptake interactions—has been investigated in solutions with acidic, neutral, or basic pH, utilizing immersion or jet erosion techniques. Most products were found to erode at a pH of less than 4,[1] with the erosion rate depending mainly on the chemical composition of the cement and the setting status. Generally, polyacrylic acid–base cements are more erosion resistant than cements based on copolymers of acrylic and maleic acids.[1] Silver cermet cements also demonstrate less erosion than do conventional materials.[10] For resin-modified materials, higher erosion resistance was found due to the presence of the polymer network.[11] Nevertheless, it has been shown that some products in this category, although they contain basic powder and polyacid components, are incapable of producing a polysalt matrix, an observation which puts in question their erosion resistance and clinical durability.[12]

The dynamic equilibrium established between glass-ionomers and the oral environment substantially affects the reactivity of the materials through ion exchange processes, resulting in the release of ionic species of important biological activity. Among these, fluoride has attracted the most interest because of its documented ability to help prevent caries when added to oral health care products. It has been postulated that glass-ionomer restorations exert an anticariogenic effect on adjacent cavity walls in the event of primary or secondary caries attack. This effect has been attributed to the fluoride released which is absorbed by hard dental tissues, increasing their resistance to demineralization, enhancing remineralization reactions, and modifying carbohydrate metabolism of plaque.[2] The complex mechanisms implemented in the development of the cariostatic effect of glass-ionomers in vitro, their in vivo relevance, and their clinical efficiency are discussed in the rest of this chapter. The approach used is intended to facilitate understanding of the importance of the enormous number of in vitro findings compared to the limited amount of existing information for in vivo conditions.

Fluoride Release

The source of fluoride ions from glass-ionomer cements are the calcium fluoride (CaF_2), strontium fluoride (SrF_2), lanthanum fluoride (LaF_2), sodium hexafluoroaluminate (Na_3AlF_6), and aluminum trifluoride (AlF_3) inclusions of the low-temperature glasses used to formulate the powder components. The primary role of these fluorides is to lower the glass fusion temperature during the manufacturing process, although they also improve handling properties and increase cement strength and translucency.[1] During setting, the fluoride ions produced form strong soluble aluminofluoride complexes like AlF^{2+} and AlF^{2+}, which prevent premature gelation of polyions by aluminum ions. In fully set cements, fluoride is located in the partially degraded glasses that form the glass core and in the polysalt matrix, primarily in the form of aluminum complexes.[1]

When a fully set glass-ionomer is exposed to neutral aqueous solutions, it absorbs water and releases ions such as sodium, silica, calcium, and fluoride.[2,13] Of the total amount of fluoride in the set cement, only a small fraction is available for release. This is not related to the total fluoride content of the cement,[14] but

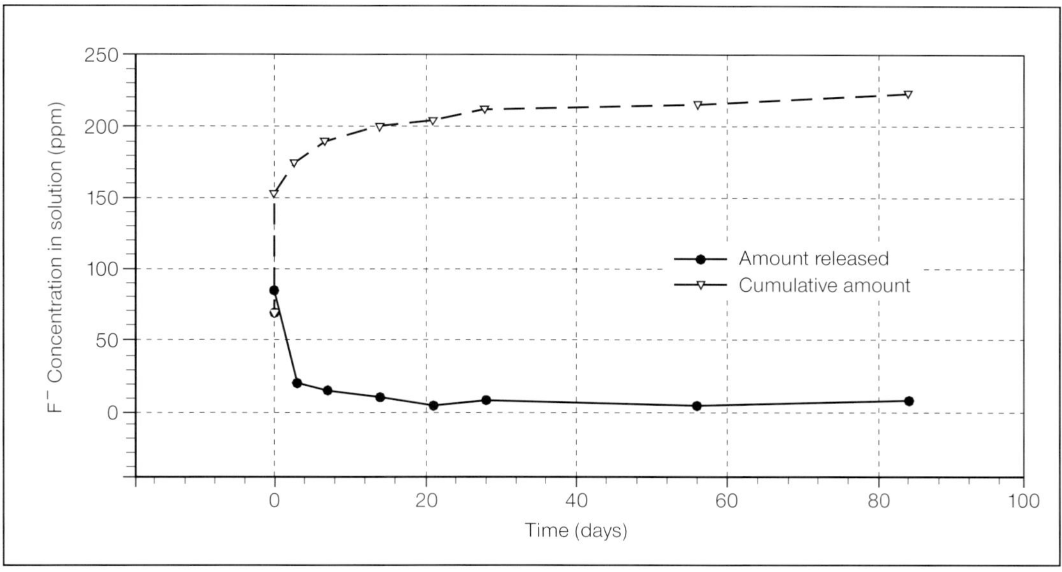

Fig 4-1 Typical graph of fluoride release from a conventional glass-ionomer cement immersed in distilled water 1 hour after setting. Note the differences between the amount released and the cumulative amount as a function of time.

depends on the amount of sodium that maintains cement electron neutrality after fluoride release.[2] Only the fluoride present in the matrix is available for elution at neutral conditions.[15]

Mechanisms of fluoride release

Although many studies have reported a sustained release of fluoride from set glass-ionomer cements in distilled water over a long period of time,[2,16,17] the mechanism of fluoride release is still not completely understood.[14] It is generally accepted that two reactions are involved: a short-term reaction of high fluoride release corresponding to initial elution due to the postsetting maturation process, and a long-term reaction of low release attributed to equilibrium diffusion processes (Fig 4-1).

A systematic investigation of the fluoride release from a series of conventional and metal-reinforced glass-ionomer cements showed that the cumulative amount of fluoride released (Fc) in distilled water at 37°C as a function of time (t) corresponds to the following equation:

$$F_c = (FI \times t) / (t + t_{1/2}) + (b \times \sqrt{t})$$

where FI is the maximum value of fluoride released during the short-term reaction period that occurs rapidly after specimen immersion in water and ceases after some days, $t_{1/2}$ is the half-life of the short-term reaction process, and b is a constant that expresses the measure of the driving force during the slow release period.[18]

The chemical composition and type of mixing were identified as the main factors affecting the kinetics of fluoride release.[18] Amalgam alloy admixed cements were found to release amounts of fluoride higher than or equal to those of conventional glass-ionomers[17–20] due to increased microporosity, which increases the effective surface area for release. For silver cermet cements, in which silver particles are sintered to glass particles, the effective contact area between the glass particles and polyalkenoic acid is reduced, leading to a reduction in fluoride release, especially during the initial elution period.[18–20] Resin-modified glass-ionomers release fluoride in distilled water at a range similar to those of conventional or metal-reinforced materials,[21,22] but increased cumulative fluoride release[23] or reduced short-term release rates have been noted in some products.[24] The fact that the fluoride released from conventional products is mostly sodium fluoride,[2,15] along with the observation that this is not a critical salt for the formation of the polysalt matrix, explains the lack of anticipated weakening of the materials following fluoride release.[25]

A significant increase in fluoride release is observed at low pH values, suggesting that an erosive mechanism is activated at these conditions from the preferential dissolution of the glass particles in the matrix.[26,27] Another factor governing fluoride release is its concentration in the immersion solution. In the presence of an inverse fluoride concentration gradient, glass-ionomers may absorb fluoride from the environment and release it again under specific conditions.[28] Thus, the concept of fluoride recharging old glass-ionomer fillings was introduced, in vitro evidence for which supports the theory that such interactions are feasible through an ion exchange process.[29,30]

Clinical relevance

The established fluoride releasing efficiency of glass-ionomers in aqueous solutions raised important questions as to the clinical relevance of this trait, and efforts were undertaken to investigate the fluoride release processes under conditions simulating the oral environment or in vivo. The first approach was to use artificial saliva.[31,32] Comparative data on the fluoride release from the same brands of glass-ionomers in distilled water and artificial saliva revealed a reduction in the release when using the latter.[32] When nonstimulated human saliva was used as an immersion medium, a significant reduction in fluoride release occurred which was mainly attributed to the adsorption of HPO_4^{2-} and saliva proteins onto material surfaces in the form of pellicle, inhibiting fluoride release.[33]

The important question of whether the fluoride released from glass-ionomer cements is adequate to increase the fluoride concentration in saliva was addressed in several studies during the early 1990s. These studies provided evidence of elevated fluoride concentration in saliva for a period of a few weeks after glass-ionomer application, implying that these materials may be effective short-term intraoral fluoride releasing devices[34–37]; however, other in vivo experiments did not reach the same conclusion.[38] In some of these studies, the comparisons made among the fluoride release profiles in saliva were not reliable because lining materials were employed as restoratives.

Some conclusions may be drawn from the results of the fluoride release experiments. The experiments performed in distilled water or in any other artificial medium should be interpreted only on a material screening basis. Given that the actual amount of fluoride required to exert a cariostatic effect has not yet been determined, the varying levels of fluoride release should not be considered primary criteria for material selection, because very often materials with high fluoride release lack hydrolytic stability. It should be clearly stated that fluoride release is an ion exchange process, and ionic species are absorbed simultaneously from the environment to maintain diffusion equilibrium. In vivo the fluoride salivary levels may be increased after glass-ionomer application, but within a few weeks are reduced to baseline levels. From an experimental standpoint, the discrepancy in the way fluoride release data are presented is noteworthy. Cumulative fluoride values are usually given as a function of time in mg F^-, ppm F^-, mg F^- per unit volume of the cement, or mg F^- per surface area unit of the cement. The rationale for expressing the results in cumulative mode is seriously questioned because the experimental procedure for measuring fluoride release involves an open system, in which partial or complete replacement of the immersion liquid occurs at specific time intervals. It should be stated that the fluoride-selective electrode measurements represent the maximum amount of ionizable fluoride available in the solution and not the actual ionized fraction, due to the addition of the total ionic strength adjustment buffer solution. In the case of fluoride units, elution is considered a surface phenomenon and the results should be expressed in mass per unit of total specimen surface area[2] to allow for direct comparisons among materials.

Fluoride Uptake

Several in vitro studies have shown that substantial amounts of fluoride released from glass-ionomer restorations are taken up by sound enamel and dentin cavity walls[22,39–42]; this release also has been confirmed by in vivo studies.[43,44] However, the results presented should be interpreted with caution, because in some approaches[39,43] where electron probe microanalysis was employed to investigate the elemental composition at interfaces between a glass-ionomer and enamel or dentin, no secondary or backscattered electron images of the analyzed regions were provided. The distributions of calcium[39,43] and silica[43] used in these studies to determine the exact position of the edge of the cavity wall lack accurate spatial resolution, especially if the high calcium concentration of the glass-ionomers used (which further complicates signal interpretation) is considered. Under these conditions it is possible that morphologic irregularities at the interface could be misinterpreted as

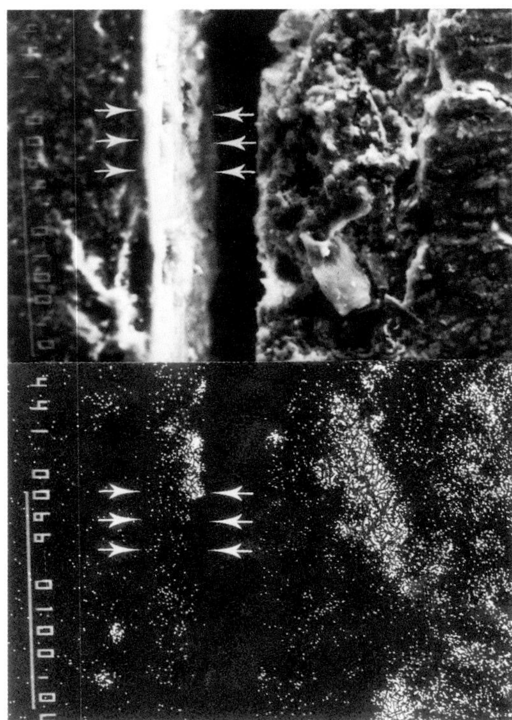

Fig 4-2 A typical electron microprobe artifact in the elemental analysis of the interface between dentin and a conventional glass-ionomer liner. The aluminum area scan image *(bottom)* implies aluminum uptake at the outermost 22 μm of dentin *(white arrows)*. However, the secondary electron image *(top)* clearly shows that the aluminum signal emerges from glass-ionomer debris left on the adjacent dentin wall after debonding of the glass-ionomer from dentin due to dehydration from the high vacuum. Note the excessive material cracking. The specimen was analyzed after storage in distilled water for 3 months. (15 kV; 20 nA; TAP crystal, original magnification ×440; bar = 100 μm)

elemental diffusion gradients, denoting selective uptake.

Another important problem when studying the interfaces of glass ionomers under the high-vacuum, high-energy incident probes required for this type of analysis is the excessive dehydration of the cements and the resulting dimensional changes. A common artifact is cracking and debonding of the material from hard tissues. In such cases residual small glass-ionomer particles attached to enamel or dentin could be considered evidence of elemental diffusion (Fig 4-2). Consequently, a high-resolution image of the interface is of critical importance for elemental characterization at this region.

The limitations of establishing the real interface in characterizing elemental gradients also apply to more sophisticated techniques. For example, a submicron resolution in depth profiling during secondary ion mass spectrometry (SIMS) measurements[41] may lack precision in determining interfacial gradients on dentin surfaces polished with 600-grit SiC paper, which creates a mean roughness at a micron scale, implicating interpretation with interfacial morphologic features. Furthermore, surface contamination during sectioning or polishing may comprise a significant source of error, especially when highly sensitive surface analysis techniques are used.

The problems encountered in such complex analytical situations have been described by Duschner et al.[45] These authors analyzed the enamel cavity walls of teeth restored with a glass-ionomer and stored in sterile filtered saliva for 6 weeks, using complementary advanced microanalytical techniques such as small-area photoelectron spectroscopy, laser ablation mass spectrometry, and confocal laser scanning microscopy. This multitechnique characterization confirmed that fluoride did not migrate into the enamel of the cavity wall. However, SIMS line scan experiments performed at glass-ionomer–dentin interfaces have clearly demonstrated fluoride uptake in dentin of 100 to 300 μm from the interface,[23,42] which overwhelms any doubts regarding interfacial interferences. Dentin pretreatment with acid etching substantially modifies dentin fluoride uptake by altering tissue permeability.[42]

An alternative experiment performed in vivo measured the amount of fluoride absorbed by the uppermost 10 μm of enamel bonded to a glass-ionomer cement at sequential micron intervals, using the biopsy technique after mechanical removal of the cement.[44] However, no information was given on the efficiency of the removal method to minimize interferences from residual glass-ionomer particles, a parameter acknowledged as a possible source of error.[40]

Based on all of these results, it is obvious that there is still no sound evidence to support fluoride diffusion from glass-ionomer restorations to the bonded enamel walls. In vivo experiments are needed to verify the in vitro findings for dentin walls. An interesting mode of fluoride uptake concerned enamel or cementum surfaces adjacent to, but not in contact with, the margins of glass-ionomer restorations. In vitro studies employing this approach have demonstrated increased fluoride concentration at these regions,[46,47] but the effect was not documented in vivo.[48]

The status of the fluoride absorbed by hard dental tissues bonded to glass ionomers is not known. The aspects concerning fluoroapatite, calcium fluoride, or nonspecifically absorbed fluoride formation are well documented in the field of topically applied fluoride agents and dentifrices,[49] but not for glass-ionomer cements. For the latter, an assumption is made that the reactivity of the fluoride released is similar to that found in oral health care products. It is reasonable to expect that the initial low pH of glass-ionomers[1,50] may induce dissolution of the adjacent apatite and redeposition of calcium salts incorporating fluoride, which is initially released at high rates. Evidence to support such an interaction has been presented in only one in vitro study, where fluoridated carbonoapatite was identified at the interface between a conventional glass-ionomer restorative and cavity walls.[51] Apparently these interactions take place at the demineralization front and not at sites distant from the interface. It is interesting to note that the only fluorinated compound identified in vitro in bulk tissue was located on dentin. Dentin demonstrates greater fluoride uptake than enamel due to the former's greater porosity, increased water content, smaller crystalline size,[52] and presence of the organic phase (which seems to be an important factor in fluoride uptake procedures). It has been shown that the organic components of dentin, such as collagen and non-collagenous proteins, take up significantly higher amounts of fluoride released from glass-ionomers than do the inorganic components and also have a high binding capacity.[53] This fraction of fluoride is believed to be involved in dentin mineralization procedures.[54] Unfortunately, no further information exists on the state of fluoride at glass-ionomer–dentin interfaces.

The concentration of fluoride in plaque, the physical in vivo barrier to fluoride elution from glass-ionomers, has been the subject of many studies during the last decade. In situ experiments have shown high levels of fluoride in plaque growing adjacent to glass-ionomer restorations,[55,56] while in vivo experiments have demonstrated that the fluoride content was greatly increased in plaque adjacent to glass-ionomers even 4 weeks after their application.[57] However, aged glass-ionomer specimens placed intraorally were found to accumulate more plaque with reduced fluoride content relative to fresh material. Still, the plaque fluoride content was higher than that of a resin composite control.[58] These findings support the theory that plaque developed on glass-ionomer restorations may act as a fluoride pool in the microenvironment of the restoration.

A critical point in understanding the role of the fluoride acquired in pellicle and plaque adjacent to glass-ionomer cements in the interfacial availability of fluoride is to identify its binding states in these integuments. So far, no studies have been published in this area. However, from the total amount of fluoride found in dental plaque, less than 1% is in an ionized state, a fraction is in the form of calcium phosphate precipitates which may be released at low pH, and the vast majority is strongly bound to macromolecules and bacteria.[59] Thus, the concept that dental plaque may act as a fluoride reservoir for adjacent hard dental tissues during remineralization periods[55] may apply only to fully fluoride saturated plaque, if such conditions can be established intraorally. The main reason is that as pH rises during remineralization, urea and amine production from plaque is increased, reaching optimum values at about pH 5.[59] These basic components demonstrate high chemical affinity to any ionic fluoride in the region, forming stable compounds. Regarding the potential of in vivo recharging of aged glass-ionomers, preliminary results indicate that recharging had no beneficial effect on the fluoride concentration of adjacent plaque.[58]

The antibacterial properties of glass ionomers documented in vitro[60–62] failed to inhibit plaque growth on their surfaces in vivo[63] (Figs 4-3 and 4-4). However, the composition of the plaque that accumulated on glass-ionomers showed a reduction in the proportion of *mutans streptococci*.[56–58,63–66] Furthermore, observations that this proportion increased as glass-ionomer restorations aged[63] implies that the short-term reaction of fluoride release is closely associated with the microbial inhibition.[61] These effects were found to be limited to the vicinity of the local environment without affecting the plaque on adjacent teeth.[67]

Fig 4-3 Microbial adsorption onto set conventional glass-ionomer (a and b) and resin composite (c and d) surfaces 1 hour after intraoral placement of freshly prepared material discs in the same patient. Note the differences in the dendritic patterns of bacteria accumulation and orientation. A more mature integument is formed on glass-ionomer during the early adsorption stages, which is probably modified later from the exertion of the antimicrobial effect.

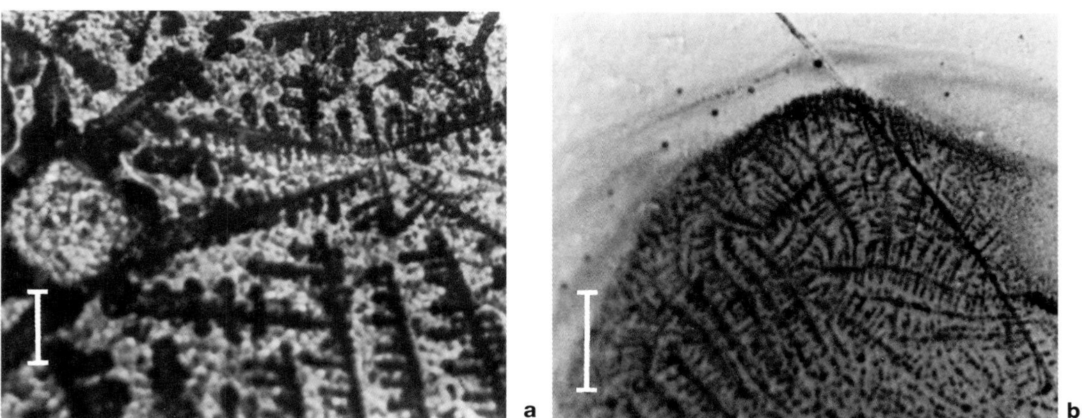

Figs 4-3a and 4-3b Bright-field reflected light images. (Original magnification ×50; bar = 100 μm.)

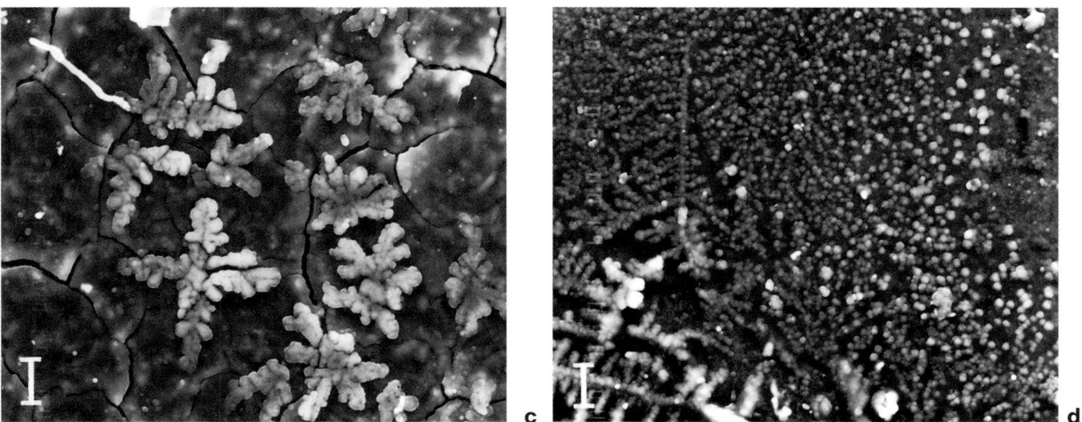

Figs 4-3c and 4-3d Secondary electron images. (Original magnification ×1,000; bar = 10 μm.)

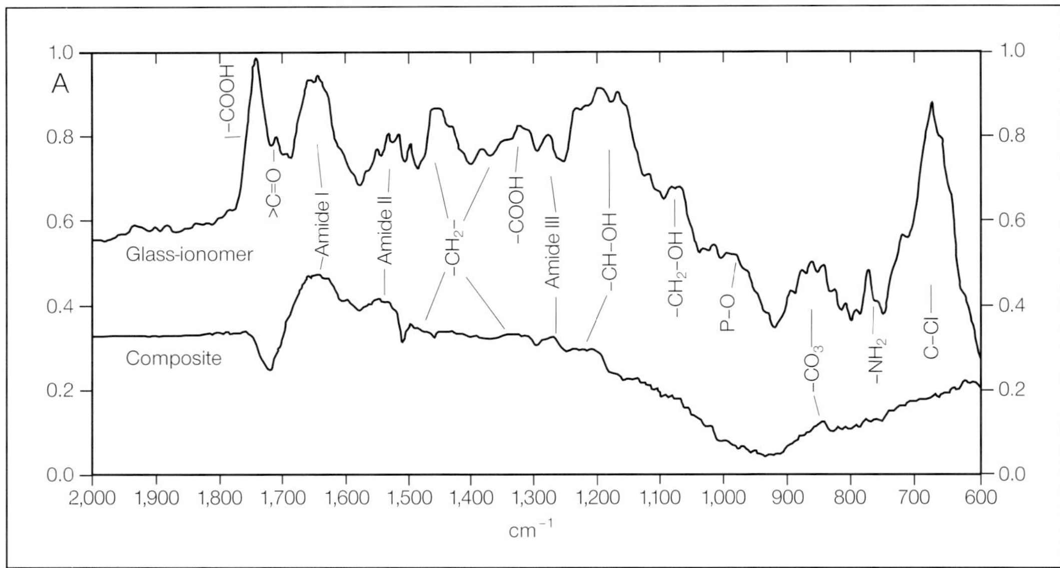

Fig 4-4 Micromultiple internal reflectance FTIR spectra showing the molecular composition of the integuments formed on set conventional glass-ionomer and resin composite surfaces 1 hour after intraoral placement of freshly prepared material disks in the same patient. More hydrophilic groups are identified on glass ionomer; these groups reflect differences in the surface properties between the restoratives. Spectra were acquired from material surfaces and subjected to sequential digital subtraction techniques to remove original material and water interferences. (KRS-5 minicrystal; 4 cm^{-1} resolution; 50 scans coaddition.)

Remineralization of Adjacent Hard Tissues

The fluoride uptake of hard dental tissues adjacent to glass-ionomer materials has been considered a fundamental factor for inhibition of secondary caries attack.[68] Today, however, it is generally accepted that fluoride uptake alone does not necessarily imply caries reduction susceptibility.[49] The determining factor is the secondary mobility of fluoride absorbed by the tissues, which reflects the ability of the fluoridated compounds formed to establish a solution equilibrium at the interface during demineralization and remineralization cycles.[49]

In vitro studies

To evaluate the performance of the fluoride released from glass-ionomer restorations under simulated conditions of secondary caries attack, a series of artificial caries experiments was conducted and showed that the frequency and extent of outer and wall lesions was reduced around glass-ionomer restorations in vitro.[69–75] The reduction in the extent of the outer lesion, which is considered to resemble primary caries, was attributed to the diffusion of fluoride ions through the artificial caries medium, whereas the reduction in the depth of the wall lesion was attributed to the low solubility of the cavity walls to the hydrogen ion diffusion gradient set at the interface, due to fluoride release and uptake procedures.[68] Limited information is available on the composition of the artificial caries lesions. Studies of artificial lesions on dentin walls in contact with glass-ionomers showed that the levels of calcium and phosphorous in lesion bodies were decreased relative to the organic component; in inhibited zones these levels were similar to those in sound dentin, but the level of fluoride was significantly higher.[76]

In several in vitro studies, demineralization and remineralization cycles were performed to better simulate intraoral pH fluctuations. These studies documented that glass-ionomers prevent demineralization of adjacent enamel[72,77] and hypermineralize dentin walls through a mechanism possibly associated with the formation of calcium fluoride deposits. These findings were consistently obtained from fresh glass-ionomer restorations, but no similar effects were documented for aged specimens.[67] The clinical relevance of these findings has not been verified. The absence of pellicle, plaque, and bacteria and the strong acidic environment used in vitro to mimic acid production by bacteria intraorally, invalidate the extrapolation of the in vitro findings to in vivo conditions.[78,79] Direct comparison is not even feasible between the in vitro reported studies because the composition of the acidified gels, the demineralizing or remineralizing solutions used, the pH, and the duration of the testing periods vary greatly.

In vivo studies

The extensive use of in vitro models to simulate the in vivo situation and the criticism of such simplified approaches established the need for controlled studies of fluoride releasing materials in the oral environment. The first approach was to design in situ experiments. Several models were developed for the study of the interfaces of enamel or dentin with fluoride releasing materials placed in partial dentures or other removable appliances worn intraorally for periods of 1 to 3 months. These models incorporated assessment of several variables, such as the presence of a standardized interfacial gap between the restoration and tissues,[80] the presence of an artificial carious lesion,[81] or the simulation of high cariogenic challenge by immersing the specimens in sucrose solution at specific time intervals.[55] The results confirmed the beneficial effects of fluoride release to the adjacent tissues for the time periods tested. Of particular importance was the finding that, in cases of interfacial discontinuities in the form of gaps, the amount of fluoride released into the liquid in the gap is of much greater importance than the amount of fluoride taken up by tissues.[80]

A modification of the standardized gap model also has been used for in vivo assessment of the enamel anticariogenic potential of glass-ionomers for orthodontic band cementation.[82] The experimental design included the development of a standardized microspace between cemented bands and enamel to accumulate plaque. Four weeks after band cementation, the mineral content of the lesion found around glass-ionomer cements was significantly higher than that around a nonfluoride-containing phosphate cement used as a control. This design, however, did not take into account the strong initial acidic challenge of a setting phosphate cement to the microspace; the pH of phosphate cements remains below 5 even 24 hours after setting, while the corresponding values for glass-ionomers range from 5.5 to 6.5.[83] Thus it is not known whether the initial acidic environment created around the phosphate cement affected the total mineral loss observed.

A common finding in the in vivo studies concerning the anticariogenic properties of glass-ionomers is that the experimental period is limited to the first few weeks after placement of the restorations. It is well established that during this period, glass-ionomers exert the highest fluoride release rate and the strongest antibacterial activity.[61] The long-term performance of the cariostatic properties of glass-ionomer cements has not been systematically investigated, and the information currently available is limited to clinical studies reporting secondary caries incidence with all the associated diagnostic limitations.[78,79]

Several clinical studies have documented a low incidence of secondary caries adjacent to glass-ionomer restorations.[84–86] However, two recently published articles, based on surveys of the reasons for restoration replacement in general dental practice, reported relatively high incidences of secondary caries in relation to glass-ionomer restoration failures.[87,88] These findings forced the authors to emphasize the urgent need for further studies to confirm the anticariogenic effect in vivo.

To investigate the anticariogenic efficiency of glass ionomers over a longer period, a study[89] was designed introducing an artificial gap model in vivo and correlating the results with the same model under artificial caries attack. Briefly, at the mid-buccal area of sound premolars to be extracted for orthodontic reasons, paired Class V cavities limited to enamel were prepared in each patient. Lesions were filled with a conventional glass ionomer and a nonfluoride-containing light-cured resin composite on contralateral sides after placing 40-μm-thick metal spacers at the incisal walls of the cavities to create artificial gaps. The incisal walls received no conditioning or priming treatments. After setting, the spacers were removed and, after 6 months, the teeth were extracted, sectioned, and studied under polarized light. The same procedure was used to restore cavities prepared at the buccal area of sound premolars extracted for orthodontic reasons, which were then subjected to an artificial caries experiment using an acidified gel (pH 4) for 4 weeks.

The in vitro findings of the study confirmed the cariostatic effect of glass-ionomers in gap-free regions, as shown in many previous studies, as well as its beneficial role in the presence of interfacial gaps. However, the in vivo findings demonstrated a different lesion pattern. No lesions were observed at gap-free restorations. In the presence of artificial gaps, the area of lesions adjacent to the glass-ionomer was greater than that adjacent to the resin composite (Fig 4-5). The depth of the enamel wall lesion, the length of the superficial mineralized enamel, and the extent of the underlying demineralized region were increased in

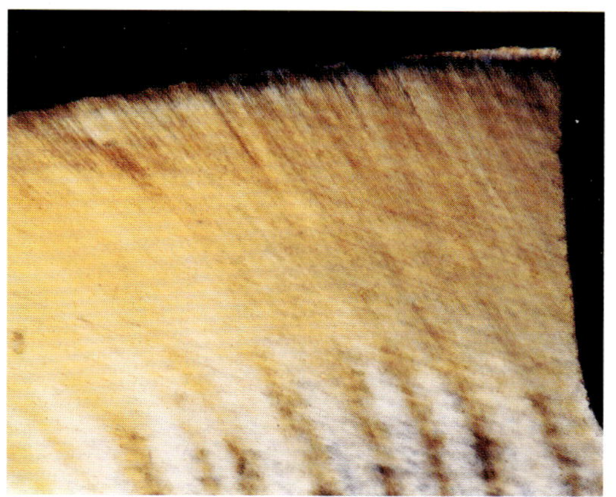
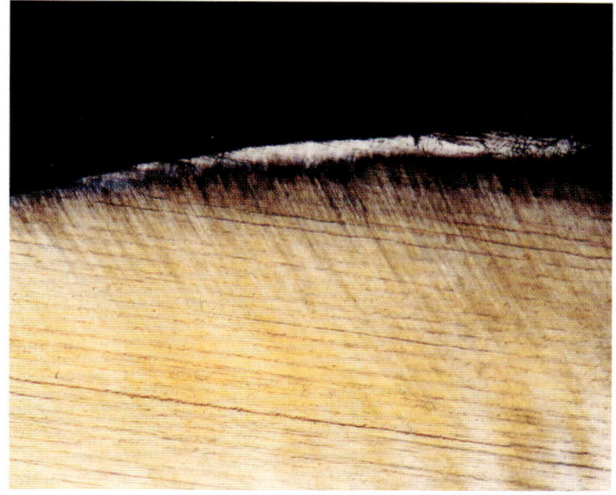

Figs 4-5a and 4-5b Transmitted polarized light images of thin sections from restorative-enamel interfaces in the presence of 40-μm interfacial gaps after 6 months in vivo. The sections were obtained from contralateral premolars of the same patient restored with (A) a glass ionomer and (B) a resin composite. Note the greater length of wall and surface lesion that has developed adjacent to the glass-ionomer. (Bright-field, crossed polarizers; original magnification ×20; sections immersed in distilled water; n = 1.33.)

cavities restored with glass-ionomer. These preliminary results show that some glass ionomers may not exert an efficient anticariogenic effect at adjacent enamel walls in vivo in the presence of an interfacial gap. They also highlight the role of gap-free restorations in reducing secondary caries incidence.

Optimization of the adhesive and sealing properties of glass-ionomer cements may provide protection against secondary caries, until the expected anticariogenic activity of the fluoride released is established in well-defined in vivo models and controlled clinical studies.[90] Unfortunately, such an effect has not yet been fully documented.[79]

References

1. Wilson AD, Nicholson JW. Polyalkenoate cements. In: West AR, Baxter H (eds). Acid-based Cements. Their Biomedical and Industrial Applications. Chemistry of Solid State Materials, vol 3. Cambridge: Cambridge University Press, 1993.

2. Wilson AD, Groffman DM, Kuhn AT. The release of fluoride and other chemical species from a glass-ionomer cement. Biomaterials 1985;6:431–433.

3. Sarkar NK, El-Mallakh B, Graves R. Silver release from metal reinforced glass-ionomers. Dent Mater 1988;4:103–104.

4. Tam LE, McComb D, Pulver F. Physical properties of proprietary light-cured lining materials. Oper Dent 1991;16:210–217.

5. Wilson AD, Crisp S. Ionomer cements. Br Polymer J 1975;7:279–296.

6. Crisp S, Lewis BG, Wilson AD. Characterization of glass-ionomer cements. 6. A study of erosion and water absorption in both neutral and acidic media. J Dent 1980;8:68–74.

7. Wilson AD. Resin-modified glass-ionomers. Int J Prosthodont 1990;3:425–429.

8. Nicholson JW, Anstice HM, McLean JW. A preliminary report on the effect of storage in water on the properties of commercial light-cured glass ionomer cements. Br Dent J 1992;173:98–101.

9. Eliades G, Palaghias G. In vitro characterization of visible light cured glass-ionomer liners. Dent Mater 1993;9:198–203.

10. Walls AWG, Adamson J, McLabe JF, Murray JJ. The properties of a glass-polyalkenoate (ionomer) cement incorporating sintered metallic particles. Dent Mater 1987;3:113–116.

11. Gao F, Matsuya S, Ohta M, Zhang J. Erosion process of light-cured and conventional glass-ionomer cements in citrate buffer solution. Dent Mater J 1997;16:170–179.

12. Kakaboura A, Eliades G, Palaghias G. An FTIR study on the setting mechanism of resin-modified glass-ionomer restoratives. Dent Mater 1996; 12:173–178.

13. Povis DR, Pioner HJ, Wilson AD. Long term monitoring of microleakage of dental cements by radiochemical diffusion. J Prosthet Dent 1988;59:651–657.

14. Meryon SD, Smith AJ. A comparison of fluoride release from three glass-ionomer cements and a polycarboxylate cement. Int Endod J 1984; 17:16–24.

15. Walls AWG. Glass polyalkenoate (glass ionomer) cements: A review. J Dent 1986; 14:231–246.

16. Swartz MC, Phillips RW, Clark HE. Long-term F release from glass-ionomer cements. J Dent Res 1984;63:158–160.

17. Forsten L. Short- and long-term fluoride release from glass-ionomers and other fluoride-containing filling materials in vitro. Scand J Dent Res 1990;98:179–185.

18. De Moor RJG, Verbeek RM, De Maeyer EAP. Fluoride release profiles of restorative glass-ionomer formulations. Dent Mater 1996;12:88–95.

19. Thorton JB, Retief DH, Bradey EL. Fluoride release from and tensile bond strength of Ketac-Fil and Ketac-Silver to enamel and dentin. Dent Mater 1986;2:241–245.

20. Hörsted-Bindslev P, Larsen MJ. Release of fluoride from conventional and metal-reinforced glass-ionomer cements. Scand J Dent Res 1990;98:451–455.

21. Hörsted-Bindslev P, Larsen MJ. Release of fluoride from light cured lining materials. Scand J Dent Res 1991;99:86–88.

22. Momoi Y, McCabe JF. Fluoride release from light-activated glass-ionomer restorative cements. Dent Mater 1993;9:151–154.

23. Mitra SB. *In vitro* fluoride release from a light cured glass ionomer liner/base. J Dent Res 1991;70:75–78.

24. Arnold A, Holmes D, Wistrom D, Swift E. Short-term fluoride release/uptake of glass-ionomer restoratives. Dent Mater 1995;11:96–101.

25. Wilson AD, McLean JW. Glass-Ionomer Cement. Chicago: Quintessence, 1988.

26. Cranfield M, Kuhn AT, Winter G. Factors relating to the rate of fluoride ion release from glass-ionomer cement. J Dent 1982;10:333–341.

27. Forss H. The release of fluoride and other elements from light-cured glass-ionomers in neutral and acidic conditions. J Dent Res 1993;72: 1257–1262.

28. Forsten L. Fluoride release and uptake by glass-ionomers. Scand J Dent Res 1991;99:241–245.

29. Seppä L, Forss H, Ögaard B. The effect of fluoride application on fluoride release and the antibacterial action of glass-ionomers. J Dent Res 1993;72:1310–1314.

30. Seppä L, Korhonen A, Nuntinen A. The inhibitory effect of s. *mutans* by fluoride treated conventional and resin reinforced glass ionomer cements. Eur J Oral Sci 1995;103:182–185.

31. De Schepper EJ, Berry EA, Cailleteau JG, Tate WH. Fluoride release from light-cured liners. Am J Dent 1990;3:397–400.

32. El-Mallakh BF, Sarkar NK. Fluoride release from glass-ionomer cements in de-ionized water and artificial saliva. Dent Mater 1990;6:118–122.

33. Rezk-Lega F, Ögaard B, Rölla G. Availability of fluoride from glass-ionomer luting cements in human saliva. Scand J Dent Res 1991;99:60–63.

34. Hallgren A, Oliveby A, Twetman S. Salivary fluoride concentrations in children with glass-ionomer cemented orthodontic appliances. Caries Res 1990;24:239–241.

35. Koch G, Hatibović-Kofman S. Glass-ionomer cements as a fluoride release system in vivo. Scand J Dent Res 1990;14:267–273.

36. Hattab FN, el Mowafy OM, Salem NS, el Badrawy WAG. An in vivo study on the release of fluoride from glass-ionomer cement. Quintessence Int 1991;22:221–224.

37. Hatibović-Kofman S, Koch G. Fluoride release from glass ionomer cement in vivo and in vitro. Swed Dent J 1991;15:253–258.

38. Forss H, Seppä L. Studies on the effect of fluoride released by glass-ionomers in the oral cavity. Adv Dent Res 1995;9:389–393.

39. Wesenberg G, Halls E. The in vitro effect of a glass-ionomer cement on dentine and enamel walls. J Oral Rehabil 1980;7:35–42.

40. Tsanidis V, Koulourides T. An in vitro model for assessment of fluoride uptake from glass-ionomer cements by dentin and its effect on acid resistance. J Dent Res 1992;71:7–12.

41. Lin A, McIntyre NS, Davidson RD. Studies on the adhesion of glass-ionomer cements to dentin. J Dent Res 1992;71:1836–1841.

42. Tam LE, Chan GP, Yim D. In vitro caries inhibition effects by conventional and resin-modified glass-ionomer restorations. Oper Dent 1997;22:4–14.

43. Skartveit L, Tveit AB, Tötdal B, Øvrebø R, Raadal M. In vivo fluoride uptake in enamel and dentin from fluoride containing materials. J Dent Child 1990;57:97–100.

44. Shimokobe H, Komatsu H, Matsui J. Fluoride content in human enamel after removal of the applied cement. J Dent Res 1982;66(special issue):131 [abstract 196].

45. Duschner H, Ernst CP, Götz H, Rauscher M. Advanced techniques of micro-analysis and confocal microscopy: Perspectives for studying chemical and structural changes at the interface between restorative materials and cavity wall. Adv Dent Res 1995;9:355–362.

46. Retief DH, Bradley EL, Denton JC, Switzer P. Enamel and cementum fluoride uptake from a glass-ionomer cement. Caries Res 1984;18: 250–257.

47. Scoville RK, Foreman F, Burgess J. In vitro fluoride uptake enamel adjacent to a glass-ionomer luting cement. J Dent Child 1990;57:352–355.

48. Seppä L, Salmenkivi S, Forss H. Enamel and plaque fluoride following glass-ionomer application in vivo. Caries Res 1992;26:340–344.

49. White DJ. The application of in vitro models to research on demineralization and remineralization of teeth. Adv Dent Res 1995;9:175–193.

50. Woolford MJ, Chadwick RG. Surface pH of resin-modified glass-polyalkenoate (ionomer) cements. J Dent 1992;20:359–364.

51. Geiger SB, Weiner S. Fluoridated carbonoapatite in the intermediate layer between glass-ionomer and dentin. Dent Mater 1993; 9:33–36.

52. Mellberg JR, Singer L. Discussion. Caries Res 1977;11(suppl 1):101–115.

53. Meryon SD, Jakeman KJ. Uptake of zinc and fluoride by several dentin components. J Biomed Mater Res 1987;21:127–135.

54. DeSteno CV, Feagin FF. Effect of matrix bound phosphate and fluoride on mineralization of dentin. Calcif Tissue Res 1975;17:151–159.

55. Benelli EM, Serra MC, Rodrigues AL Jr, Cury JA. In situ anticariogenic potential of glass-ionomer cement. Caries Res 1993;27:280–284.

56. Forrs H, Jokinen J, Spets-Happonen S, Seppä L, Luoma H. Fluoride and mutans streptococci in plaque grown on glass-ionomer and composite. Caries Res 1991;25:454–458.

57. Hallgnen A, Oliveby A, Twetman S. Fluoride concentration in plaque adjacent to orthodontic appliances retained with glass-ionomer cement. Caries Res 1993;27:51–54.

58. Forss H, Näse L, Seppä L. Fluoride concentration, mutans streptococci and lactobacilli in plaque from old glass-ionomer fillings. Caries Res 1995;29:50–53.

59. Jenkins NG. The Physiology and Biochemistry of the Mouth, 4th ed. Oxford: Blackwell, 1978: 486–487.

60. Meryon SD, Johnson SG. The modified model cavity method for assessing antibacterial properties of dental restorative materials. J Dent Res 1989;68:835–839.

61. Palenik CJ, Behnen MJ, Setcos JC, Miller CH. Inhibition of microbial adherence and growth by various glass ionomers in vitro. Dent Mater 1992;8:16–20.

62. Loyola-Rodriguez JP, Garcia-Godoy F, Lindquist R. Growth inhibition of glass ionomer cements on mutans streptococci. Pediatr Dent 1994;16: 346–349.

63. Forss H, Seppä L, Alakuijala P. Plaque accumulation on glass-ionomer filling materials. Proc Finn Dent Soc 1991;87:343–350.

64. Svanberg M, Mjör IA, Ørstavik D. Mutans streptococci in plaque from margins of amalgam, complete and glass-ionomer restorations. J Dent Res 1990;69:861–864.

65. Hallgren A, Olivery A, Twetman S. Caries associated microflore in plaque from orthodontic appliances retained with glass-ionomer cements. Scand J Dent Res 1992;100:140–143.

66. Van Dijken J, Persson S, Sjöström S. Presence of streptococcus mutans and lactobacilli in saliva and on enamel, glass-ionomer cement and complete resin surfaces. Scand J Dent Res 1991;99:13–19.

67. Forss H, Seppä L. Studies on the effect of fluoride released by glass-ionomers in the oral cavity. Adv Dent Res 1995;9:389–393.

68. Swift EJ. Effects of glass-ionomers on recurrent caries. Oper Dent 1989;14:40–43.

69. Kidd EAM. Cavity sealing ability of composite and glass-ionomer cement restorations. Br Dent J 1978;144:139–142.

70. Dezand T, Johansson B. Experimental secondary caries around restorations in roots. Caries Res 1984;18:548–554.

71. Swift EJ. In vitro caries inhibitory properties of a silver cermet. J Dent Res 1989;68:1088–1093.

72. Forss H, Seppa L. Prevention of enamel demineralization adjacent to glass-ionomer filling materials. Scand J Dent Res 1990;98:173–175.

73. Wesenberg G, Hals E. The structure of experimental in vitro lesions around glass-ionomer restorations in human teeth. J Oral Rehabil 1980;7:175–184.

74. Hicks MJ, Flaitz CM, Silverstone LM. Secondary cavities formation in vitro around glass-ionomer restoratives. Quintessence Int 1986;17:527–532.

75. Hattab FM, Mok NYC, Agnew EC. Artificially formed caries-like lesions around restorative materials. J Am Dent Assoc 1989;118:193–197.

76. Erickson RL. Elemental analysis of artificial caries lesions adjacent to fluoride releasing materials. J Dent Res 1995;74 (special issue): 440 [abstract 915].

77. Ten Cate JM, Buijs MJ, Dawen JM. The effects of GIC restoration on enamel and dentin demineralization and remineralization. Adv Dent Res 1995;9:384–388.

78. Özer L, Thylstrup A. What is known about caries in relation to restoration as a reason for replacement? A review. Adv Dent Res 1995;9:394–402.

79. Hörsted-Bindslev P. Fluoride release from alternative restorative materials. J Dent 1994;22(suppl 1):S17–S20.

80. Dijkman GEHM, Arends J. Secondary caries *in situ* around fluoride releasing light-curing composites. A qualitative model investigation on four materials with a fluoride content between 0 and 26%. Caries Res 1992;26:352–357.

81. ten Cate JM, van Duinen RN. Hyper-mineralization of dentinal lesions adjacent to glass-ionomer cement restoration. J Dent Res 1995; 74:1266–1271.

82. Rezk-Lega F, Øgaard B, Arends J. An in vivo study on the merits of two glass-ionomers for the

cementation of orthodontic bands. Am J Orthod Dentofacial Orthop 1991;99:162–167.

83. Charlton DG, Moore BK, Swartz ML. Direct surface pH determinations of setting cements. Oper Dent 1991;16:231–238.

84. Tyas MJ. Cariostatic effect of glass-ionomer cement: A five-year clinical study. Aust Dent J 1991;36:236–239.

85. Svanberg M. Class II amalgam restorations, glass ionomer tunnel restorations and caries development on adjacent tooth surfaces: A 3-year clinical study. Caries Res 1992;26:315–318.

86. Mjör IA, Jokstad A. Five year study of class II restorations in permanent teeth using amalgam, glass polyalkenoate (ionomer) cement and resin-based composite materials. J Dent 1993;21: 338–343.

87. Mjör IA. Glass-ionomer cement restorations and secondary caries: A preliminary report. Quintessence Int 1996;27:171–174.

88. Wilson NHF, Burke FJT, Mjör IA. Reasons for replacement and replacement of restorations of direct restorative materials by a selected group of practitioners in the United Kingdom. Quintessence Int 1997;28:245–248.

89. Kakaboura A, Papagiannoulis L, Eliades G. *In vitro* vs in vivo anticariogenic potential of esthetic restorative materials. [abstract 209]. J Dent Res 1998;77 (Special issue B):658.

90. Erickson RL, Glasspoole EA. Model investigations of caries inhibition by fluoride-releasing dental materials. Adv Dent Res 1995;9:315–323.

Chapter 5

Biocompatibility of Glass-Ionomer Cements

Michel Goldberg, Lena Stanislawski, Eric Bonte, Xavier Daniau, and Jean-Jacques Lasfargues

Glass-ionomer cements seem to be beneficial from a clinical point of view because of their continuous release of fluoride which reduces the rate of secondary caries both in filled teeth and on the enamel surfaces of adjacent teeth.[1,2] Fewer microorganisms are found in remaining carious dentin subjacent to glass-ionomer restorations,[3] and there is actually a fluoride uptake in human dentin.[4] Another great advantage of glass-ionomers is the continuous uptake of fluoride,[5] which may greatly extend the beneficial effects of these materials.

The first group of glass-ionomers on the market had a low pH during the initial setting period and therefore had adverse effects on pulpal tissues when the residual dentin was thin. Although improvements have been made to these materials, especially with the addition of resins, there are still some questions with respect to the biocompatibility of glass-ionomer cements.

Biocompatibility and Cytotoxicity of Dental Biomaterials

It is well documented that some dental biomaterials are harmful and others are not. Months or years after cavities are treated and filled with cements or resins, the pulp may react and undergo degeneration. When oxyphosphate cements containing orthophosphoric acid were used for luting or filling, the reaction was acute and painful; pulp necrosis sometimes followed pulpitis. With other biomaterials the reaction was gradual and almost silent, but pulp degeneration still occurred. In many cases, no reaction was observed, and dentin deposition in the pulp chamber together with a living pulp or surviving tissue was considered as a success.

Even with the development of new materials such as adhesive and resin composites, glass-ionomer cements, and mixtures of glass-ionomer and resin composite, there are still reactions. However, they are less frequent and those that occur escape the attention of clinicians, with asymptomatic pulp apoptosis.

There is no legal requirement for a systematic study of pulp status after the introduction of new dental biomaterials. Therefore, the continuous influx of new materials to the market does not allow in vivo evaluations and in vitro tests of the biocompatibility or toxicity of these materials. The evolution of dental products is so rapid that as soon a new material is put in the market, it is outdated, with another version appearing within weeks or months and claiming to be extensively improved. As a consequence, no systematic studies are carried out on the pathology induced by recent adhesives, composites, or glass ionomers.

Bergenholtz[6] has shown that the presence of bacteria between the cavity surface and the restorative material is responsible for pulp reaction. In this context, a clear relationship was drawn between the presence of bacteria and the diffusion of exotoxins in dental tubules toward the pulp. This phenomenon was especially true for many products available in the 1980s. At that time, there was always a crevice between the wall of the cavity and the filling. Some contraction of the filling was due to dehydration during preparation of samples, and shrinkage was enhanced by the high vacuum used when samples were observed with scanning electron microscopy (SEM). It is widely accepted that the gap between the biomaterial and dental tissue was about 10 to 25 μm, a width which allowed hundreds of microorganisms to penetrate the interface simultaneously.

New adhesives have since been developed and, from the literature, it is clear that no gaps exist between fillings and cavity walls that might be colonized by bacteria. The formation of a hybrid layer also prohibits the formation of such gaps.[7,8] Therefore, two possibilities exist: *(1)* bacteria located at the resin–dentin interface are responsible for the harmful reactions and the problem should be solved by improving the adhesives and biomaterials, or *(2)* the diffusion of uncontrolled components of the biomaterials induces pulp alterations. It may be derived from this that many biological problems still need to be solved to avoid pulp reactions from dental biomaterials.

Pulp Biology

The embryonic pulp develops together with the dental lamina and enamel organ in the first branchial arch. In mammals, early emigrating midbrain crest cells migrate to the dental mesenchyma.[9] These cells appear in the condensing mesenchyme and in the dental papilla. After a fixed number of mitotic divisions, they appear at the surface of the embryonic pulp either as postmitotic odontoblasts, which differentiate, polarize, and acquire all the biological properties of dentin-forming cells, or as daughter cells that have no direct contact to the basement membrane, or Höhl layer.[10] The participation of cells originating from the para-axial mesenchyme has still not been determined, but it is highly probable that some pulp components are not of neural crest origin. Cells migrate from the dental sac and adjacent mesenchyma and remain in the central part of the pulp. In this context, the sprouting of endothelial cells and axon growth during pulp morphogenesis leads to the development of vascularization and innervation.

After the onset of tooth formation, any replacement of postmitotic odontoblasts can damage or destroy these cells. Cells from the Höhl layer have the same embryonic origin as the odontoblasts; therefore, it can be hypothesized that they have the potential to differentiate and become replacement cells acting as odontoblasts. In adult pulp, no cell population can differentiate, polarize, and act as second-generation odontoblasts, but some precursor cells contribute to the deposition of reparative dentin.[11] The normal histology of pulp and dentin is shown in Fig 5-1.

Cell differentiation in adult pulp

Some undifferentiated cells located in the central pulp—called mesenchymal stem cells, pericytes, endothelial cells, or fibroblasts—keep the potential for differentiation and become mitotic. In the case of experimental pulp capping, after a first mitosis, they migrate toward a wounded zone and a second mitosis occurs. The daughter cells then differentiate into replacement cells capable of producing a mineralized layer of what seems to be osteodentin.[12]

Vascularization and innervation both play essential roles in pulp biology, including the provision of nutrients to the tissue.[13–15] In addition, pulp cells have their own specificities.

Specialized pulp cells

Pulp fibroblasts, or pulpoblasts, exhibit specific differences from other cells. They are never isolated but are linked one to another by intercellular (desmosome-like and gap) junctions. This relationship implies a continuity in the cell network inside the pulp, from the center where they emerge and differentiate toward the outer pulp beneath the Höhl layer[10] and the odontoblasts.

It is interesting to note that mitosis is hardly detected in adult pulp for unknown reasons. It is hardly conceivable that mitotic cells can be present during the whole life of the tooth as neurons are. In noncarious teeth, the percentage of cells bearing the proliferating cell nuclear antigen is low compared with cells derived from periodontal ligament, bone stroma, and muscular tissue. There is increased labeling only in cases of advanced caries. Labeling with the silver-binding nucleolar organizer region (AgNOR) stain provides the same type of information. In addition, it has been shown that there is no difference between the coronal and radicular areas of the pulp in this respect. They both display low labeling, except in response to caries.[16]

There is a population of immunocompetent cells in normal dental pulp. Dendritic cells, T lymphocytes, and macrophages have been identified in rat incisor pulp.[17–20] The hypothesis that these cells are present in case of aggression is unacceptable. In an investigation carried out on the pulp of essential fatty acid–deficient (EFAD) rats, cell density in EFAD rats was double that in control rats.[21] One possible explanation of this phenomenon may be that the influence of the deficiency on arachidonic metabolism (less than half the value found in control rats) interferes with the synthesis of prostaglandins and leukotriens. In such circumstances, deregulation of apoptosis, a phenomenon known to be prostaglandin dependent and involved in the control of cell number, can lead to the increase in density that was noted.[21] When three methods—TUNEL staining, anti-transglutaminase, and characteristic morphology—were used to identify apoptotic cells, most pulp cells did not react, with the exception of a few located in the outer pulp beneath the Höhl layer and odontoblasts.[22]

All together, the distribution and labeling of cells show that undifferentiated cells appear in the central pulp. As soon as they differentiate into pulpoblasts, they establish strong links due to the presence of junctional complexes and form a dense network. Cells are further transported subjacent to odontoblasts, where immunocompetent cells act as killers to control the cell population. Cells move toward the outer pulp where killer cells such as dendritic cells, T lymphocytes, and cells expressing Class II antigen are present. As is usual in apoptosis, intercellular junctions are disrupted. Individual cells are subjected to specific chromatin changes in the nuclei and disintegrate. Residual apoptotic bodies are easily observed in the pulp. Cell remnants are destroyed by macrophages. If this interpretation is correct, it implies that immunocompetent cells are not involved in normal pulp defense processes, nor in rescuing the pulp in case of aggression. However, these cells are implicated in the control of pulp cell populations. In this context, the mechanisms of cytotoxicity can be considered the deregulation of a normal cell control mechanism.

Results of in vivo studies are difficult to compare because of the many parameters involved, including legal restrictions and extrapolation from young, healthy teeth to carious, older teeth and from animal models to human specimens. Thus, research must be carried out using in vitro systems to study biological reactions.

Pulp cells in culture

When pulp from neonatal mice with intact odontoblasts was isografted to spleen, tubular dentin was produced. In contrast, ectomesenchymal cells of dental papilla transplanted in isogenic mouse spleen produced only osteodentin-like material and not orthodentin. Assuming that the culture model is representative of the exposed pulp in vivo, cells were cultured from human pulp explants. These specimens were different from fibroblast-like cells. At the beginning, the young cells were round or elongated with thin spinous processes, were highly mobile, and contained numerous lipid vesicles as evidenced with Oil Red O stain under a light microscope and by osmium-imidazole electron-dense lipid droplets seen on ultrathin sections under an electron microscope. These lipids probably originated from pinocytotic activity because no active synthesis was revealed by 1-[^{14}C]palmitic acid incorporation.[23] It is known that marrow cells can differentiate, under some culture conditions, into adipocytes that convert along the osteogenic pathway.[24] Pulp cells display strong alkaline phosphate staining and are able to form mineralized nodules.[23] This formation of nodules can be used as a model to study either pathologic pulp mineralizations or the formation of what has been called *reparative dentin*.[25–27] This type of cell culture has been widely used for in vitro investigations on the biocompatibility of dental biomaterials, including glass-ionomer cements.

In Vivo Studies on Humans and Animals

The original composition of glass-ionomer powders was based on a formulation of silicon dioxide, aluminum oxide, calcium fluoride, aluminum phosphate, and sodium hexafluoroaluminate.[28] This allowed a possible toxic reaction from aluminum. Other components, such as fluoride, corundum, strontium, barium, lanthanum, zinc oxide, and zirconium oxide, are now used to increase opacity. Some glass-ionomers use a copolymer of acrylic acid to control the viscosity of the polyacrylic acid. Some of these acids are not biocompatible. Stronger glass-ionomer cements are produced by the addition of 2-hydroxyethylmethacrylate (HEMA), which is capable of free radical polymerization. Developments in the formulation of resin-modified glass-ionomers also have enhanced their properties and are widely used. Metal particles, fibers, or powders in cermet cements have significantly improved resistance to abrasion. This adds another parameter to the potential cytotoxicity of glass-ionomers. Thus, three groups of components of glass-ionomer cements can induce adverse reactions: the glass-ionomer itself, metals that are added to the cement, and nonpolymerized resin components. Each of these components presents its own problems and may contribute to adverse reactions.

Tissue reactions can be ranked from moderate to severe,[29] although in some reports pulp reactions have been evaluated as none, slight, moderate, or severe.[30] Moderate responses exhibit a predominant population of lymphocytes, and sometimes giant cells and macrophages; capillary proliferation; and fibroblasts and fibrocytes. Severe responses are characterized by a mixture of granulocytes and lymphocytes, predominant capillary proliferation, and a large number of giant cells and macrophages.

The initial acidity of glass-ionomer cements (close to pH 2 at 5 minutes after placement and pH 3 at 10 minutes) may contribute to pulp reaction. This was the case for the first generation of glass-ionomers, especially when they were used as luting agents. Pameijer and Stanley[31] observed pulpal abscesses and intense hemorrhage when a glass-ionomer was used under continuous pressure and the remaining dentin thickness was 0.5 mm or less. This was also the case when the study involved a full crown preparation. Some pulpal reaction, including abscesses and hemorrhage, persisted even after 60 days.[31] Stanley[32] concluded that when the remaining dentin thickness is less than 1 mm, there is a need for pulpal protection before glass-ionomer cements are used.

In cell culture, initial tests indicate that traditional glass-ionomer cements are cytotoxic, but no adverse response is

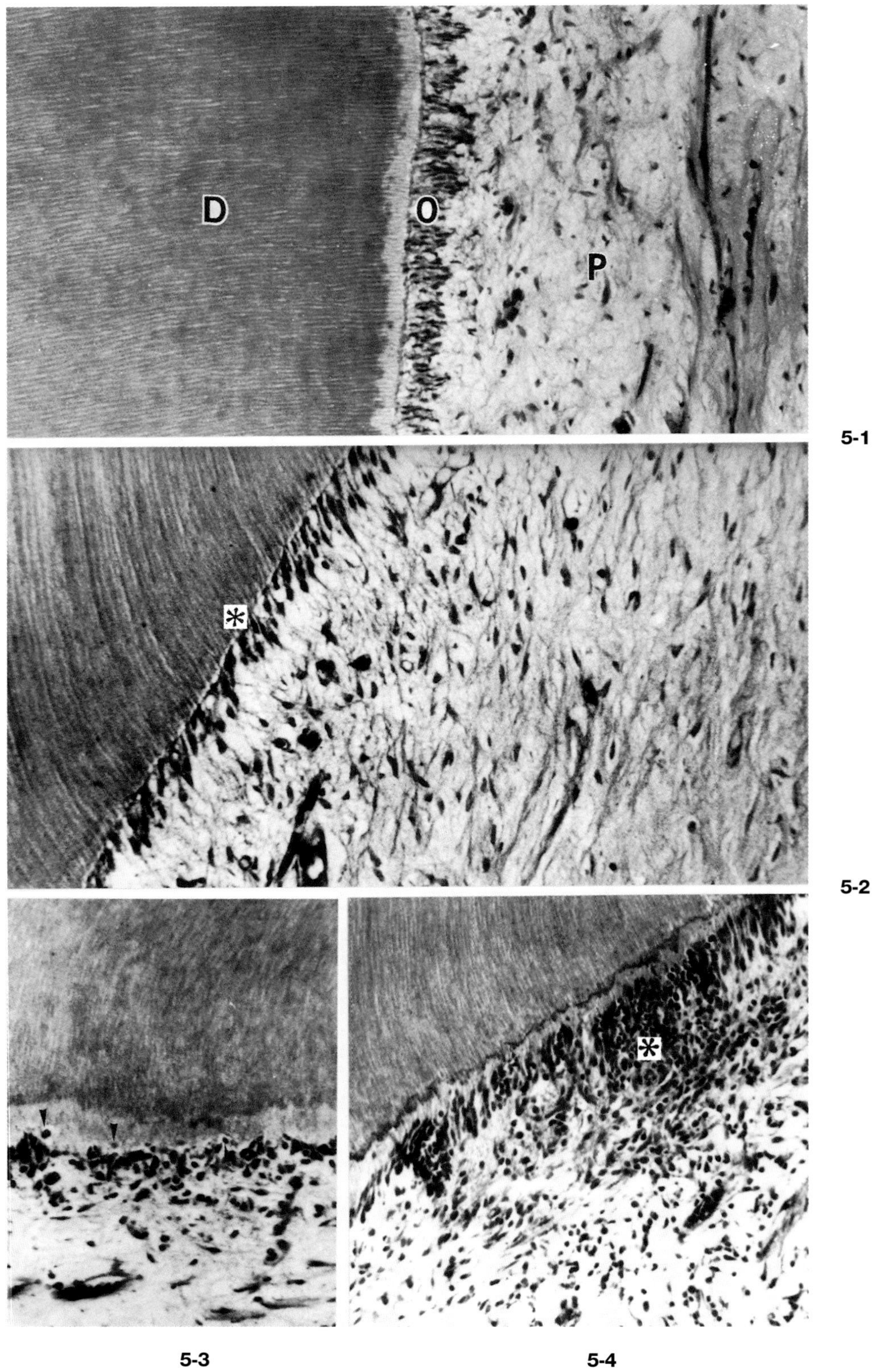

5-1

5-2

5-3

5-4

found with light-cured glass-ionomers. Animal experiments have shown that direct contact of cements with pulp tissues causes necrosis and should be avoided. Human studies of glass-ionomer restorations in Class I sites in premolars have shown inflammation in 5% of the pulps.[33] Correlation between pulpal inflammation and bacterial microleakage was found by Browne et al.[34] This group concluded that the potential chemical inflammation was of only minor importance. Sensitivity after Class III and Class V restorations was minimal with glass-ionomer fillings.[35]

When Class V cavities were prepared in 170 adult dog teeth and 20 Class I cavities in human teeth, it was concluded that a combination of glass-ionomer and light-cured composite was superior to the composite restoration alone because fewer microorganisms were present with the former. No correlation was found between pathologic results and remaining dental thickness, but there was a correlation between bacteria and inflammation.[36]

The present authors carried out human studies several years ago following Class V preparations on premolars of 12- to 14-year-old patients. Teeth were prepared and filled with a light-cured glass-ionomer cement that is no longer commercially available. After 8 days, 1 month, or 3 months they were extracted and treated according to the Recommended Standard Practices for Biological Evaluation of Dental Biomaterials (ISO Technical Report 7405, 1984) and further processed for examination by light microscope. The results of pulpal reaction were ranked from slight to moderate after 1 month (Figs 5-2 to 5-4). However, after 3 months the pulp in 8 of 10 teeth was seriously damaged (Figs 5-5 and 5-6). Large areas in the pulp had been destroyed (Fig 5-7), but the odontoblast layer had not. At the time, the authors were unfamiliar with apoptotic degeneration of tissues and were unable to provide a clear-cut explanation of the results. Because odontoblasts are located adjacent to the dentinal tubules, it seemed logical that reactions would occur in this layer first and subsequently in the pulp. However, it is now well documented that apoptosis occurs more often in cells undergoing mitosis than in postmitotic cells. Thus, the

Plate 1 From normal to slight reaction in human teeth (hematoxylin-eosin stain).

Fig 5-1 Control section. A layer of predentin is located between odontoblasts (O) and dentin (D). Normal pulp (P). (Original magnification ×250.)

Fig 5-2 Slight pulpal reaction. After the preparation of a cervical cavity and placement of a filling material, there is no more evidence of predentin *(asterisk)*. Odontoblasts are slightly disturbed, and there is a slight increase of cells in the pulp. (Original magnification ×250.)

Fig 5-3 An early stage of osteodentin formation. Round-cell infiltration is seen inside the predentin *(arrowheads)*. Odontoblasts are present, and the palissade organization has been disrupted. (Original magnification ×320.)

Fig 5-4 Slight reaction in the subodontoblastic area. Predentin is present, as are odontoblasts. There is a localized accumulation of small round cells in the pulp *(asterisk)*. (Original magnification ×250.)

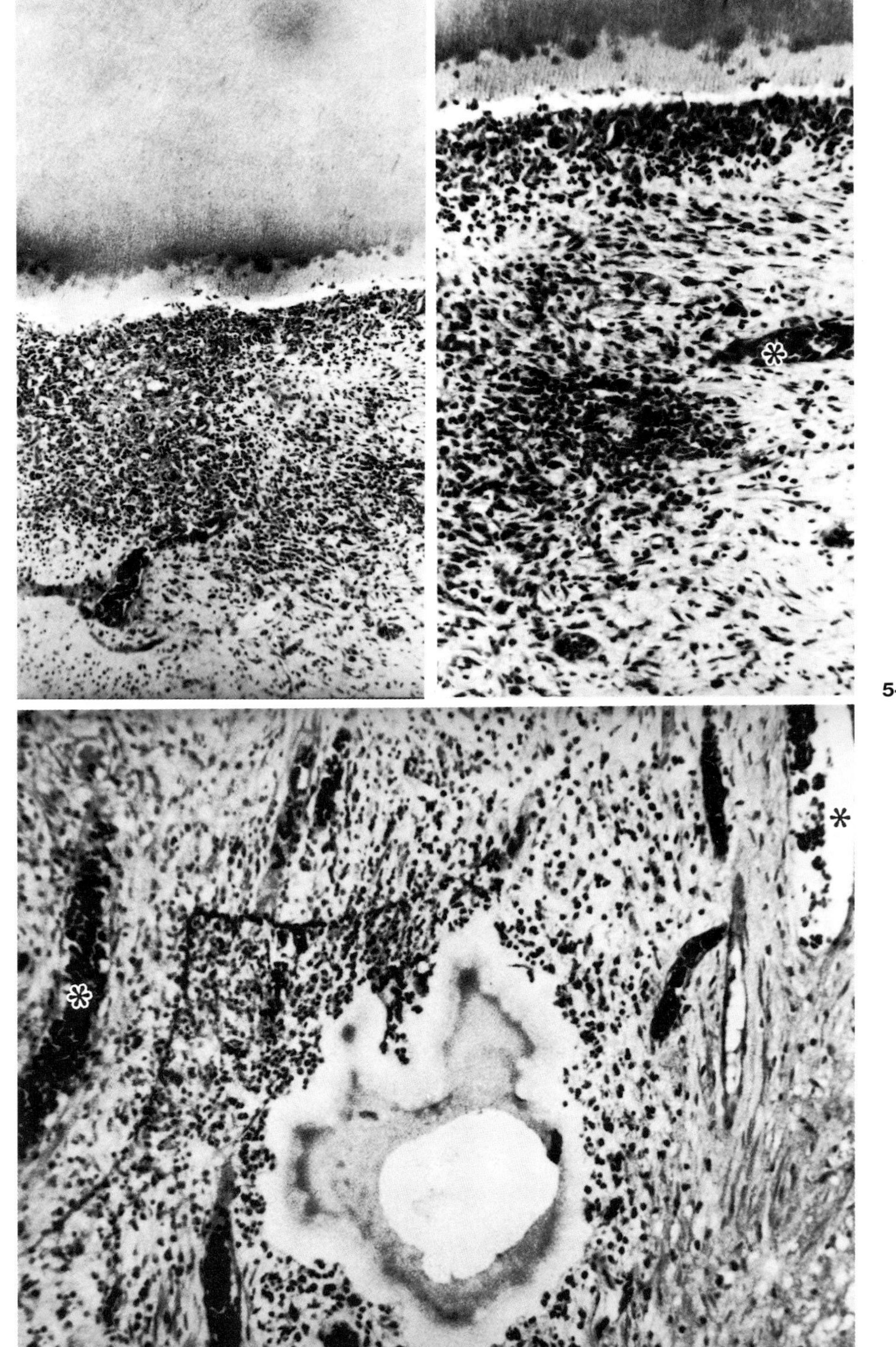
5-5
5-6
5-7

fact that odontoblasts are postmitotic cells and that pulp cells keep this potential property may be relevant. The reactions seen in this study were not limited to light-cured glass-ionomer cements. Less dramatic phenomena occurred with some adhesives and resins.

The authors obtained different results with another light-cured glass-ionomer (Fuji II LC). The biocompatibility of this glass-ionomer cement was good, most teeth displaying reactions ranking from none to moderate. When this cement was used to restore Class V cavities in sound dentin, tubular orthodentin was deposited adjacent to a marked calciotraumatic line (Figs 5-8 to 5-10). This finding is worth noting because in most cases, after the placement of adhesive, resin, or cement fillings, reparative dentin is of the osteodentin type, often without tubules and comprising cell inclusions within the mineralized tissue (Figs 5-11a and 5-11b).

Despite the specificity of the model and the small size of the animals, the authors next developed a rat model. Rats were anesthetized intraperitoneally with 6% chloral. After electosurgery of the gingiva and using a stereoscopic microscope at ×16 magnification, two cavities were prepared on the mesial aspect of each of the maxillary molars in 1 to 2 seconds with a high-speed contra-angle handpiece working at 120,000 rpm. Round cavities were prepared through half the thickness of the dentin. The tungsten carbide bur (0.05 ISO) was changed after every fourth cavity. No water cooling was used; cavities were rinsed with a wet cotton pellet and dried with a gentle blast of air. Sixteen cavities were filled with a light-cured glass-ionomer, five with Compoglass, and eight with Dyract. As controls, cavities with no retention were left unfilled. After demineralization of block sections of the teeth, 7-μm-thick sections were stained with Masson's, hematoxylin-eosin, and Brown and Brenn for bacterial demonstration (Figs 5-12a and 5-12b).

In most cases, no adverse pulp reaction was seen, and the worst reactions that did occur were moderate. Results for the glass-ionomers were compared to those for two adhesives and two resin composites. In sections prepared from rats allowed to survive 8 days following the placement of the filling material, a severe reaction was seen in each section of the 6 teeth treated with one adhesive (Figs 5-13a and 5-13b).

Plate 2 From moderate to severe reactions in human teeth. (Hematoxylin-eosin stain.)

Fig 5-5 Extensive accumulation of cells in the peripheral part of the pulp. (Original magnification ×320.)
Fig 5-6 Severe reaction with small round-cell infiltration near the predentin. These cells also are present in the odontoblast layer. There is severe reaction in the deeper pulp as well. Accumulation of coagulated blood has occurred in the capillaries *(asterisk)*. (Original magnification ×320.)
Fig 5-7 A severe reaction inducing the formation of a structureless area of destruction in the pulp. Round cells and cell debris are seen in the pulp. Nearby blood vessels display dilatation and accumulation of coagulated blood *(asterisks)*. (Original magnification ×640.)

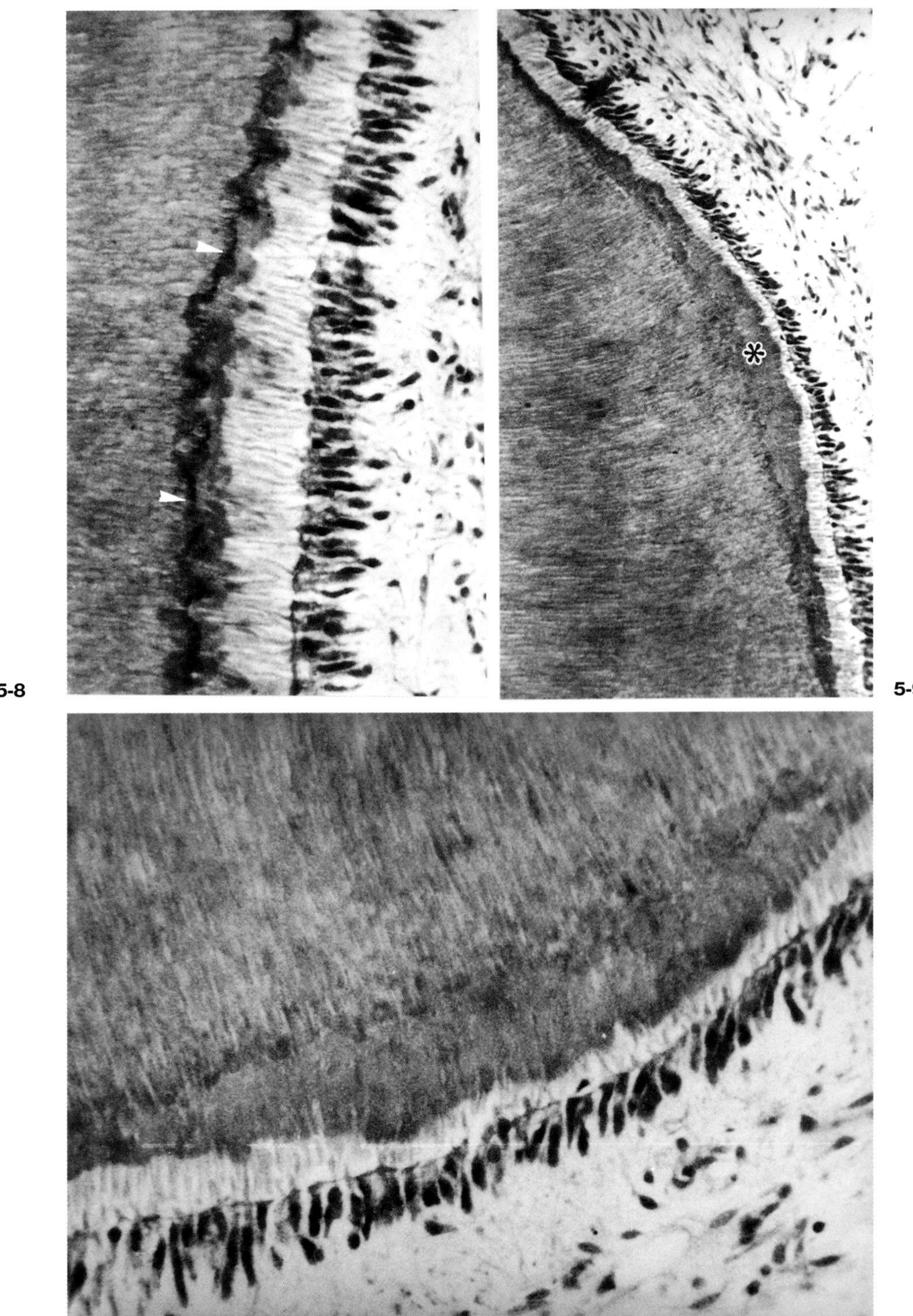

5-8

5-9

5-10

TUNEL labeling detected apoptosis in a group of cells in the zone connected with the tubules emerging from the lower cervix (Figs 5-14a and 5-14b). Odontoblasts were not damaged. Osteodentin was seen in both experimental and control specimens. No clear relationship could be established between the presence of bacteria and the adverse reactions. In some cases, a thin red layer was present at the interface between the biomaterial and the cavity wall. In other cases, microorganisms were seen in the dentinal tubules. Brown and Brenn stained slides revealed that, in this animal model, bacteria were not present when the cavity was left unfilled. This is probably due to the fact that food intake has a self-cleaning effect on the surface of the open cavity. In contrast, in cavities filled with either glass-ionomers or resin composites, bacteria were present at the filling–dentin interface and, in many cases, inside the lumen. This finding limits the conclusions that can be reached with this model, dealing with the specificity of the animal model versus actual human clinical studies. However, in most cases using this model, glass-ionomer cements were found to be biocompatible.

In Vitro Studies

Due to the lack of confidence in animal models and to the complexity of in vivo or clinical studies, in vitro approaches have been proposed. There are a few reports on the cytotoxicity and components of conventional and light-cured glass-ionomer cements. Imazato et al[37] showed that VitreBond lining cement is extremely cytotoxic, while the toxicity of Fuji Lining LC and Ketac-Bond is negligible. This investigation was carried out on L-929 mouse fibroblasts. According to the findings, the concentration of zinc in the cement seems to affect the degree of toxicity, whereas concentrations of silicon, aluminum, calcium, and strontium do not. Although the eluate for VitreBond contained about 6.9 times the HEMA concentration of Fuji Lining LC, the implication of this molecule in cytotoxicity is still uncertain. Using MTT assay, Kan et al[38] detected minimal reduction in percentage absorbance values for the four materials evaluated. Resin composite and Fuji II LC eluate exhibited close to 100% cell growth 1 day after extraction, whereas with conventional glass-ionomer and Vitremer the percentage of control

Plate 3 Formation of reparative dentin in human teeth. (Hematoxylin-eosin stain.)

Fig 5-8 Initial formation of reparative dentin beneath a calciotraumatic line *(arrowheads)*. Calcospherites are seen in the predentin. Odontoblasts are apparently undisturbed. (Original magnification ×1,000.)
Fig 5-9 Interruption of dentinogenesis by the preparation of a cavity. This is followed by placement of a biomaterial, leading to the formation of osteodentin *(asterisk)*. (Original magnification ×250.)
Fig 5-10 Enlarged view of the reparative dentin. Note the irregular structure of the tubular dentin. (Original magnification ×1,000.)

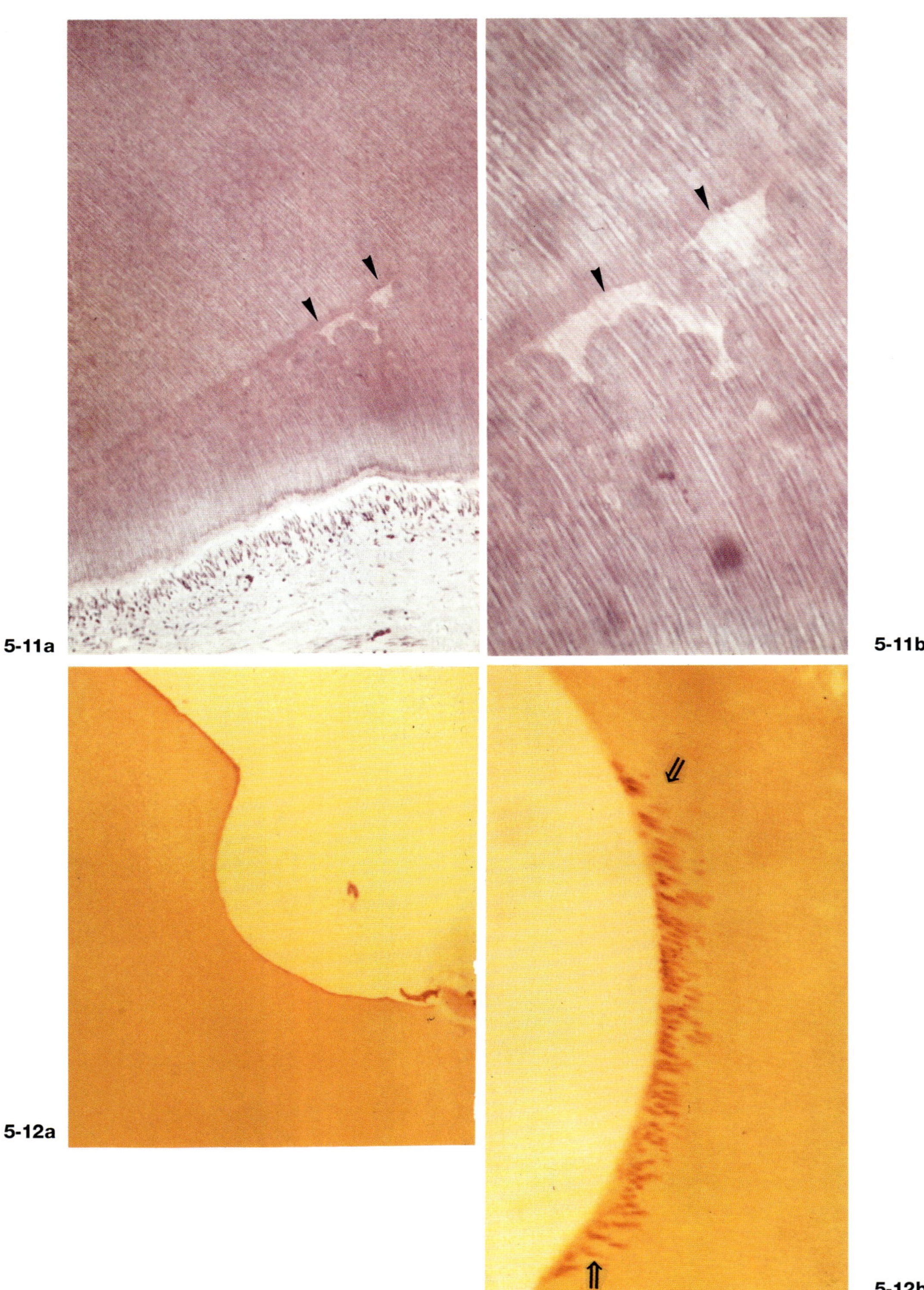

5-11a

5-11b

5-12a

5-12b

was 85.7 and 73.6, respectively. The conclusion was that fluoride release did not account for the cytotoxicity observed. From this study and others[39] it can be concluded that the cytotoxicity of glass-ionomer cements is not due to fluoride release, but to unidentified toxic components diffusing into the culture medium or components of resins.[40]

On a clone of L-929 mouse fibroblasts, Chem-Fil, Ketac-Fil, and Ketac-Silver gave excellent results in percentage of control growth with the MTT test, whereas the percentage of cell growth for VitreBond was low. Results obtained following surgical implantation into bone did not conflict with the results from direct cell contact.[41]

In another experiment, five glass-ionomer cements were put in direct contact with cultured human osteoblastic cells. The plating efficiency, adhesion, osteocalcin production, and morphology of the cells were tested. The results indicated that four of the five cements (Ketac-Fil Aplicap, Fuji II, Fuji II LC, and Ionocem Ionocap) are biocompatible when they are put in contact with this biological material, whereas Vitremer exhibits a marked toxicity toward the cells. Oliva et al[42] attributed the adverse reaction to the leaching of HEMA from the cement. The addition of pure HEMA at the same concentration found by protonic magnetic resonance analysis. The adverse reaction was attributed by these authors to the leaching of HEMA. The concentration of HEMA was evaluated by protonic magnetic resonance analysis. When pure HEMA was added to the culture medium at the same concentration, the same toxic effects were observed. This conclusion corroborates the assumption that unpolymerized and leachable resin components, such as Bis-GMA, urethane dimethacrylate (UDMA), triethylene glycol dimethacrylate (TEGDMA), and Bis-phenol A, have major cytotoxic effects.[40] These monomeric resin components are not only toxic to fibroblasts in culture but can evoke immunosuppression or immunostimulation on mitogen-driven proliferation of purified T lymphocytes.[43]

In vitro studies were carried in the present authors' laboratory with eluates obtained from standardized cylinders of material (1.9 mm in diameter and 1 mm

Plate 4 Formation of secondary orthodentin.

Fig 5-11 Formation of orthodentin in a treated human tooth. The preparation of the cavity has induced slight irregularities, including enlarged interglobular spaces *(arrowheads)*. Tubular orthodentin was formed after filling the cavity with a glass ionomer.
Fig 5-11a Original magnification ×250. (Hematoxylin-eosin stain.)
Fig 5-11b Original magnification ×750. (Hematoxylin-eosin stain.)
Fig 5-12a Cavity drilled in a rat molar. The surface of the cavity stains red, but no staining is detected inside dentin tubules. (Original magnification ×500; Brown and Brenn stain.)
Fig 5-12b Rat molar. After preparation of the cavity and filling with a glass-ionomer cement, staining is seen inside the lumens *(arrows)*. This reveals the presence of bacteria in the dentin. (Original magnification ×500; Brown and Brenn stain.)

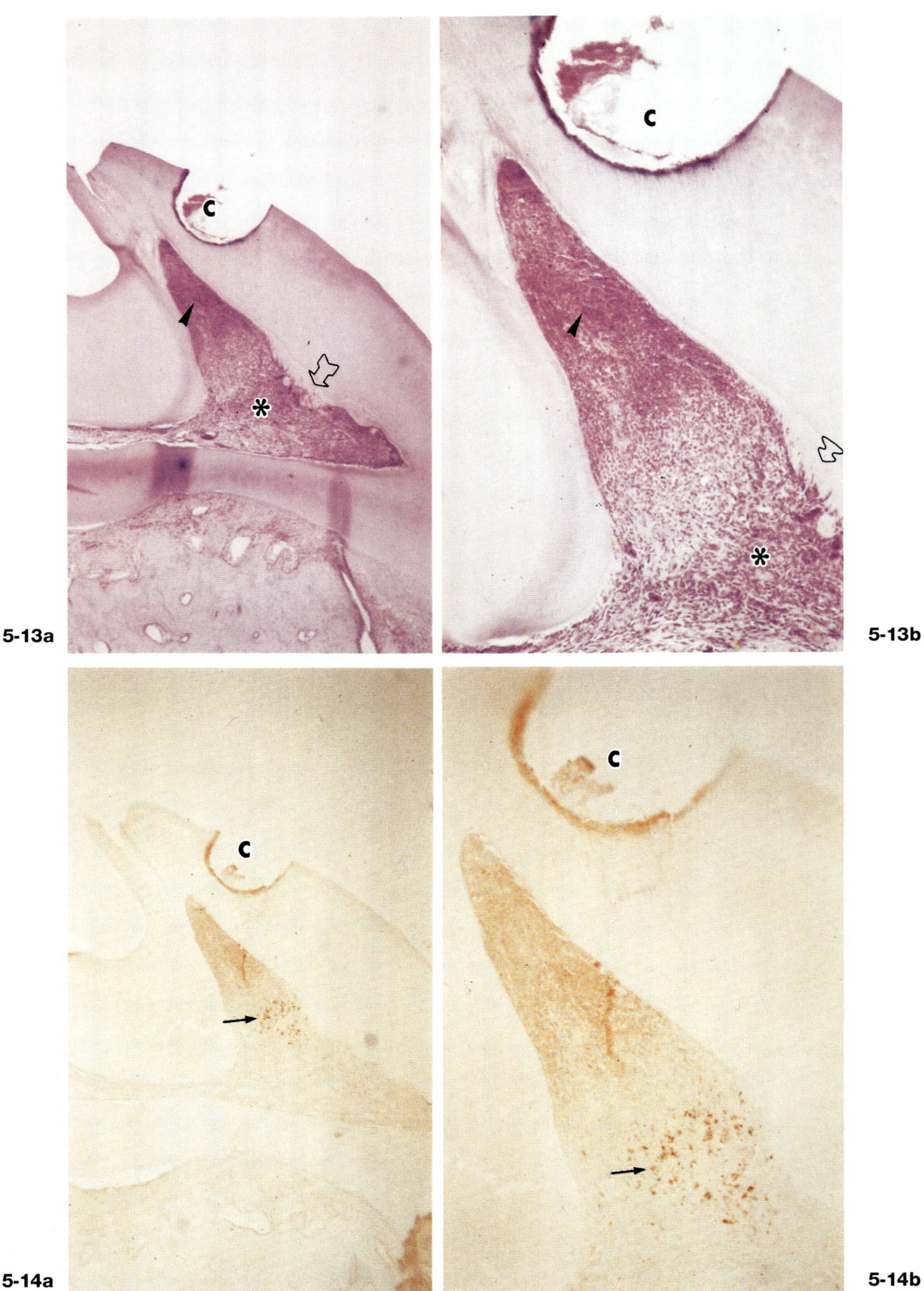

5-13a
5-13b
5-14a
5-14b
c
c
c
c
*
*

high) of Photac-Fil Aplicap, Vitremer, Fuji II LC, Dyract, and Compoglass. The eluates were tested on cultures of confluent pulp cells (second subculture) and on gingival and dermal cells (sixth and seventh subcultures). The following conclusions were reached:

- The most highly cytotoxic effect is obtained from eluates obtained within the first 3 days after extraction. The toxicity of the eluates decreased after 3 days for Vitremer and after 2 days for Hi-Dense, Fuji II LC, and Dyract. Eluate obtained with Compoglass was less cytotoxic than eluates obtained from other biomaterials.
- The concentration of the eluate plays a role in cytotoxicity. For example, Hi-Dense eluate is always cytotoxic, whatever the concentration. In contrast, Vitremer and Fuji II LC are cytotoxic at concentrations above 5%. Eluates from Photac-Fil, Dyract, and Compoglass are cytotoxic at concentrations above 5% and strongly cytotoxic at 10%.
- Only slight differences appear between the reactions observed in pulp cells and gingival cells. However, in some circumstances, pulp cells react very specifically.
- Preabsorption of the eluate on dentin powders firmly reduces the cytotoxicity of eluates.
- Because some cytotoxic components can be absorbed on dentin powder, potential agents were checked. The pHs of all the eluates were between 7.5 and 8, except for Hi-Dense and Vitremer, which were 5.9 and 6.3, respectively, for a 100% concentration. Hence, the pH was not related to the reaction.
- Fluoride and aluminum concentrations exerted a severe influence on pulp cells, but only above 1 mM. Fluoride release by the biomaterials varied. At 100% concentration of the eluate, Compoglass did not release any fluoride. The same quantity was released by Photac-Fil, Vitremer, Fuji II LC, and Dyract, but Hi-Dense released twice as much.
- Zinc was toxic at concentration in the order of 0.01 mM. Strontium was never cytotoxic at any concentration.

These conclusions indicate that none of the parameters listed earlier are involved in cell cytotoxicity and therefore it is possible that some unpolymerized and leachable resin components are responsible for the cytotoxic reactions.

Plate 5 Pulp reaction to a biomaterial in a rat molar with evidence of apoptosis.

Fig 5-13 A cavity (C) prepared in the mesial aspect of a rat maxillary molar and filled with an adhesive biomaterial. Cells have increased in number in the mesial pulp horn *(arrowheads)*. In the lower pulp near a zone of reparative dentin formation *(open arrows)*, there is also increased cellular accumulation *(asterisks)*.
Fig 5-13a Original magnification ×60. (Hematoxylin-eosin stain.)
Fig 5-13b Original magnification ×120. (Hematoxylin-eosin stain.)
Fig 5-14 Apoptotic reaction seen with the TUNEL method. Apoptotic cells are stained in the lower mesial pulp horn (see Figs 5-13a and 5-13b), but not in the upper condensation. In control molars, where cavities were left unfilled, pulp cells did not stain.
Fig 5-14a Original magnification ×60.
Fig 5-14b Original magnification ×120.

Summary

Dental materials continue to evolve, and which material will finally prove optimal is unknown. It might be glass-ionomer cements or new materials formed from biological molecules that will heal wounded tissue at great speed or induce biological mineralization. At the moment, glass-ionomer cements are useful materials, especially those whose physical properties have been improved by the addition of resins. However, if these materials are going to replace others, it will first be necessary to have a better understanding of what happens in their interaction with pulp cells.

References

1. Forss H, Seppa L. Prevention of enamel demineralization adjacent to glass-ionomer filling materials. Scand J Dent Res 1990;98:173–178.

2. Benelli EM, Serra MC, Rodrigues AL Jr, Cury JA. In situ anticariogenic potential of glass-ionomer cement. Caries Res 1993;27:280–284.

3. Weerheijm KI, de Soet JJ, van Amerongen WE, de Graaff J. The effect of glass-ionomer cement on carious dentine: An in vivo study. Caries Res 1993;27:417–423.

4. Mukai M, Ikeda M, Yanagihara T, Hara G, Kato K, Nakagaki H, Robinson C. Fluoride uptake in human dentine from glass-ionomer cement in vivo. Arch Oral Biol 1993;38:1093–1098.

5. Creanor SL, Carruthers LMC, Saunders WP, Strang R, Foye RH. Fluoride uptake and release characteristics of glass-ionomer cements. Caries Res 1994;28:322–328.

6. Bergenholtz G. Relationship between bacterial contamination of dentin and restorative success. In: Rowe N (ed). Proceedings of Symposium on Dental Pulp: Reaction to Restorative Materials in the Presence or Absence of Infection. Ann Arbor: University of Michigan 1982:93–107.

7. Van Meerbeek B, Inokoshi S, Braem M, Lambrechts P, Vanherle G. Morphological aspects of the resin-dentin interdiffusion zone with different dentin adhesive systems. J Dent Res 1992; 71:1530–1540.

8. Van Meerbeek B, Dhem A, Goret-Nicaise M, Lambrechts P, Vanherle G. Comparative SEM and TEM examination of the ultrastructure of the resin-dentin interdiffusion zone. J Dent Res 1993;72:495-501.

9. Imai H, Osumi-Yamashita N, Ninomiya Y, Eto K. Contribution of early-emigrating midbrain crest cells to the dental mesenchyme of mandibular molar teeth in rat embryos. Dev Biol 1996;176:151–165.

10. Ruch JV. Determinisms of odontogenesis. Revis Biol Celular 1987;1–81.

11. Lesot H, Bëgue-Kirn C, Kubler MD, Meyer JM, Smith AJ, Cassidy N, Ruch JV. Experimental

induction of odontoblast differentiation and stimulation during reparative processes. Cell Mater 1993;3:201–217.

12. Fitzgerald M, Chiego DJ, Heys DR. Autoradiographic analysis of odontoblast replacement following pulp exposure in primate teeth. Arch Oral Biol 1990;9:707–715.

13. Takahashi K. Vascular architecture of dog pulp using corrosion resin cast examined under a scanning electron microscope. J Dent Res 1985;64:579–584.

14. Kim S. Regulation of pulpal blood flow. J Dent Res 1985;64:590–596.

15. Hildebrand C, Fried K, Tuisku F, Johansson CS. Teeth and tooth nerves. Prog Neurobiol 1995;45:165–222.

16. Kobayashi I, Izumi T, Okamura K, Matsuo K, Ishibashi Y, Sakai H. Biological behavior of human dental pulp cells in response to carious stimuli analyzed by PCNA immunostaining and AgNOR staining. Caries Res 1996;30:225–230.

17. Jontell M, Gunraj MN, Bergenholtz G. Immunocompetent cells in the normal dental pulp. J Dent Res 1987;66:1149–1153.

18. Jontell M, Bergenholtz G, Scheynius A, Ambrose W. Dendritic cells and macrophages expressing class II antigens in the normal rat incisor pulp. J Dent Res 1988;67:1263–1266.

19. Jontell M, Eklof C, Dahlgren U, Bergenholtz G. Difference in capacity between macrophages and dendritic cells from rat incisor pulp to provide signals to concanavalin-A-stimulated T lymphocytes. J Dent Res 1994;73:1056–1060.

20. Okiji T, Kosaka T, Kamal AMM, Kawashima N, Suda H. Age-related changes in the immunoreactivity of the monocyte/macrophage system in rat molar pulp. Arch Oral Biol 1996;41:453–460.

21. Vermelin L, Ayanoglou C, Septier D, Carreau J-P, Bissila-Mapahou P, Goldberg M. Effects of essential fatty acid deficiency on rat molar pulp cells. Eur J Oral Sci 1995;103:219–224.

22. Vermelin L, Lècolle S, Septier D, Lasfargues J-J, Goldberg M. Apoptosis in human and rat dental pulp. Eur J Oral Sci 1996;104:547–553.

23. Stanislawski L, Carreau J-P, Pouchelet M, Chen ZHJ, Goldberg M. In vitro culture of human dental pulp cells: Some aspects of cells emerging early from the explant. Clin Oral Invest 1997;1:131–140.

24. Bennett JH, Joyner CJ, Triffitt JT, Owen ME. Adipocytic cells cultured from marrow have osteogenic potential. J Cell Sci 1991;99:131–139.

25. Nakashima M. Establishment of primary cultures of pulp cells from bovine permanent incisors. Arch Oral Biol 1991;36:655–663.

26. Tsukamoto Y, Fukutani S, Shin-Ike T, Kubota T, Sato S, Suzuki Y, Mori M. Mineralized nodule formation by cultures of human dental pulp-derived fibroblasts. Arch Oral Biol 1992;37:1045–1055.

27. Kasugai S, Shibata S, Suzuki S, Susami T, Ogura H. Characterization of a system of mineralized-tissue formation by rat dental pulp cells in culture. Arch Oral Biol 1993;38:769–777.

28. Bowen RL, Marjenhoff WA. Dental composites/glass-ionomers: The materials. Adv Dent Res 1992;6:44–49.

29. Kallus T, Gjerdet NR, Syrjanen S, Mjör IA. Ranking of histologic tissue response in biologic evaluation of dental materials. Scand J Dent Res 1988;96:265–274.

30. Mjör IA, Tronstad L. Experimentally induced pulpitis. Oral Surg 1972;34:102–108.

31. Pameijer CH, Stanley HR. Primate response to anhydrous Chembond. J Dent Res 1984;63:171.

32. Stanley HR. Local and systemic responses to dental composites and glass-ionomers. Adv Dent Res 1992;6:55–64.

33. Plant CG, Jones DW. The damaging effects of restorative materials. Part 2. Pulpal effects related to physical and chemical properties. Br Dent J 1976;140:406–412.

34. Browne RM, Tobias RS, Crombie IK, Plant CG. Bacterial microleakage and pulpal inflammation in experimental cavities. Int Endod J 1983; 16:147–155.

35. Bayne SC. Dental composites/glass-ionomers: Clinical reports. Adv Dent Res 1992;6:65–77.

36. Ohsone T. Histopathological studies on a combined restoration technique with a visible light

cured composite resin and a glass-ionomer cement. Shikwa Gakuho 1991;91:341–378.

37. Imazato S, Yokota W, Torii Y, Torii M, Tsuchitani Y. Studies on light-cured glass-ionomer cements. J Jpn Prosthod Soc 1991;34:840–847.

38. Kan KC, Messer LB, Messer HH. Variability in cytotoxicity and fluoride release of resin-modified glass-ionomer cements. J Dent Res 1997; 76:1502–1507.

39. Muller J, Bruckner G, Kraft E, Horz W. Reaction of cultured pulp cells to eight different cements based on glass-ionomers. Dent Mater 1990; 6:172–177.

40. Hanks CT, Strawn SE, Wataha JC, Craig RG. Cytotoxic effects of resin components on cultured mammalian fibroblasts. J Dent Res 1991; 70:1450–1455.

41. Sasanaluckit P, Albustany KR, Doherty PJ, Williams DF. Biocompatibility of glass-ionomer cements. Biomaterials 1993;14:906–916.

42. Oliva A, Della Ragione F, Salerno A, et al. Biocompatibility studies on glass-ionomer cements by primary cultures of human osteoblasts. Biomaterials 1996;17:1351–1356.

43. Jontell M, Hanks CT, Bratel J, Bergenholtz G. Effects of unpolymerized resin components on the function of accessory cell derived from the rat incisor pulp. J Dent Res 1995;74:1162–1167.

Chapter 6

Bonding Glass-Ionomer Cements to Tooth Structure

Timothy F. Watson

Ten years ago it would have been relatively straightforward to write about the mechanisms of attachment of glass-ionomer cements to tooth tissue, but the same cannot be said today. In the intervening years, the field's understanding of the strengths and weaknesses of dental hard tissues has not changed greatly, but the range of materials related to the ionomeric setting reaction has greatly diversified. The characterization and classification of these new systems are covered in chapter 1 of this book. Briefly, the available glass-ionomer materials now range from highly water-sensitive acid-base cements to materials with setting reactions that are almost entirely resin based. Not surprisingly, the way they bond to tooth tissue may be profoundly affected by their resin content. To gain a full appreciation of their adhesive–substrate interactions it is first necessary to understand the relevant anatomy and physiology of the substrate itself.

The Substrate: Enamel and Dentin

To grossly simplify the situation, enamel is dry and brittle, dentin is wet and resilient. Enamel is an immensely strong biomaterial but does have inherent planes of weakness, a fact not often appreciated in the literature for adhesive dental materials.

The basic structural unit of enamel is the hydroxyapatite crystal. Approximately 10,000 of these long, slender crystals are packed closely together to form a 7-μm-diameter prism or rod.[1] This unit extends from the enamel-dentin junction (EDJ) to the surface of the tooth, a distance of up to 2.5 mm. The hydroxyapatite crystals can be very long in comparison to their width, behaving rather like the fibers in a rope; this, in conjunction with the complexity of the prism shape and course, leads to an extremely tough and hard-wearing material. Such strength is, however, highly directional in this anisotropic material.[2] The prism unit is very difficult to pull and break on its long axis because of the crystal orientation. The optimal enamel prism orientation for bonding is therefore on the long axis. Attachment to the sides of prisms is less satisfactory. Prisms can, however, be bent laterally and ruptured by weaker forces than are required for breakage on the long axis.[2,3] Such prism orientations are readily encountered in the lateral walls of proximal cavities.

A major structural unit of dentin is the dentin tubule, running from the EDJ to the pulp. This 1- to 2-μm-diameter tubule conveys pulpal fluid from the pulp to the enamel, maintaining the hydration of the tooth and other physiologic functions.[4] The inherent outward flow of fluid profoundly reduces the penetration of adhesives into the tubules and may have an effect on water-sensitive cements.[5–8] Tubule density at the EDJ is 19,000/mm^2 and increases toward the pulp to 45,000/mm^2. The diameter of the tubule also increases from 0.8 μm at the EDJ to 2.5 μm at the pulp.[9] It is therefore self-evident that deeper dentin is much "wetter" than that at the periphery of the tooth, affecting the performance of water-sensitive restorative materials.

In the outer two thirds of the dentin, the tubule itself is surrounded by a thin coating of highly mineralized peritubular dentin. The bulk of this coating consists of a matrix of type 1 collagen embedded in hydroxyapatite crystals to form the intertubular dentin.[10] Hypermineralization of dentin occurs as a normal response to caries and tooth wear and, by reducing permeability, confers a protective function by preventing noxious substances from entering the pulp.[11]

Dentin is neither strong nor weak in any particular direction; compared to enamel it is isotropic. It can therefore be appreciated that dentin is a multiphase material which presents many problems for bonding due to its water content, its resilience and its inhomogeneity.

Enamel and dentin are intimately related to each other with a scalloped interface at the EDJ. The enamel protects the dentin from wear, and the dentin supports the brittle enamel. Without adequate support from the dentin, the enamel shell is easily lost: examples of this are situations in which the dentin structure is defective, as in dentinogenesis imperfecta or dentinal caries. Many of the crack-stopping features within enamel, such as prism decussation and the sinuous nature of the prisms in the inner two thirds of the enamel, commence at the EDJ.

Cutting these hard tissues produces a structure called the *smear layer* (< 20 μm thick) on both the enamel and dentin. This is more or less well attached to the tooth surface and consists of cutting debris which is pressure-welded to the tooth.[12] It has the effect of reducing fluid outflow from the dentin by plugging the tubular openings.[13] Due to its brittleness, cutting enamel introduces subsurface cracks and fault lines which can lead to structural weakness if adhesive materials are bonded to this damaged substrate.[14,15]

Nondestructive microscopic imaging

Scanning optical, or confocal, microscopy offers many advantages for imaging tooth tissue and glass-ionomer cements, because of the ability of the investigator to control their water content and also to examine undisturbed structures below the section surface. Further information can be gained by consulting specific references.[16–18]

General Requirements for Adhesion

The general perceived requirements for adhesion are expounded in many dental textbooks. Good substrate wetting, a low contact angle, and a clean substrate are normally considered essential. The surface tension of the liquid adhesive must always be less than the surface energy of the enamel or dentin. The contamination of the tooth surface by saliva, blood, or other proteinaceous substances reduces the surface energy of the substrate and impairs wetting by the liquid adhesive. Put simply, the first thing to touch a "clean" tooth surface, whether saliva or bonding resin, makes the strongest bond.

The most likely mechanisms of bonding to tooth structure are as follows:[19]

- Mechanical theories that involve the concept of interlocking the solidified adhesive with the irregularities of the adherent surface.
- Adsorption theories that comprise all the explanations involving chemical bonding and similar forces between the adhesive and adherent. The forces involved may be primary (ionic and covalent) and secondary (hydrogen, dipole interaction, or Van der Waals') valence forces.
- Diffusion theories that involve the concept of bonding between mobile molecules across the interface.

Following these criteria, it would be easy to appreciate that the enamel–composite bond falls into the first category: the tooth surface is etched and dried, and free-flowing fluid resin is placed and cured. A viscous glass-ionomer cement may fall into the second and third categories because, even without acid etching of the tooth, conventional glass-ionomer cements are inherently adhesive restorations compared with the resin composites. It would appear that there must be other mechanisms at work.

Adhesion can be achieved in a number of different ways and much of the literature has speculated on the attachment of conventional glass-ionomers to teeth. Much of this is based on concepts of polar dispersion, ionic diffusion, and alterations to surface topography and surface energies.

Adhesion Mechanisms of Conventional Glass-Ionomer Cements

The development of the tooth–glass-ionomer bond evolves over time. Unlike resin-based systems, the bond strength increases to become eventually limited by the cohesive tensile strength of the cement rather than by its adhesive strength alone.

The initial attraction between the cut tooth and freshly placed cement is mainly due to polar attraction, with weak hydrogen bonds predominating. At this stage, the acidity of the cement allows it to act as a self-etching agent on the tooth smear layer. The hydrogen ions are rapidly buffered by the phosphate ions from the hydroxyapatite crystals, but widespread exposure of collagen is limited because of the weakness of the acids involved. Even if the cement is relatively viscous, the watery environment of the tooth and the free water in the cement

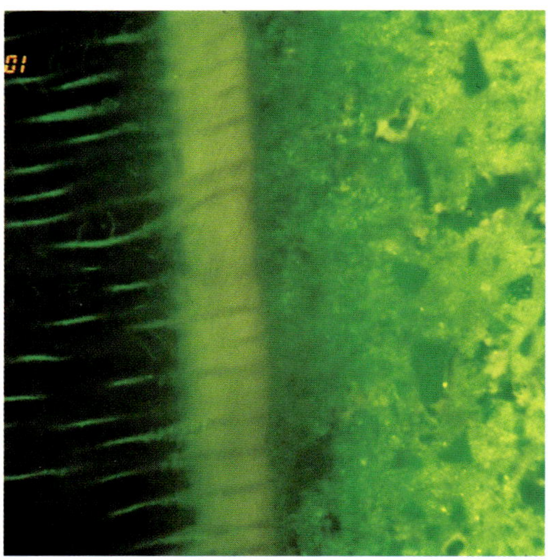

Fig 6-1 Fluorescent yellow band just below the cavity surface following placement of a conventional glass-ionomer labeled with rhodamine in the water used to rehydrate the cement. Notice that the fluorescent band is traversed by dentin tubules. A tandem scanning confocal microscope (TSM) with a 1.4 numerical aperture oil immersion (NA OI) lens was used with 546 (green excitation) and no barrier filter (/-). (Original magnification ×60; field width = 120 μm.)

should ensure an ionic exchange at the interface. In this way, good wetting of the substrate by the adhesive is achieved. Water flux at the dentin interface is indicated by the transfer of dye from the cement as a fluorescent band, as imaged using confocal microscopy (Fig 6-1).[8]

The continuing development of the bond is thought to be caused by further movement of ionic species in the interface, perhaps due to diffusion as the phosphate ions are displaced by the polyalkenoic acids.[20] This theory suggests that to maintain an electrolytic balance it is necessary for each phosphate ion to take with it a calcium ion. These are then taken up by the cement adjacent to the tooth to produce an ion-enriched layer that is firmly bound to both enamel and dentin. The strength of both the ion-enriched layer and its union to the tooth have yet to be measured.

Maximum achievable bond strength for glass-ionomers is only reached after the cement has undergone its maturation process. On addition of the liquid to the powder, hardening occurs due to attack of the glass surface by hydronium ions (hydrated protons of the acid), causing the release of calcium and aluminum ions. The ions form salt bridges between carboxyl groups of the polyacid, resulting in a gel matrix surrounding the intact glass particles.[21] The maturation of glass-ionomer restorations is relatively slow. In the initial stages of the setting reaction, divalent calcium ions are released rapidly and form primarily calcium salt bridges between polyacrylate chains within the cement. Such salt bridges also form at the interface with hydroxyapatite in the tooth. At this stage, both water uptake and water loss can occur, with the attendant clinical problems of contamination and dehydration. Provisions must be made to maintain the water balance of restorations for the first 24 hours. In later stages of the setting reaction, cross-linking by trivalent aluminum ions gives greater stability to the matrix structure.[22]

At full maturation, the cement at the interface will have become very viscous and its initial reactions with the tooth substrate will have ensured a close adaptation. Minimal setting movements of the cement, if it is kept fully hydrated,[8,23] will also maintain the close approximation of tooth and cement to allow further ion exchange to occur over the lifetime of the restoration.

Acid etching

Glass-ionomer cements are appropriate for restoring cavities such as abrasion or erosion cavities where little or no cavity preparation is required. The tooth is, however, coated with a pellicle and other surface debris, so some sort of cleaning or conditioning treatment is required. The use of acid etchants with glass-ionomer cements has been advocated for many years.[24] As the adhesion to tooth tissue is primarily mediated by the mineral component, the use of strong acids cause exposure of a collagen network in the dentin and a reduced bonding potential. Strong acids have been investigated extensively with the resin-based adhesive systems.[25,26] Polyacrylic acid has a minor effect on the dentin, removing the smear layer and surface contaminants without opening the dentin tubules too widely.[24] It has therefore become the etchant of choice for conventional glass-ionomers. There are two advantages in using polyacrylic acid for etching the dentin. First, because it is the acid used in the cement itself, any residue inadvertently left behind does not interfere with the setting reaction. Second, it enhances the wettability of the tooth surface to a water-containing cement and preactivates the calcium and phosphate ions in the dentin, rendering them more available for ion exchange with the cement.[20]

Enamel bonding

The conventional glass-ionomer cements have very different interfacial characteristics with tooth tissue compared to those of resin composites and dentin bonding agents. As previously outlined, their adhesive mechanisms are restricted essentially to surface attraction. This restriction has severe implications if the materials become dimensionally unstable, which may happen as a result of excess water uptake or desiccation.[8,23,27] Drying problems are most pronounced in relation to enamel, where the cement is adherent to the surface alone and where dehydration first appears clinically.

Dehydration can happen quickly intraorally with the placement of a rubber dam, or during impression-taking procedures: the first sign of drying in the cement is a chalky white appearance on its surface. There usually are cracks below the enamel surface from previous cutting operations, so any shrinkage of the cement on drying causes cohesive failure of the substrate.[14] The bond between glass-ionomer and enamel is stronger than is often realized; indeed, it can be stronger than the bond between enamel prisms, especially when these are running parallel with the cavity surface (Fig 6-2). This form of enamel fracture can be observed readily in any test sample where the material has not been maintained in a sufficiently hydrated form. Examination of fracture surfaces with

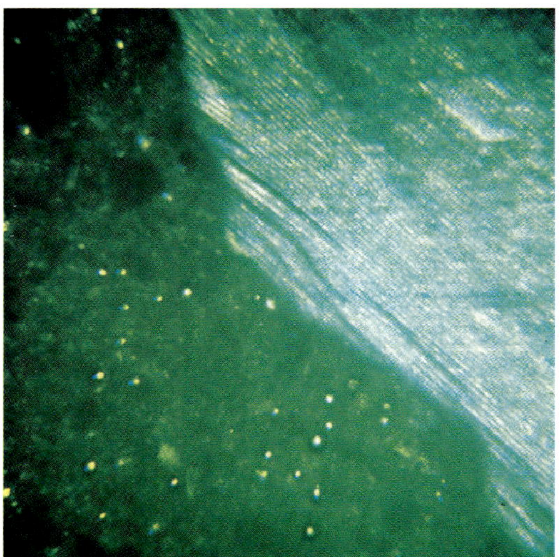

Fig 6-2 Cracking of an enamel margin following dehydration and shrinkage of a chemically setting glass-ionomer cement. The water used to rehydrate this cement was labeled with rhodamine, highlighting the glass particles within the matrix. (Original magnification ×20; TSM with 0.8 NA OI, 546/-; field width 450 μm.)

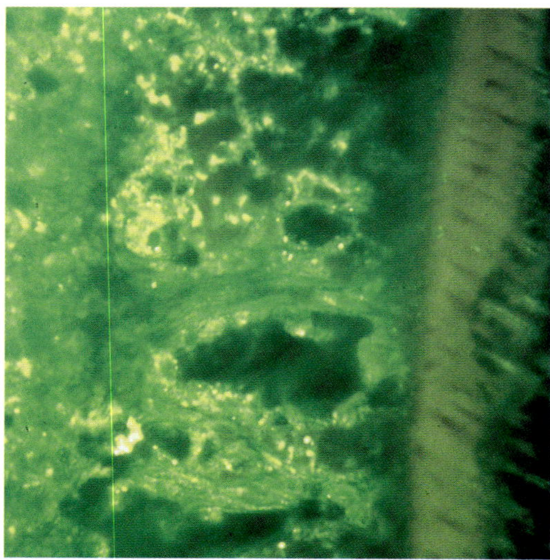

Fig 6-3 Dentin interface with a poorly mixed, sloppy conventional glass-ionomer cement. The material has shrunk on setting, showing arcades within the matrix. Fluorescent dye (rhodamine) has leached from the cement to form a yellow band in the dentin (see Fig 6-1). (Original magnification ×60; TSM with 1.4 NA OI, 546/-; field width = 120 μm.)

scanning electron microscopy (SEM) can make it difficult to delineate enamel from cement, a difference which is seen easily with fluorescent labels and confocal microscopy.

Dentin bonding

The inherent wetness of the dentin interface may reduce the strength of the matrix close to the tooth by effectively reducing the powder–liquid ratio of the water-setting cements. Microcracks can often be seen in this region.[8] The net result may be cohesive failure of the cement in this region; an observation frequently reported in the literature.

Figure 6-3 shows a cement where the powder–liquid ratio has been greatly decreased from the manufacturer's recommendations to make a very fluid mix. The arcading within the matrix indicates the stresses imparted to the interface by the fluorescent labeled cement "dehydrating" and shrinking on setting. The band of fluorescent dye within the dentin is characteristic of any of the acid-base cements; even phosphate cement. Following etching with polyacrylic acid, the tubular openings may be exposed, making it is possible to see 2- to 3-μm-long plugs of glass-ionomer cement matrix occupying these openings, especially if the cement is labeled with 0.2-μm-diameter titanium dioxide parti-

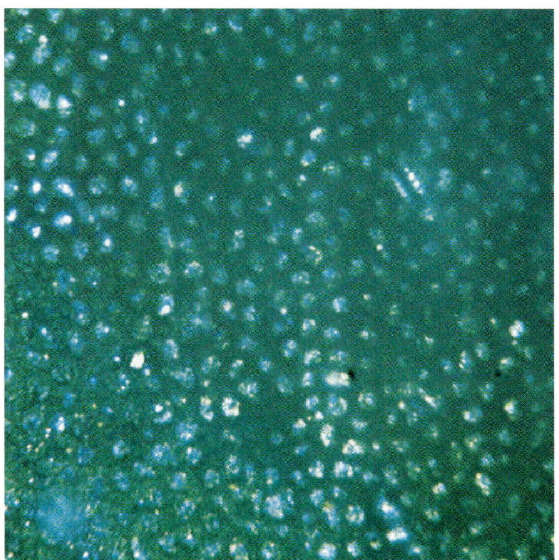

Fig 6-4 Reflection image of a glass-ionomer matrix forming plugs in acid-etch dentin tubule openings. The matrix was labeled with reflective titanium dioxide particles (0.2 μm in diameter). The sample is imaged *en face* looking into the cement from the cavity floor. The dentin was polished gently to leave a very thin layer next to the restoration. Remnants of this can be seen on the lower left. The microscope was focused below the surface of the remaining dentin to show the plugs of glass-ionomer matrix. (Original magnification ×60; TSM with 1.4 NA OI, 546/-; field width = 180 μm.)

cles and a reflection image made with a confocal microscope (Fig 6-4).[28] These plugs may impart some mechanical interlocking to the adhesive interface but are in no way equivalent to the long tags seen with resin-based dentin bonding agents (DBAs).[23]

Resin-Modified Glass-Ionomer Cements

Lining materials

The resin-modified cements were first introduced as lining materials, being unsuitable as restorative materials because of the marked polymerization shrinkage imparted by their high resin content. This resin component can be encouraged to act in a manner similar to that of DBAs with the use of suitable conditioning/priming systems.[29] The light-curing capabilities of these liners offer some advantages in terms of increased resistance to acid dissolution when used with the acid-etch composite/"sandwich" technique, but the high resin content allows particularly severe polymerization shrinkage. The fact that the liners are normally placed as thin layers also makes them more prone to dehydration, in much the same way as conventional glass-ionomers.

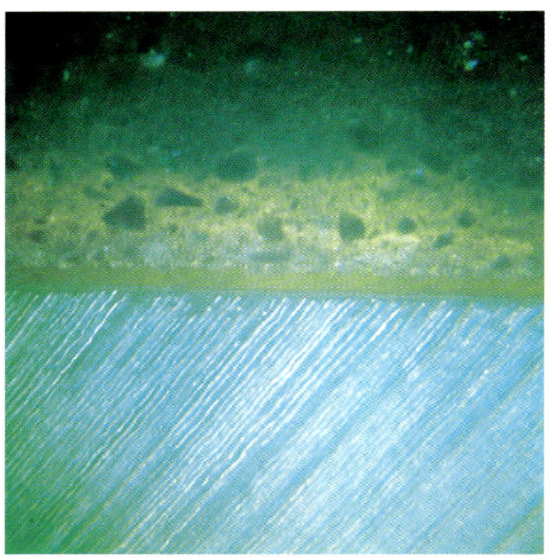

Fig 6-5 Resin-modified cement subjected to dye uptake from dentinal fluid. The material has formed an absorption layer within the interface, showing as the fluorescent band in the center of this combined reflection-fluorescence image. Some movement of dye into the cement also has occurred and highlights the glass particles in the cement. (Original magnification ×20; TSM with 0.8 NA OI, field width = 450 μm.)

Restorative materials

Development of resin-modified glass-ionomers into restorative materials produces an interesting mixture of properties.[30] The use of conditioners or primers containing 2-hydroxyethylmethacrylate (HEMA) produces interfacial appearances very similar to those of resin composites when the latter are used in conjunction with a DBA, an effect first noted with resin-modified lining materials.[29]

Dynamic interactions can still occur with these new materials after the initial set. Resin-modified glass-ionomer cements can be porous to pulpal fluids, as indicated by dye uptake in the interfacial region of the cement (Fig 6-5).[31,32] Examination of many samples suggests that a nonparticulate, easily stained layer of solid material (< 30 μm thick) often forms between the bulk of the cement and the dentin within 24 hours. This layer only forms next to dentin tubules that communicate with the wet pulp cavity and has been observed with Fuji II LC, Fuji Bond LC, and Photac-Fil Quick (see Fig 6-5). Its presence with Vitremer is less discernible and may be doubtful. It is particularly obvious when fluorescent labeled solutions are placed in the pulp cavity, but it is not simply a contraction gap in which fluid has accumulated.

The solid interfacial layer is superficial to the cavity surface and is not a function of the acid etchants used, being present in interfaces where the smear layer has been removed by the use of an air abrasive stream.[31,32] When the cut sample surface is imaged, it is seen to be intact and solid, which would be the appearance detected with conventional

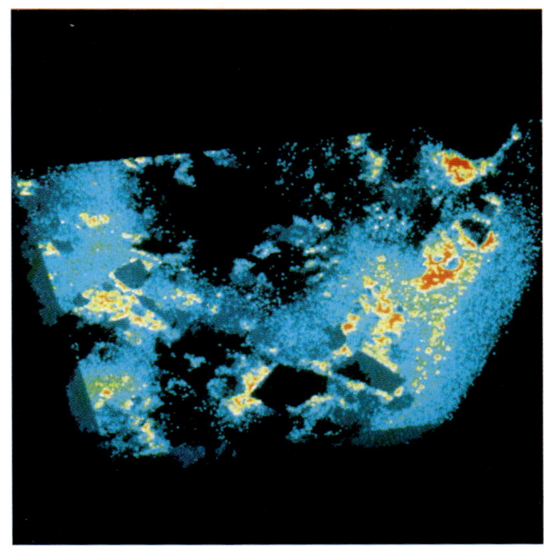

Fig 6-6 A resin-modified glass-ionomer adhesive, labeled with APSS[18], which has been dosed with the liquid component of the cement. This dye has a great affinity for HEMA. Particulate distribution can be seen close to the dentin interface (diagonal margin of reconstruction) with the glass particles displaced from the cavity surface by a swelling of the matrix component of the system, or the absorption layer. The dye shows fluorescence around the glass particles, which may be related to its fluorescence being strongest in an alkaline localized environment. This dye was originally developed for two-photon imaging, and when this technique is used, high-resolution images can be produced up to 80 μm below the surface of dense materials. Volume reconstruction (20 μm thick) color rendered. (Original magnification ×60; 1.4 NA OI, 800 μm excitation giving 400 μm fluorescence emission; field width = 100 μm.)

imaging techniques such as radiographs and SEM. Long tags of resin infiltrating dentin tubules are *not* a characteristic feature of resin-modified glass-ionomer cements. The term *absorption layer* has been applied to this structure[31,32]; it may be important in the maintenance of the fit of the restoration to compensate for the contraction of the resin on polymerization. This feature may be a resin layer at the restoration interface that has taken up fluid and swelled. It is not seen on the free outer surface of the restoration when it is soaked in dye-containing solutions, nor is it associated with enamel or a desiccated dentin surface.[31,32]

Adhesives

The absorption layer is particularly marked in materials with a high HEMA–resin content, such as Fuji Bond LC, where labeling with special dyes and two-photon confocal imaging have shown HEMA distribution and the associated absorption layer next to the tooth interface (Fig 6-6).[18,33] This type of material is marketed as a stress-relieving bonding system for composites, in which the interfacial stresses from a shrinking, polymerizing composite restoration are dissipated by a resin-modified glass-ionomer cement that sets or polymerizes at a slower rate. Time lapse studies of restoration–tooth interfaces conducted in this laboratory indicate that the mechanism to counteract the polymerization shrinkage of the composite is one of swelling and

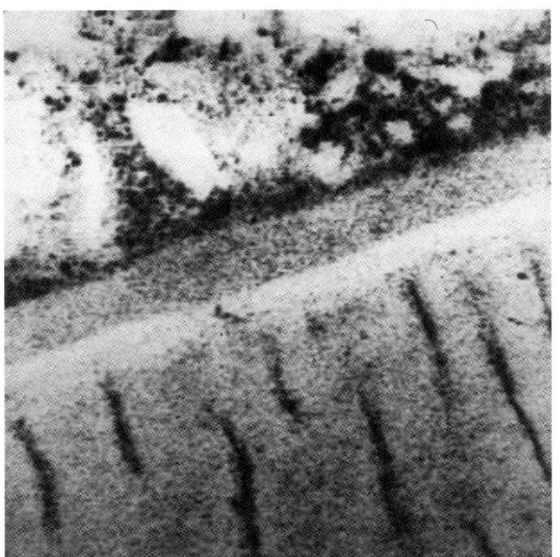

Fig 6-7 Polyacid-modified resin composite and adhesive at the dentin interface. Notice the alteration in the appearance of the dentin adjacent to the restoration. (Original magnification ×60; reverse-contrast CLSM reflection image, with 1.4 NA OI; field width = 80 μm.)

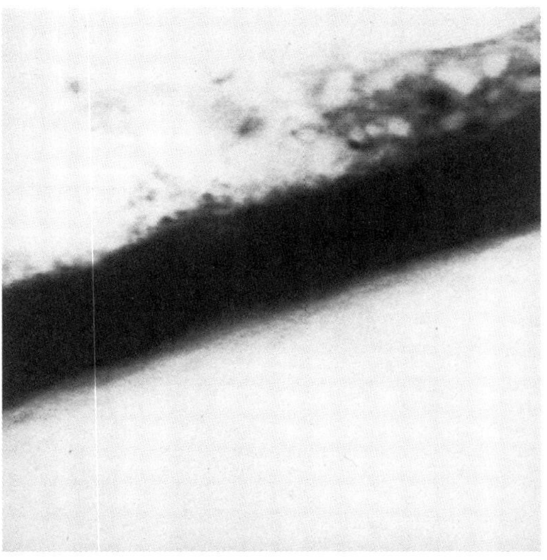

Fig 6-8 Same sample as Fig 6-7 with fluorescence image of rhodamine-labeled adhesive. Virtually no penetration into dentin tubules has occurred, but there is some penetration into the dentin corresponding to the altered region in Fig 6-7. (Original magnification ×60; reverse-contrast CLSM image with 1.4 NA OI, 514/600 μm; field width = 80 μm.)

movement within the immature cement as it takes up fluid from the dentin.

Dehydration shrinkage is still present with resin-modified cements. This happens very quickly and, after a few minutes, considerable gaps can open up in immature cements.[34] When failure is seen adjacent to the dentin, it is often in the absorption layer, whereas restorations with enamel margins often fail with structural cohesive failure of the enamel in a manner similar to that of conventional glass-ionomers.

Polyacid-Modified Resin Composites

The development of the polyacid-modified resin composites, or compomers, effectively completes the transition from materials with a water-based setting reaction to those that are almost entirely resin based. In contrast to resin composites, these materials are designed to be water tolerant in that they are required to absorb water for the development of the acid-base setting reaction after polymerization of the light-cured resin. In conventional glass-ionomers, the availability of free water to bound water decreases as the material matures over a period of months.[20] Polyacid-modified composites

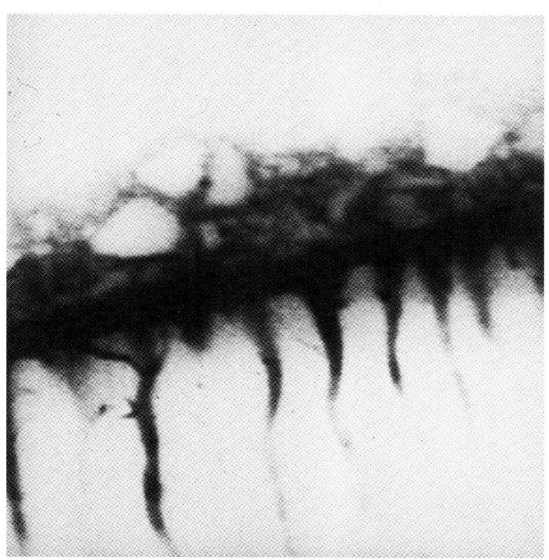

Fig 6-9 Dentin–adhesive interface following phosphoric acid etching. The adhesive has been labeled with rhodamine. Resin tag and hybrid zone formation is more apparent than in Fig 6-7, but the occurrence of full sealing depends on the penetrating capabilities of the adhesive into the heavily etched and demineralized dentin. (Original magnification ×60; reverse-contrast CSLM image with 1.4 NA OI, 514/600 μm; field width = 80 μm.)

also show an increase in bound versus free water as they mature, giving some evidence that they may have a limited glass-ionomer–type setting reaction.[35]

Despite some evidence of such setting reactions, there is no inherent adhesion of polyacid-modified composites to tooth tissue. It is essential, therefore, that an intermediary adhesive be applied to the tooth. Most of the adhesives that have been produced for use with polyacid-modified composites are of the self-etching variety, so as to simplify handling. The manufacturers claim that etching with phosphoric acid is unnecessary. The low pH of the adhesive is sufficient to remove the smear layer and produce a resin infiltration zone in dentin (Figs 6-7 and 6-8). However, penetration into the dentin tubules is considerably reduced when compared with the same adhesive applied following phosphoric acid etching of the dentin (Fig 6-9). The penetration of resin tags into the enamel also is greatly reduced. There is therefore a risk of failure in both dentin and enamel at these interfaces when roughness of the substrate surface and penetration of the adhesive is reduced. However, a counterargument states that a "self-contained" primer-etchant system will give penetration of the resin only as far as the etchant effect. This has been shown with one of the commercial adhesives available, with which excellent sealing of the interface is produced.[36]

Hybrid zone formation

The concept of hybridization and micromechanical interlocking has become a popular explanation for the adhesion of resin-based DBAs when used for attaching resin composites.[37,38] It is considered the major mechanism of attachment for the fluid hydrophilic resins often carried in volatile solvents, which impregnate the etched dentin surface and mediate the bond for the polyacid-modified composites. Much of the popularity for this concept stems from the relative ease of imaging these tough resin–tooth interfaces using SEM and transmission electron microscopy (TEM). However, the infiltration achieved may be only partial, with unfilled spaces in the acid-etched dentin interface.[36] High-vacuum imaging techniques, such as SEM and TEM, cause great difficulty for observing water-containing cements. Therefore, despite the availability of environmental SEM, the concept of a hybrid zone has seldom been applied to conventional glass-ionomers, because it is difficult to produce interfacial images that are not seriously affected by the dehydration artifact.[39]

The ion exchange that probably occurs at the tooth interface with glass-ionomer cements certainly yields a region with intermediate properties of both materials so in those terms it is a hybrid zone. However, the mechanisms involved are undoubtedly more subtle, relating more closely to the adsorption and diffusion theories of adhesion mentioned earlier than to the relatively macroscopic mechanical retention effects seen with resin infiltration.

Interfacial fracture

The failure of an adhesive joint involves three possible mechanisms which may or may not occur in combination: cohesive failure in the substrate, cohesive failure within the adhesive, and adhesive failure. It is possible to image interfacial fracture of adhesive systems subjected to shear bond testing.[17] Conventional glass-ionomers show deformation of the cement as load is applied, with slow propagation of cracks and flaws until catastrophic failure which often leaves a thin layer of residual cement, the ion-enriched layer on the tooth substrate (Fig 6-10). Resin-modified cements also can show significant flexibility, but this is usually most apparent in the absorption layer, especially in cements designed to act as an adhesive system for composite restorations.[40]

Much of the published literature on dental adhesives uses load testing to rank effectiveness. The difficulty of making comparisons between different test centers because of variable specimen geometries and test configurations is well known.[41] Making comparisons between different classes of material also is problematic because tough materials such as resin composites may perform well in a simple shear bond test; conventional glass-ionomers seldom perform as well because of their inherent weakness which leads to their cohesive failure under these conditions. However, conventional glass-ionomers have other desirable properties such as limited setting shrinkage, good elasticity, and the ability to show self-repair mechanisms once cracks have appeared within them, as reported by Watson et al[23] and Feilzer

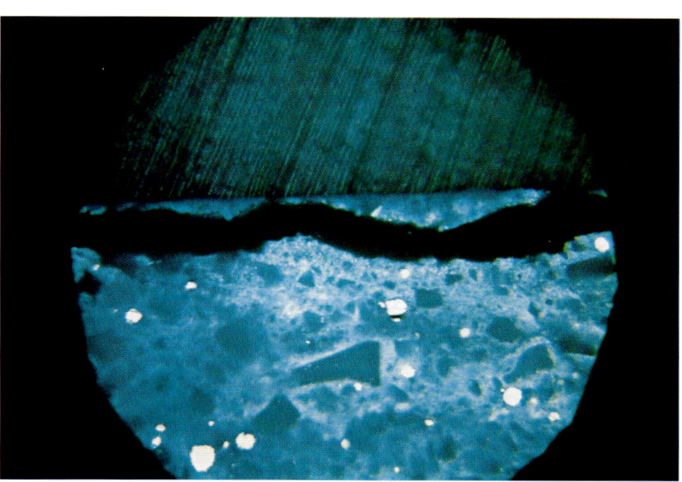

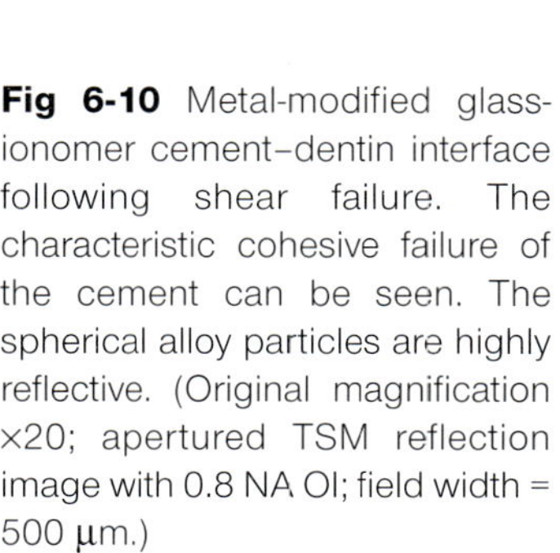

Fig 6-10 Metal-modified glass-ionomer cement–dentin interface following shear failure. The characteristic cohesive failure of the cement can be seen. The spherical alloy particles are highly reflective. (Original magnification ×20; apertured TSM reflection image with 0.8 NA OI; field width = 500 μm.)

et al.[41] All these factors help in the survival of restorations in the oral environment.

Resin-modified glass-ionomers exhibit greater bonding strengths than do conventional glass-ionomers in shear bond testing.[42] Polyacid-modified composites perform in a manner similar to that of conventional composites, their bond strength being related mainly to the effectiveness of the DBA used rather than their inherent adhesive properties.

Conclusion

The sensitivity of glass-ionomer cements to water loss presents a significant challenge for the microscopic assessment of both their interfacial morphology and the chemical composition of the interface. Glass-ionomer cements cover nearly the whole spectrum of bonding mechanisms and, although much is already known about their interfacial characteristics with tooth tissue, there is still much to explore.

Acknowledgments

The author would like to thank Briggitte Griffiths, Mohamad Naasan, Peter Pilecki, Martyn Sherriff, Sharan Sidhu, and Ian Small for helpful discussions during the writing of this chapter. The work has been supported by the EPSRC GRJ/01035, MRC G9619537, the BDA Shirley Glasstone Hughes Memorial Fund, and the Special Trustees of Guy's Hospital.

References

1. Boyde A. Enamel. In: Oksche A, Vollrath L (ed). Handbook of Microscopic Anatomy, vol 6. Berlin: Springer-Verlag, 1989:309–473.

2. Spears IR. A three-dimensional finite element model of prismatic enamel: A re-appraisal of the data on the Young's modulus of enamel. J Dent Res 1997;76:1690–1697.

3. Watson TF. Tandem scanning microscopy of slow-speed enamel cutting interactions. J Dent Res 1991;70:44–49.

4. Brännström M. Dentin and Pulp in Restorative Dentistry. London: Wolfe Medical Publishers, 1982.

5. Pashley DH, Pashley EL. Dentin permeability and restorative dentistry: A status report for the American Journal of Dentistry. Am J Dent 1991;4:5–9.

6. Watson TF, Wilmot DM. A confocal microscopic evaluation of the interface between syntac adhesive and tooth tissue. J Dent 1992;20:302–310.

7. Griffiths BM, Watson TF. A confocal microscopic study of the handling characteristics of Scotchbond Multi-Purpose dentin adhesive. Am J Dent 1995;8:212–216.

8. Watson TF, Billington RW, Williams JA. The interfacial region of the tooth/glass-ionomer restoration: A confocal optical microscope study. Am J Dent 1991;4:303–310.

9. Garberoglio R, Brannstrom M. Scanning electron microscopic investigation of human dentinal tubules. Arch Oral Biol 1976;21:355–362.

10. Jones SJ. The pulp-dentine complex. In: Elderton RJ (ed). The Dentition and Dental Care. Oxford: Heinemann Professional Publishing, 1990:49–73.

11. Mjör IA. Reaction patterns of dentin. In: Thylstrup A (ed). Dentine and Dentine Reactions in the Oral Cavity. Oxford: IRL Press, 1987:27–31.

12. Boyde A. Physical effects of clinical procedures on the hard dental tissues. In: Elderton RJ (ed). The Dentition and Dental Care. Oxford: Heinemann Professional Publishing, 1990:325–347.

13. Pashley DH. Smear layer: Physiological considerations. Oper Dent 1984;9:13–29.

14. Watson TF, Cook RW. The influence of bur blade concentricity on high speed tooth cutting interactions: A video-rate confocal microscopic study. J Dent Res 1995;74:1749–1755.

15. Xu HHK, Kelly JR, Jahanmir S, Thompson VP, Rekow ED. Enamel subsurface damage due to tooth preparation with diamonds. J Dent Res 1997;76:1698–1706.

16. Watson TF. Applications of scanning optical microscopy to dentistry. Br Dent J 1991; 171:287–291.

17. Watson TF. Applications of high speed confocal imaging techniques in operative dentistry. Scanning 1994;16:168–173.

18. Watson TF. Fact and artefact in confocal microscopy. Adv Dent Res 1997;11:433- 441.

19. Allen KW. Theories of adhesion. In: Packaham DE (ed). Handbook of Adhesion. Essex: Longman Scientific and Technical, 1992:473–475.

20. Wilson AD, McLean JW. Glass-Ionomer Cement. London: Quintessence, 1988.

21. Nicholson JW, Brookman PJ, Lacy OM, Wilson AD. Fourier transform infrared spectroscopic study of the role of tartaric acid in glass-ionomer cements. J Dent Res 1988;67:1451–1454.

22. Blagojevic B, Mount GJ. A laboratory study of glass-ionomer cement in relation to clinical dentistry. Aust Dent J 1988;33:320–321.

23. Watson TF, Pagliari D, Sidhu SK, Naasan M. Confocal microscopic observation of structural changes in glass-ionomer cements and tooth interfaces. Biomaterials 1998;19:581–588.

24. Powis DR, Folleras T, Merson SA, Wilson AD. Improved adhesion of a glass-ionomer cement to dentin and enamel. J Dent Res 1982; 61:1416–1422.

25. Gwinnett AJ. Quantitative contribution of resin infiltration/hybridization to dentin bonding. Am J Dent 1993;6:7–9.

26. Watson TF, Griffiths BM. Handling of bonding agents: Clinical procedures. In: dall'Oroglio GD, Prati C (eds). Factors Influencing the Quality of

Posterior Restorations: Theory and Practice. Bologna: Kuraray, 1997.

27. Watson TF, Bannerjee A. The effectiveness of glass-ionomer surface protection treatments: A scanning optical microscope study. Eur J Prosthodont Rest Dent 1993;2:85–90.

28. Naasan M, Watson TF. Glass ionomer plugs in conditioned dentine surfaces. In: Proceedings of First European Conference on Glass-Ionomer Cements. London: I[st] European Union Conference on Glass-Ionomers 1996:92.

29. Watson TF. A confocal microscopical study of some factors affecting the adaptation of a light-cured glass-ionomer to tooth tissue. J Dent Res 1990;69:1531–1538.

30. Sidhu SK, Watson TF. Resin-modified glass-ionomer materials: A status report for the American Journal of Dentistry. Am J Dent 1995;8:59–67.

31. Sidhu SK, Watson TF. Fluid permeability and other interfacial characteristics of light-cured glass-ionomer restorations. J Dent Res 1994;73:183 [abstract 651].

32. Sidhu SK, Watson TF. Interfacial characteristics of resin-modified glass-ionomer cements. J Dent Res 1998;77:1749–1759.

33. Watson TF, Sidhu SK, Cheng PC. Confocal and 2 photon microscopic imaging of a resin-modified glass-ionomer adhesive. J Dent Res 1997;76:1032 [abstract 105].

34. Sidhu SK, Sheriff M, Watson TF. The effects of maturity and dehydration shrinkage on resin-modified glass-ionomer cements. J Dent Res 1997;76:1495–1501.

35. Small ICB, Watson TF, Chadwick AV, Sidhu SK. Water sorption in resin-modified glass-ionomer cements: An in vitro comparison with other materials. Biomaterials 1998;19:545–550.

36. Griffiths BM, Watson TF, Sherriff M. The influence of dentine bonding systems and their handling characteristics on the morphology and micropermeability of dentine adhesive systems. J Dent 1998.

37. Nakabayashi N, Kojima K, Masuhara E. The promotion of adhesion by the infiltration of monomers into tooth substrates. J Biomed Mater Res 1982;16:265–273.

38. Van Meerbeek B, Inokoshi S, Braem M, Lambrechts P, Vanherle G. Morphological aspects of the resin interdiffusion zone with different dentin adhesive systems. J Dent Res 1992;71:1530–1540.

39. Gwinnett AJ. Chemically conditioned dentin: A comparison of conventional and environmental scanning electron microscopy findings. Dent Mater 1994;10:150–155.

40. Van Noort R, Cardew GE, Howard IC, Noroozi S. The effect of local interfacial geometry on the measurement of the tensile bond strength to dentin. J Dent Res 1991;70:889–893.

41. Feilzer AJ, Kakabour A, De Gee AJ, Davidson CL. The influence of setting shrinkage and water sorption on the development of stresses in traditional and light-curing glass-ionomer cements. J Dent Res 1994;73:655.

42. Sidhu SK, Watson TF. Failure mechanism of a new modified glass-ionomer bonding system. J Dent Res 1997;76:1156 [abstract 22].

Chapter 7

Use of Glass-Ionomers as Bondings, Linings, or Bases

Marco Ferrari

Because glass-ionomer cements were designed to adhere directly to tooth structures, the nature of the substrate is as important as the quality of the cement. The mechanism by which polyalkenoic acids react with cation-releasing materials to form insoluble structures through ion exchange has been covered in the preceding chapters. In this chapter, attention is given to the condition of the substrate for bonding, particularly to the dentin surface.

Bonding

Prerequisites for good bonding are a large, clean area and good wetting by the adhesive. Because freshly cut dentin is covered by a rather structureless smear layer, fixation or removal of that layer is recommended.[1,2] Clinically, the complete removal of the smear layer can be performed by etching the cavity walls with polyacrylic or phosphoric acid. Several other acids or conditioning agents also are recommended for this purpose.

As discussed in earlier chapters, not only ionic bonds are believed to be responsible for the adhesion of glass-ionomers to dentin; some sort of hybridization of the substrate has been demonstrated (Fig 7-1). It is essential to realize that both mechanisms of bonding can proceed under wet conditions, which gives glass-ionomers a great advantage over resin composites when employed under clinical circumstances. Even if the addition of a resinous component to the original glass-ionomer formulation partially prevents chemical bonding, the hydrophilic compomers can create a sort of interdiffusion layer in natural "wet" dentin.[3]

When bonding conventional glass-ionomer cements to enamel, etching with polyacrylic acid cleans the substrate, creates a rough surface, and reduces its surface energy, allowing both micromechanical and chemical bonding.[4,5] When a compomer is used, additional etching of the cavity walls with phosphoric acid creates a better seal than that obtained when only an application of priming adhesive solution is used.[6] The application of a hydrophilic bonding system permits effective infiltration of the resin into the demineralized dentin, forming a hybridized area and creating a mechanical interlock between the two substrates (Fig 7-2). At the enamel site of

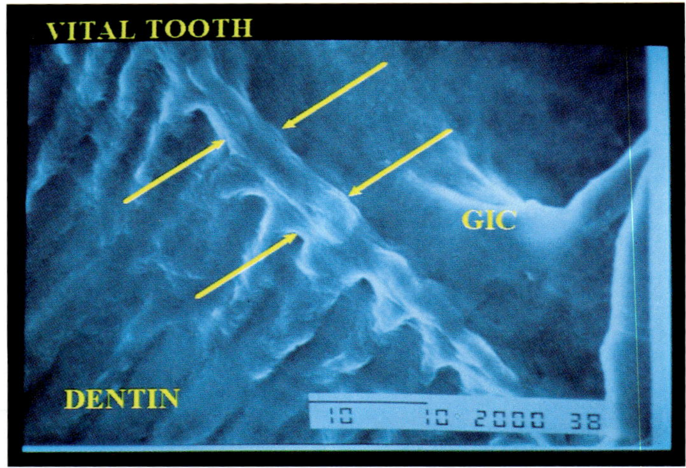

Fig 7-1 The interdiffusion of traditional glass-ionomer cement into vital conditioned dentin. Both mechanical and chemical bonding mechanisms can be formed between the two substrates. (Scanning electron microscopy; original magnification ×2,000.)

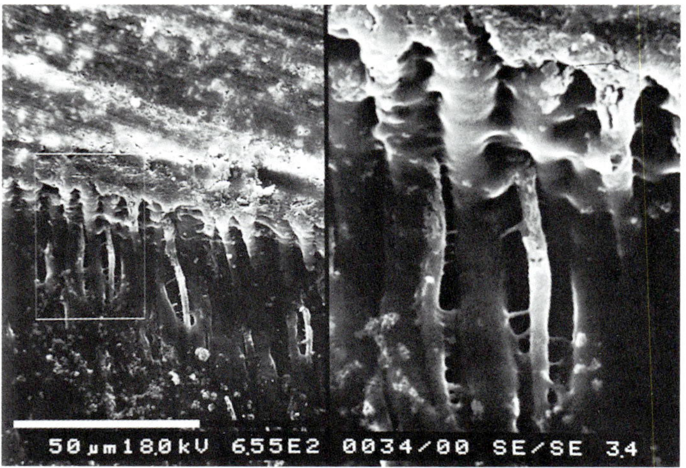

Fig 7-2 The use of compomers combined with phosphoric acid etching of dentin to create a strong mechanical bond by resin tags and hybrid layer formation. (Scanning electron microscopy; original magnification ×655 *[left]*, ×3,400 *[right]*.)

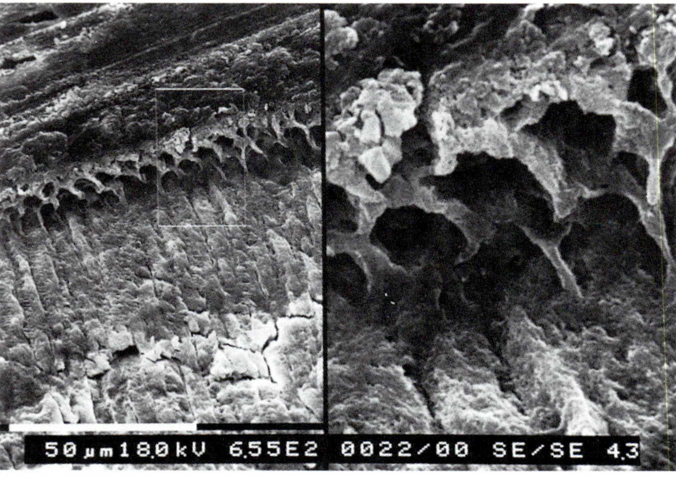

Fig 7-3 Etching with phosphoric acid on enamel margins to develop a mechanical interlock by resin tag formation. (Scanning electron microscopy; original magnification ×655 *[left]*, ×4,300 *[right]*.)

compomer restorations, acid etching and the use of an enamel-dentin bonding system permits the formation of traditional mechanical interlocking by resin tag formation (Fig 7-3).

Another proof of infiltration is found in the control of postoperative sensitivity after the application of conventional or resin-modified glass-ionomers to vital dentin. To achieve such control, dentin tubules are normally sealed by resin tags (see Fig 7-3).[7,8] The observation of cohesive failure within the glass-ionomers, rather than an adhesive type of detachment of acid-etched tooth structure from glass-ionomers, is explained by the fact that a sufficiently strong bond to the substrate is achieved.[4,9]

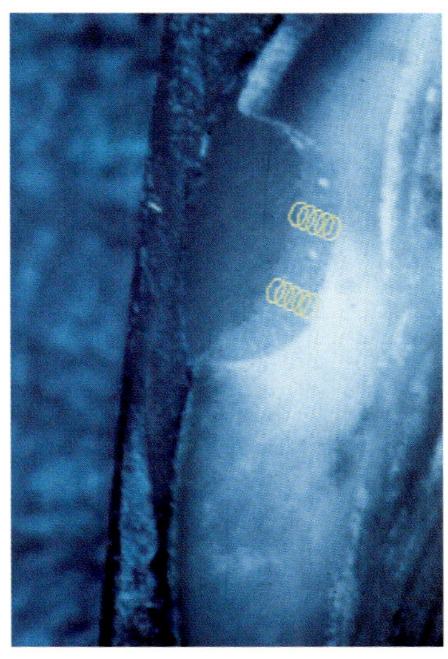

Fig 7-4 The liner absorbs mechanical and thermal stresses, maintaining the bonding between the restoration and the cavity wall.

Stress absorption

Another reason glass-ionomers are used as adhesive materials is that they can directly contribute to a reduction of shrinkage stress. Setting stress, functional loading, and temperature fluctuations deform restorations and stress the margins. Any mismatch at the interface of the restoration and cavity wall causes separation of the bond. Adding special mechanical properties to an adhesive so it can act as an elastic buffer can reduce interfacial stress concentration. To reproduce the physical characteristics of enamel and dentin, two different restorative materials are needed: one must be hard and rigid like enamel and the other resilient like dentin. The material used to replace lost dentin also can serve as a lining. The ideal liner must be sufficiently flexible to completely absorb mechanical and thermal stress in order to maintain bonding at the tooth structure–restoration interface during clinical procedures (Fig 7-4). A study by Kemp-Scholte and Davidson[10] showed that in adhesive composite Class V restorations, a strong correlation exists between marginal con tinuity and flexibility of the filling material when only one sort of bonding is employed. It was suggested that microfilled resin composites or compomers perform better than the stiff hybrid composites when marginal seal is the main target.

Setting stress can be controlled by proper selection of restorative materials and creative handling (Figs 7-5 to 7-8). When the restorative material can flow and contract freely, the shrinkage stress of the restoration is reduced; thus, the clinician has to adapt the restorative procedure to the properties of the se-

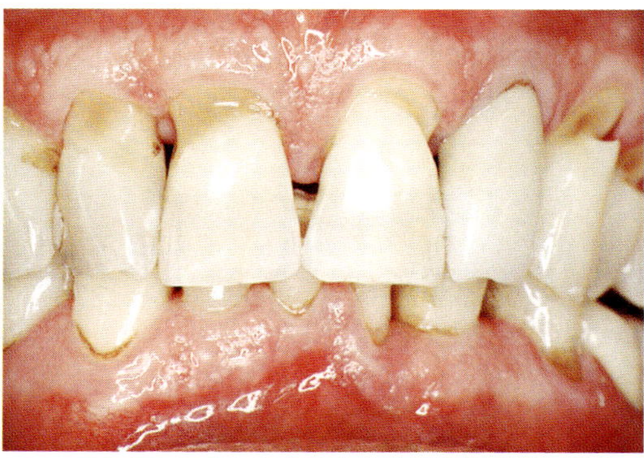

Fig 7-5 Proper selection of restorative materials based on the knowledge and handling of the operator. This patient presented with a number of Class V lesions and an old porcelain crown on the left second incisor which needed to be replaced.

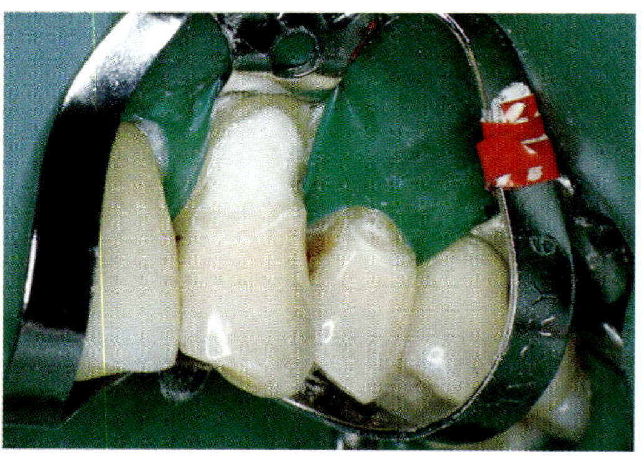

Fig 7-6 Application of a conventional glass-ionomer material as a base. The material is placed at the proper thickness to fill the deepest area of the cavity, to reduce the configuration factor, and to act as an elastic buffer to absorb stresses.

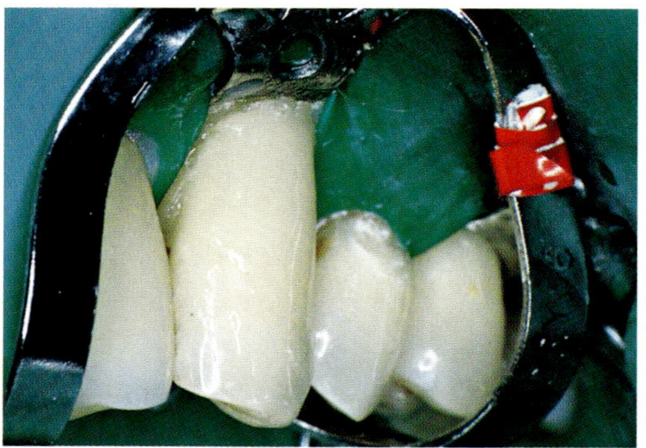

Fig 7-7 Incremental layering technique to reproduce the original anatomic shape of the tooth.

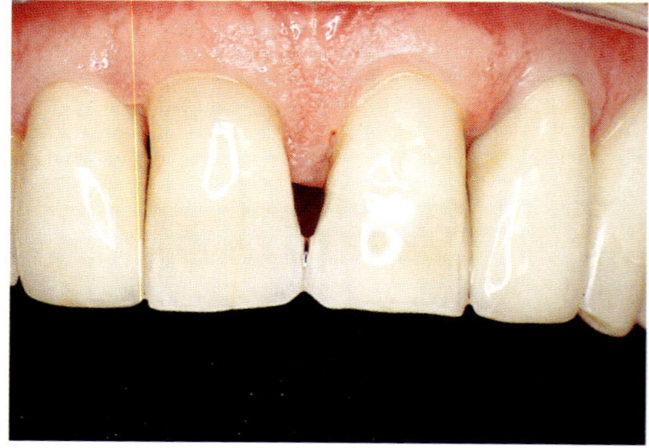

Fig 7-8 Final appearance. Two single-unit all porcelain crowns have been luted to the second incisors, and all cervical lesions have been restored using the sandwich technique.

lected materials,[6,11] the cavity shape,[11,12] the site of the restoration, and the cavity substrates.[13]

Several intrinsic factors of conventional glass-ionomer cements can reduce setting stress. Because of their low and delayed shrinkage rates, glass-ionomer cements flow during their pre-gel phase. In the postgel phase, their flow capacity decreases and they harden slowly.[14] The longer the setting time, the better the restoration can adapt to shrinkage. For this reason light-activated materials, which harden quickly, create more interfacial mismatch than self-curing materials.[15,16]

Another favorable factor of glass-ionomers is their intrinsic porosity. The presence of microcracks, voids, and bubbles in these materials permits the volume and form of the restoration to change during setting, allowing for load compensation. A glass-ionomer cement can modify its shape without breaking the bond at the interface with the cavity wall. It is well known that, under restricted conditions, microcracks appear in the cement during setting.[11] However, when sufficient water is available, the material swells rapidly, closing the cracks. Due to the relatively long reaction time, some of the cracks are repaired through chemical reaction.[11]

To act as a stress-absorbing liner, the glass-ionomer material must be applied in a substantial thickness, and the thickness must be adequate for each restoration (Fig 7-6). The thickness of the liner/base material is important to balance the occlusal forces on cervical restorations.[17] Other materials, such as self-curing and flowable resin composites and resin-modified glass-ionomer cements, also can be used as linings.

Sealing ability

The evaluation of restorations placed in vital teeth that are subsequently extracted after a period of clinical service are useful because dehydration shrinkage may occur with glass-ionomer restorations placed under laboratory conditions. Shrinkage occurs quickly after placement, and considerable gaps may open up in immature cements.[18] If the restoration is kept fully hydrated, minimal setting movement of the cement maintains the close adaptation of tooth and cement, allowing further ion exchange to occur during the lifetime of the restoration.

In contrast to the usual studies on the sealing ability of glass-ionomer cement, in which restorations are placed under laboratory conditions,[19,20] the leakage studies described in this chapter were performed mainly on vital teeth. Although in vivo studies on sealing ability are rare, it appears that the in vitro protocol is of only limited value in predicting the clinical performance of Class II restorations.[21,22]

Marginal seal studies of in vitro and in vivo Class II restorations, made with a conventional glass-ionomer cement (Fuji IX) in combination with acid etching (GC Cavity Conditioner), revealed that 80% of the fillings remained free from cervical margin leakage (Fig 7-9).[23] This supports the use of glass-ionomer cement as a (long-term temporary) filling material in Class II cavities (Fig 7-10), when an observation period is needed before making the final treatment planning, and as a final restorative material for Class V lesions when esthetics are not of primary importance.

A variety of adhesive restorative material combinations were tested in

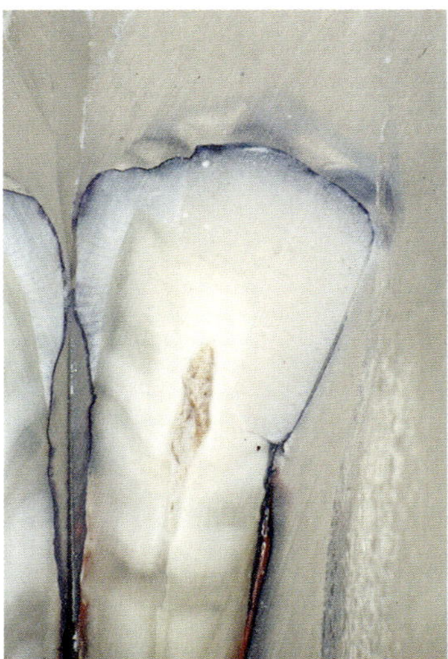

Fig 7-9 A Class II restoration made with a conventional glass-ionomer cement under clinical conditions after evaluation for leakage. No dye penetration was found at either the cementum-dentin or enamel margins.

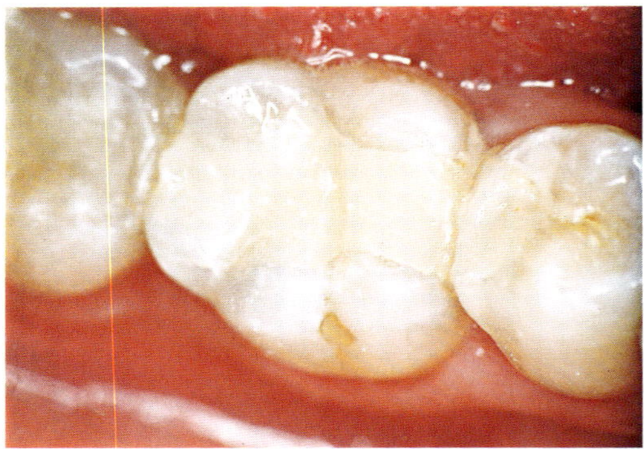

Fig 7-10 A Class II conventional glass-ionomer restoration placed as a long-term temporary filling in a sensitive molar. After 5 months, no post-operative sensitivity and/or pain was reported. The glass-ionomer cement was prepared, partially left in the cavity, and used as a base for the final restoration.

Class V cavities by Davidson and Abdalla.[23] Mason and Ferrari[24] evaluated the "sandwich" technique using a resin-modified glass-ionomer cement (Vitrebond) as a liner at the base of the cavity; no leakage was observed. Ferrari and Davidson[25] tested the sealing capacity of another resin-modified glass-ionomer (Fuji II LC) versus a resin composite (Z100) and found that more than 30% of the restorations in both groups exhibited cervical leakage, although no statistically significant difference between the two groups could be found. In a study on two compomers (Compoglass and Dyract) used in conjunction with proprietary enamel-dentin bonding agents, the effects of etching the enamel and dentin simultaneously with phosphoric acid was investigated.[26] When the compomers were used without acid etching, the leakage was significantly higher than when the full bonding procedures were applied. From this study it may be concluded that compomers should be bonded in a manner similar to that for resin composites.

The need for adequate etching and bonding with a suitable agent also may be demonstrated with another compomer (F2000). Although a compomer contains hydrophilic components, the resin apparently does not spontaneously infiltrate the dentin substrate in the same way an enamel-dentin bonding agent can; therefore, it is not self-bonding. This must be regarded as a step backward in the evolution of glass-ionomers. Yet all glass-ionomers, including compomers, have proved capable of improving the seal of a restoration.

Sandwich Technique

Due to their favorable flow characteristics, glass-ionomer cements show superior sealing capacity to resin composites. However, during mechanical loading of the restoration, the modulus of elasticity of the restorative material once more plays an important role. Ideally, the restorative material and the tooth structure should undergo similar changes to avoid mismatch at the interfaces. Thus there would be no need for a stress-absorbing interfacial layer.[27]

Unfortunately, resin materials deform differently than dentin under thermal and mechanical stress; consequently, an inhomogeneous deformation might damage the interface and the coherence of the restored tooth material.[28] If an interfacial layer with a low modulus of elasticity is applied with sufficient strain to compensate for the mismatch in deformation to the volume and shape of both the restoration and the cavity wall, the bond can be maintained. Because of its low modulus of elasticity and its capacity for self-repair of eventual cohesive microcracks,[11] conventional glass-ionomer cement is indicated as a restorative material for lining in the sandwich technique.

If separation of the restoration from the cavity wall is still a possibility, the fluoride release from the glass-ionomer may have the potential to prevent secondary caries. Because one can never be sure that leakage has been completely prevented, the further insurance of a glass-ionomer material as a possible cariostatic agent at the existing margins is desirable.

In practice, the sandwich technique involves replacing the lost dentin with a glass-ionomer cement and the enamel with a resin composite. This clinical procedure involves using a base of either chemically set or light-cured glass-ionomer, which is then covered with a resin composite to improve the physical and esthetic characteristics. The use of the sandwich technique can help those clinicians who consider the placement of full resin composite restorations in posterior teeth an unpredictable and somewhat risky procedure. The placement of glass-ionomer cement as a base also can decrease the configuration factor value, reducing the stress during shrinkage of the resin composite.[29,30]

The sandwich technique can be used in restoring Class V and Class II lesions. When a glass-ionomer cement is used as a liner in Class V cavities, an appropriate shade must be selected to avoid the unesthetic appearance of glass-ionomer showing through the final restoration. To act as an elastic buffer, the liner material must be applied in an appropriate (visible) thickness of at least 0.4 mm in Class V cavities and 1.5 to 2 mm in Class II cavities (Figs 7-6 and 7-11 to 7-13). When the Class V cavity is due to abrasion or erosion, occlusion must be checked carefully.[17,31] The eccentric loads applied to the occlusal surfaces can concentrate the stress in the cervical region, provoking disruption in natural teeth and detachment or breakage of the restorations.[32] To avoid a premature failure when wear facets are present, the clinician must adjust the occlusion before restoring the cervical lesion. When abfraction lesions are present, careful lining and nightguard use are particularly indicated.

Different sandwich techniques can be performed to restore Class II cavities

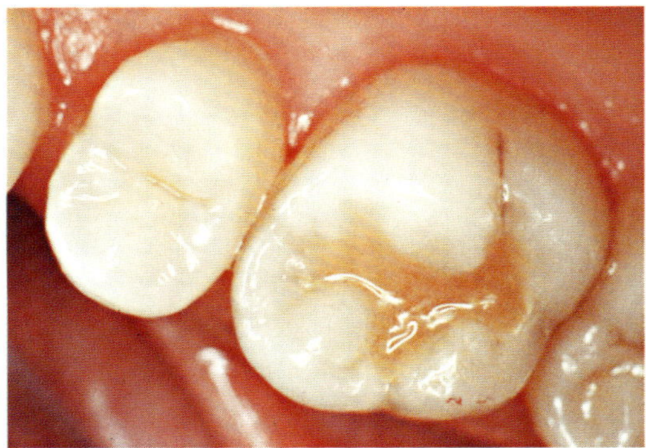

Fig 7-11 A mandibular first molar with interproximal distal decay.

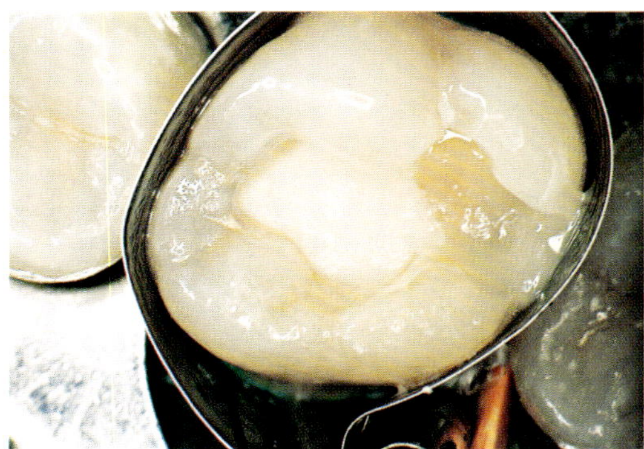

Fig 7-12 Placement of the restoration. After preparation of the cavity, a thick base of conventional glass-ionomer material is placed in the deepest area of the cavity.

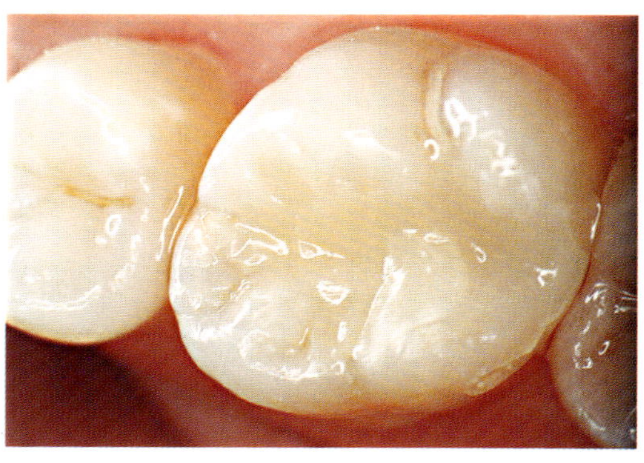

Fig 7-13 The final restoration 10 months after placement.

(Figs 7-14 and 7-15). The "delayed," or "closed", sandwich technique consists of first completely restoring the cavity with glass-ionomer cement and, between a few days and 2 to 3 weeks later, repreparing the restored tooth, leaving a thick glass-ionomer base and creating sufficient space to make a resin composite veneer. The sandwich technique also can be performed in one appointment (the "open" sandwich technique). In this case, the clinician fills the interproximal box with glass-ionomer cement and completes the occlusal restoration with resin composite material.[5]

An enamel-dentin bonding agent is usually applied between the glass-ionomer base and the resin composite. Before coating the cavity wall with the adhesive, the occlusal enamel margins and eventually the base material are acid etched. To avoid weakening and detachment of the glass-ionomer cement from the cavity wall, it has been suggested that

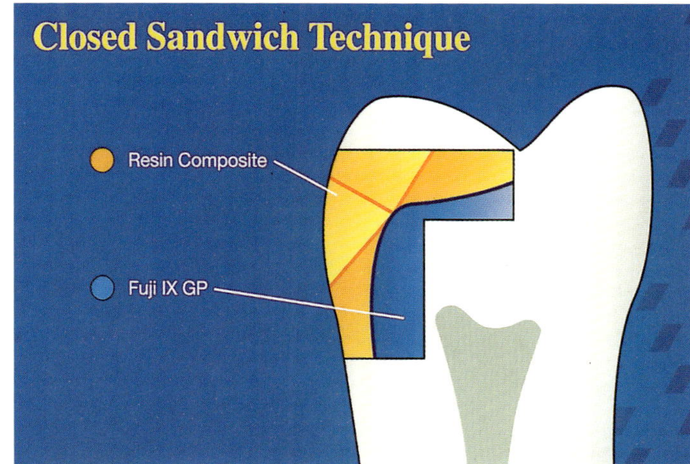

Fig 7-14 Closed sandwich technique. The Class II cavity is partially restored with a base of glass-ionomer material, then covered and sealed at the margins with a resin composite.

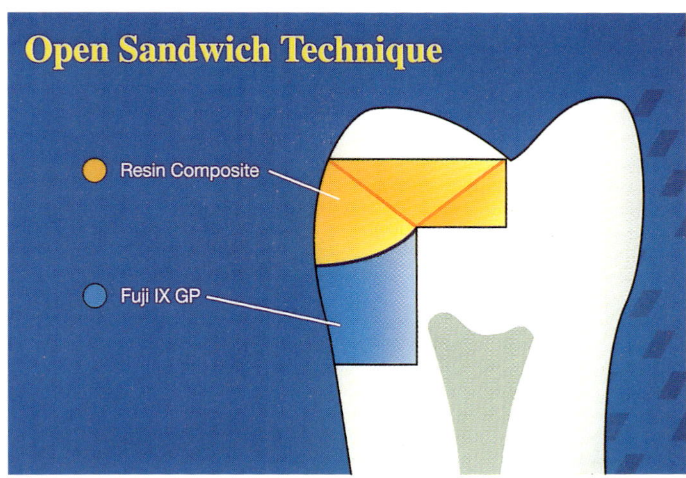

Fig 7-15 Open sandwich technique. The Class II interproximal box is filled with a conventional glass-ionomer material. The restoration is completed with a resin composite layered on top.

acid etching of the glass-ionomer be delayed until the cement is completely hardened.[5,24] It has been shown that the etching pattern presented by the glass-ionomer surface is appropriate for good micromechanical attachment for lamination.[9,33] In fact, the bond between conventional glass-ionomer cement and resin composite is mainly micromechanical and requires micropores in the glass-ionomer surface into which the resin composite or, preferably, a bonding resin can penetrate. Recently, it has been shown that acid etching and subsequent application of resin composite on a thick (2-mm) glass-ionomer base did not result in a gap formation between the cementum-dentin margins and the restorative materials.

Wassell et al[34] observed no evidence of dissolution of a glass-ionomer base, even when it extended to the cervical margins, yet many authors still suggest using glass-ionomer cement only as a

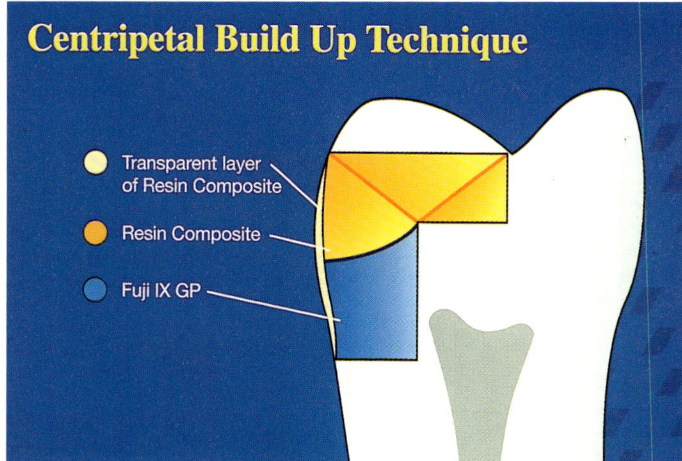

Fig 7-16 Centripetal build-up technique. A thin transparent layer of resin composite is applied toward the proximal surface of the matrix to modify the original Class II cavity to a Class I cavity. The lesion is filled with a conventional glass-ionomer material. Finally, a resin composite veneer is applied over the glass-ionomer base to recreate the original anatomic form and esthetic appearance of the tooth.

fully internal base. Clinical experience shows that dissolution of glass-ionomers can be related to the level of oral hygiene. In patients with poor oral hygiene, the pH of the saliva goes down and the acidic environment can attack the exposed surface of the glass-ionomer cement, dissolving it over time. To diminish the risks of base dissolution in the oral environment, a coating of unfilled bonding resin can be applied (Fuji LC). Such an external coating also can be created using a resin composite layer applied in the interproximal area of a Class II sandwich restoration, a procedure called the "centripetal build-up" technique (Fig 7-16).[35] This latest technique is, in principle, a closed sandwich technique; the proximal wall is reestablished by adapting a small increment of semi-transparent posterior composite toward the matrix band using a condenser and light curing it. This procedure modifies the original Class II cavity to a Class I cavity. The cavity is then filled with a glass-ionomer cement, leaving at least 1.5 mm unfilled occlusally to permit coating with resin composite. The veneer creates a natural appearance for the final restoration, completes the occlusal margins, and protects the glass-ionomer material from occlusal wear and dissolution.

Summary

From a clinical point of view, glass-ionomer materials can be useful in improving the physical and esthetic characteristics of restorations: they can be used as direct fillings, as long-term temporary fillings, and as linings. Glass-ionomer cements can act as "intelligent" materials because they have the potential to self-repair microcracks that occur during setting, minimize leakage damage through fluoride release at filling margins, and replace lost dentin in sandwich restorations.[25] Thus, glass-ionomer cements can not only permanently seal cavities and restore lost anatomy, but when deformation or cohesive failure occurs, they can to some extent automatically repair the defective function.

References

1. Eick JD, Robinson SJ, Byerley TJ, Chappelow CC. Adhesives and nonshrinking dental resins of the future. Quintessence Int 1993;24:632–640.

2. Mount GJ. Glass-ionomer cements: Past, present and future. Oper Dent 1994;19:82–90.

3. Ferrari M, Davidson CL. Interdiffusion of a traditional glass-ionomer cement into conditioned dentin. Am J Dent 1997;10:295–297.

4. Mount GJ. Adhesion of glass-ionomer cement in the clinical environment. Oper Dent 1991; 16:141–148.

5. McLean JW. Dentinal bonding agents versus glass-ionomer cements. Quintessence Int 1996; 27:659–667.

6. Erickson RL, Glasspoole EA. Bonding to tooth structure: A comparison of glass-ionomer and composite-resin systems. J Esthet Dent 1994; 6:227–244.

7. Cox CF, Hafez AA, Akimoto N, Otsuki M, Suzuki S, Tarim B. Biocompatibility of primer, adhesive and resin composite systems on non-exposed and exposed non-human primate teeth. Am J Dent 1998;11(special issue):S55–S63.

8. Tay FR, Gwinnett AJ, Pang KM, Wei SHY. Resin permeation into acid-conditioned, moist, and dry dentin: A paradigm using water-free adhesive primers. J Dent Res 1996;75:1034–1044.

9. Ngo H, Mount GJ, Peters MCRB. A study of glass-ionomer cement and its interface with enamel and dentin using a low-temperature, high-resolution scanning electron microscopic technique. Quintessence Int 1997;28:63–69.

10. Kemp-Scholte CM, Davidson CL. Complete marginal seal of class V resin composite restorations effected by increased flexibility. J Dent Res 1990;69:1240–1243.

11. Davidson CL. Glass-ionomer bases under posterior composites. J Esthet Dent 1994; 6:223–226.

12. Feilzer AJ, De Gee AJ, Davidson CL. Curing contraction of composites and glass-ionomer cements. J Prosthet Dent 1988;59:297–300.

13. Cagidiaco MC. Bonding to dentin. Mechanism, morphology and efficacy of bonding resin composites to dentin in vitro and in vivo. Ph.D. thesis, University of Amsterdam, 1995.

14. Davidson CL, Davidson-Kaban SS. Handling of mechanical stresses. Dent Update 1998;25:31–34.

15. Garberoglio R, Coli P, Brännström M. Contraction gaps in class II restorations with self-cured and light-cured resin composites. Am J Dent 1995;8:303–307.

16. Ferrari M, Mannocci F, Cagidiaco MC, Kugel G. Short term assessment of leakage of class V composite restorations placed in vivo. Clin Oral Invest 1997;1:61–64.

17. Lee WC, Eakle WS. Stress-induced cervical lesions: Review of advances in the past 10 years. J Prosthet Dent 1996;75:487–494.

18. Sidhu SK, Watson TF. Failure mechanism of a new modified glass-ionomer bonding system. J Dent Res 1997;76:1156 [abstract 22].

19. Taylor MJ, Lynch E. Microleakage. J Dent 1996;20:3–10.

20. Hilton TJ, Schwartz RS, Ferracane JL. Microleakage of four class II resin composite insertion techniques at intraoral temperature. Quintessence Int 1997;28:135–144.

21. Abdalla AI, Davidson CL. Comparison of the marginal integrity of in vivo and in vitro class II composite restorations. J Dent 1993;21:158–162.

22. Ferrari M, Davidson CL. Sealing performance of Scotchbond Multipurpose plus-Z 100 in class II restorations. Am J Dent 1996;9:145–149.

23. Davidson CL, Abdalla AI. Effect of occlusal load cycling on the marginal integrity of adhesive class V restorations. Am J Dent 1994;7:111–114.

24. Mason PN, Ferrari M. In vivo evaluation of glass-ionomer cement adhesion to dentin. Quintessence Int 1994;25:499–504.

25. Ferrari M, Davidson CL. Sealing capacity of a resin-modified glass-ionomer and resin composite placed in vivo in class 5 restorations. Oper Dent 1996;21:69–72.

26. Ferrari M, Vichi A, Cagidiaco MC. Sealing ability of Fuji IX in class II restorations in vivo and in vitro. J Dent Res 1998;77: [abstract 8].

27. Davidson CL. Lining and elasticity. In: Dondi dall'Orologio G, Prati C (eds). Proceedings of International Symposium on Factors Influencing the Quality of Composite Restorations, Theory and Practice. Bologna: Isasan, 1996.

28. Davidson CL. Glass ionomer cement, an intelligent material. Bull Group Int Rech Sci Stomatol Odontol 1998;40:38–41.

29. Davidson CL, De Gee AJ, Feilzer AJ. The competition between the composite-resin bond strength and the polymerization contraction stress. J Dent Res 1984;63:1396–1399.

30. Kemp-Scholte CM, Davidson CL. Marginal integrity related to bond strength and strain capacity of composite resin restorative systems. J Prosthet Dent 1990;64:658–664.

31. Lee WC, Eakle WS. Possible role of tensile stress in the etiology of cervical erosive lesions of teeth. J Prosthet Dent 1984;52:374–380.

32. Braem M, Lambrecths P, Van Doren V, Vanherle G. The impact of composite structure on its elastic response. J Dent Res 1986;65:648–653.

33. Subrata G, Davidson CL. The effect of various surface treatments on the shear strength between composite resin and glass-ionomer cement. J Dent 1989;17:28–32.

34. Wassell RW, Walss AWG, McCabe JF. Direct composite inlays versus conventional composite restorations: Three-year clinical results. Br Dent J 1995;179:343–349.

35. Bitchacho N. The centripetal build-up for composite resin posterior restorations. Pract Periodontics Aesthet Dent 1994;6:17–23.

Chapter 8

Glass-Ionomer Luting Cements

Dorothy McComb and Dan Nathanson

Luting cements comprise a broad category of materials used to attach and seal dental restorations and appliances to teeth, including cementation of fixed partial dentures, attachment of orthodontic bands and brackets, and root canal cementation. The choice of a luting agent is dependent on the clinical conditions combined with the physical, biological, and handling properties of the agent. In the last two decades there has been considerable interest in luting materials with adhesive capabilities and therapeutic potential. This chapter focuses on the scientific information available concerning glass-ionomer luting cements and their use in restorative dentistry.

Restoration Cementation

Final permanent cementation is a critical last step in the placement of dental restorations. Conventional inlays, onlays, and crown-and-bridge units, the vast majority of which involve metal castings, use a luting agent to secure retention and to seal the microscopic gap between the restoration and tooth structure for function. The cement lute must allow complete seating, not irritate the pulp, retain the restoration, and resist dissolution in the hostile oral environment (Box 8-1). These qualities are important because the presence of exposed cement at the restoration margin can be the weakest link in the final restoration (Fig 8-1).

The cementation of restorations has increased in complexity in recent years due to rapidly evolving technology that has provided a greater variety of materials and some new restorative options, particularly in the area of esthetics. Similarly, there is now a greater choice of luting materials covering a wider variety of clinical scenarios and with an increased emphasis on adhesion. None of the available cements provide all the ideal requirements for every clinical situation. The choice of luting agent is decided by the clinical circumstances and the restorative material being used.

For more than a century, zinc-phosphate cement has been the most common cementation material for restorations involving metal, whether cast inlays or onlays, crowns, or partial dentures. Zinc-phosphate has been successful, mainly because it provides a rigid luting cement from a fluid, easy-to-handle consistency and allows simple removal of excess. It is based on a zinc oxide

Box 8-1 Luting cement requirements

Ease of use
- Adequate working time
- Ease of seating; low film thickness
- Easy removal of excess cement

Biocompatibility
- Nonirritating to pulp and periodontium
- Optimum sealing ability
- No systemic toxicity

Physical attributes
- Adequate strength, rigidity, and toughness
- Insoluble in oral fluids
- Adhesion to tooth structure and restoration

powder–phosphoric acid reaction, which allows dissolution over time in unfavorable environments, particularly if restoration margins are less than ideal. However, this cement provides no adhesive or sealing properties with tooth structure, has no therapeutic properties, and can be irritating to the vital pulp due to the material's initially low pH and slow rise to neutrality. Optimal results with all luting cements are achieved using meticulous clinical and laboratory techniques that ensure good marginal fit, contour, retention, pulp protection, and occlusion. Many clinicians continue to use zinc-phosphate cement, and survival of optimal restorations for over 20 years in patients with good oral hygiene has been documented.[1] However, many failures still occur, and there has been a shift toward the use of cements that have better physical attributes and can provide additional therapeutic and adhesive properties.

Causes of crown-and-bridge failure

Although individual treatments with various types of restorations may be successful over two decades or more, average survival periods are often far lower. Several investigators have established that the leading cause of failure by far is recurrent decay at the cervical junction of the restoration and tooth. In an early study by Schwartz et al,[1] a mean longevity of 10.3 years was recorded for the 791 crown-and-bridge units studied. Caries accounted for 36.8% of the failures, but this tended to happen after many years of service with a mean occurrence at just over 11 years. Decemented crowns were the second leading cause of failure (12.1%) at a mean of 6.8 years, which emphasizes the need for adequate crown preparation retention design. It is well established that traditional cements can only secure the inherent retention form provided by optimal length, minimal taper, and the presence of a ferrule on sound tooth structure. Other causes of failure were deficient margins and periodontal problems (approximately 11% each) and periapical involvement (2.9%).

Glantz et al[2] documented a 98.5% survival over five years for 498 fixed prosthodontic abutment crowns placed in Sweden; however, only 65.1% of surviving crowns were still judged satisfactory. Approximately one third required some adjustment or repair, but would likely remain in service. A small number (4%) were in such a poor state that they required removal. Secondary caries was the most common reason for replacement. A 7-year follow-up involving more

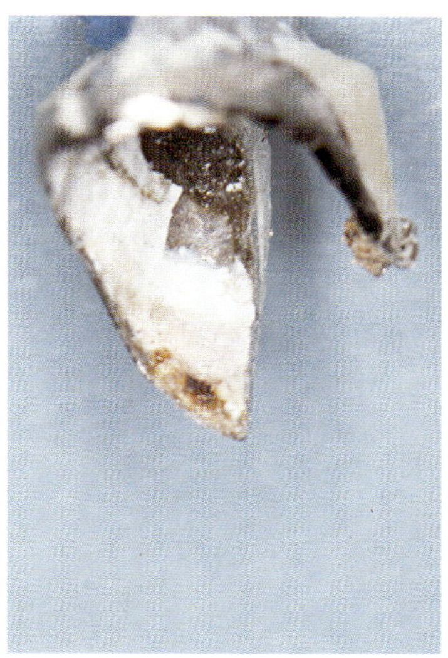

Fig 8-1 Interior of a sectioned crown that failed due to recurrent marginal decay. Cement dissolution is evident at the crown periphery.

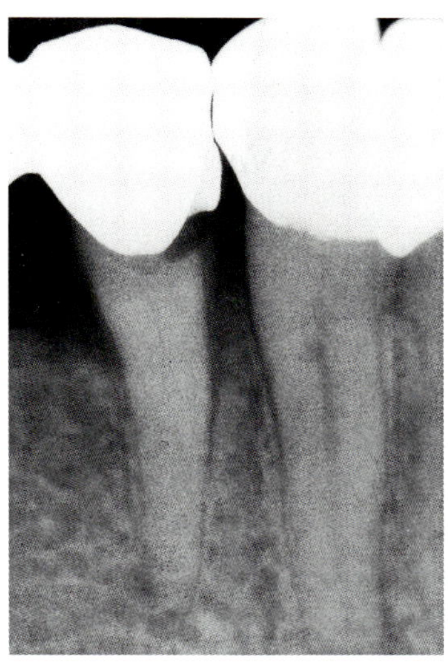

Fig 8-2 Radiograph showing recurrent decay at the cervical margin of a crown abutment.

complex fixed partial dentures, including cantilever designs, again found that dental caries was the most common complication, with a mean cumulative frequency of 26%.[3] When cantilever units were excluded, this figure was reduced to 20.9%. One in five restorations, therefore, failed after 7 years. It can be concluded that carefully crafted partial dentures involving castings can be successful for many years, but that relatively high rates of secondary caries are associated with those that fail prematurely (Fig 8-2). The causes of recurrent decay involve myriad factors, including in particular the quality of the restorative work performed, the materials used, the ability of the patient to maintain a clean marginal milieu, and the inherent resistance of the adjacent tooth structure. Zinc-phosphate luting cement was used in all the longevity studies described. The marginal areas of restorations are clearly susceptible to decay; therefore, improved luting materials, particularly those with potential caries-inhibiting properties, are considered desirable.

Adhesive luting cements

The quest for improved alternative cementation materials that are better able to withstand oral function and the oral environment over many years has resulted in the development of luting forms of both glass-ionomer (polyalkenoate) cements and resin composite. Both classes of material provide adhesive capabilities but have very different properties and usage. Fundamental attributes of glass-ionomer cements include fluoride release,[4] adhesion,[5] and biocompatibility.[6] Well-placed glass-ionomer restorations are known to provide two distinguishing and effective characteristics: sustained fluoride release and intrinsic adhesion to tooth structure.[7] Glass-ionomer luting cements therefore provide the following advantages over zinc-phosphate cement: *(1)* documented fluoride content and continuing release[4] with the potential for caries inhibition; *(2)* improved strength;[8] *(3)* better resistance to dissolution when fully set;[9] and *(4)* adhesion to tooth structure[5] with the potential for improved sealing and retention. These materials are indicated for use on all routine restorations involving metals, including all-metal inlays and onlays, and metal-ceramic or all-metal crown-and-bridge units.

Resin composite luting agents are currently the agents of choice for cementation of all-ceramic inlays, onlays, and full crowns, because they provide the optimum strength and bonding capability required as the foundation for these otherwise brittle restorative materials. Resin composite bonding and luting technology is considered an inherent part of state-of-the-art all-ceramic or all-porcelain restorations.[10] These cements provide high strength, good micromechanical bonding, and extremely low solubility. However, they are more technique sensitive and difficult to clean up intraorally than other cements. They are not intended for universal use with restorations involving metal and are reserved for low-retention clinical situations.

Recent development has resulted in a relatively new category of resin-modified glass-ionomer luting cements, a hybrid of glass-ionomer and resin composite technology. With a combination of properties from both parent groups, these materials comprise an interesting new class of luting agents. Resin-modified materials provide comparable fluoride release[11] and improved adhesive properties[12] over conventional glass-ionomer luting forms. They also exhibit reduced initial moisture sensitivity,[13] increased resistance to oral dissolution,[14] improved mechanical properties,[15] and good pulpal compatibility.[16] The possibility of resin-modified glass-ionomer luting materials replacing conventional cements or providing a simplified alternative for some uses of resin composites is addressed later in this chapter.

Conventional Glass-Ionomer Luting Cements

A glass-ionomer (polyalkenoate) cement suitable for use as a luting material was first described in 1977 by Wilson et al.[17] Commercial forms became available to dentists in the early 1980s. The powder is a fine-grained calcium fluoroalumino-silicate glass, and the liquid is an aqueous solution of a polyacrylic acid with or without the addition of various long-chain copolymers (polyitaconic or polymaleic acids). The setting reaction is complex and varies with composition but is generally represented as an acid-base reaction between the polyacid liquid and the glass.[18] Calcium and aluminum ions are released by attack on the surface of the glass particles and ultimately cross-link the polyacid chains into a network. Initial setting is due to chain entanglement plus weak ionic cross-linking. As the cement matures over the first 24 hours and beyond, progressive cross-linking occurs and the set cement becomes stronger and less moisture sensitive.[6] The increasing stability and strength of glass-ionomer cements over time is consistent with progressive aluminum cross-linking. The gradual setting mechanism ultimately results in a hard, translucent cement that adheres to both enamel and dentin. Strength and rigidity can increase for up to 1 month as the cement matures.[19] The cement is susceptible to moisture contamination and dehydration in the early stages.

Two forms are available: in one, the polyalkenoate polymers are provided as the liquid component for mixing with the powder; in the other, they are vacuum-dried and combined with the glass to provide a single powder that is activated by mixing with water or a solution of tartaric acid to initiate cement formation.[20] Tartaric acid facilitates the initial calcium and aluminum ion release from the surface of the glass particles and is particularly effective in both prolonging the working time and increasing the setting rate of glass-ionomers. Up to 10% tartaric acid is incorporated in most glass-ionomer compositions.[6]

Physical parameters of conventional glass-ionomer luting cements are favorable, with increased compressive and diametral tensile strengths over zinc phosphate.[8] The modulus of elasticity for glass-ionomer cements is lower than that for zinc phosphate, indicating less brittle characteristics. Luting versions of the cement have actually shown less solubility than analogous restorative glass-ionomers, with polyacrylic acid–based materials being more erosion resistant than those based on polymaleic acid.[21]

Handling properties

Few clinical studies have reported on glass-ionomer luting cements, but one of the first concluded that the clinical handling properties of these materials were satisfactory and similar to those of zinc polycarboxylate luting cements.[22] Removal of excess glass-ionomer cement was found to be a little more difficult, because of the material's ability to adhere to tooth structure and soft tissue. Working time for a film 25 μm thick is somewhat shorter than that for zinc phosphate, and the end of the working time is more abrupt.[19] A thin film is, however, easily achieved for all cements and the working time can be increased significantly by the use of a cold slab. The handling properties of conventional glass-ionomer luting cements are satisfactory for most routine clinical uses. Øilo[19] stated that using a slab at a temperature just above the dew point almost doubles the working time for the cement, when required for more complicated procedures.

Firm seating pressure is necessary and saliva contamination of marginal cement must be prevented until the material has set. This helps provide a secure marginal seal and avoid production of weak, moisture-contaminated, leachable cement at the restoration margin. Excess cement should not be removed before the material has reached the first setting stage and shows brittle properties. Hard-to-reach interproximal areas should be addressed first, ensuring that all excess is removed before the material has achieved a rock-hard set when it can be extremely difficult to dislodge.

Retention

Traditional zinc-phosphate cement secures the retention of cast restorations by *(1)* a mechanical interlocking of irregularities in the prepared tooth surface and casting, and *(2)* strength parameters capable of securing only those restorations that have adequate built-in retention and resistance for the particular clinical scenario. The dynamic and repetitive forces associated with oral function provide a great challenge to any luting cement; dislodged, inadequately retained crown-and-bridge units are a common cause of failure. Factors affecting retention design include tooth height, preparation taper and geometry, surface texture, and the presence of a ferrule, as well as the type of cement used. Loss of retention can be disastrous, particularly if the restoration is an abutment and micromovement is not noticed until significant caries has developed, destroying the internal tooth structure. More retentive cements are therefore considered desirable, especially in certain clinical situations where appropriate retention is difficult to achieve.

An increase in the retention capabilities of glass-ionomer cement over zinc-phosphate in vitro was shown for cast gold inlays in 1982[23] and was later documented for crowns.[24–26] Dahl and Øilo[24] found a 20% to 30% increase, and Omar[25] a 50% increase, in the force necessary to remove crowns cemented with conventional glass-ionomer luting cement over zinc-phosphate, though Gorodovsky and Zidan[27] found little difference between them. Overall, the retention properties of glass-ionomer luting cements in laboratory studies are intermediate between those of zinc-phosphate and resin composite luting materials.

Surface roughness seems to have little effect on the materials' adhesive properties. Tooth preparation finalized with cross-cut carbide burs, which produced a mean groove depth of 25 μm in dentin, increased the retention of in vitro cast crowns cemented with zinc phosphate by 46%, whereas this type of instrumentation had little effect on glass-ionomer or resin composite luting agents.[26] This minimal influence of surface roughness has generally been taken as evidence of the presence of some physicochemical bonding in glass-ionomers. No dentin pretreatment was carried out in the studies reported. Polyacrylic acid has been suggested[28] as an etchant to increase wettability of the dentin surface and possibly increase ion exchange. Such treatment can increase bond strength but may affect dentin permeability and pulpal response to acidic cements.[29,30] Conditioners should therefore be used judiciously. Biological considerations for the vital tooth generally outweigh retentive needs.

It can be concluded that conventional glass-ionomer luting cements provide higher retentive capabilities than zinc-phosphate cement in vitro, but the clinical significance of this has not yet been documented. Clinical studies have shown excellent retention of castings with glass-ionomers, but there have been no reports of a difference between zinc-phosphate and glass-ionomers in this regard. It is generally recognized that the better adhesion attained with glass-ionomer luting cement cannot provide substantially increased clinical retention for short, unduly tapered crown-and-bridge preparations or posts with inadequate tooth support. Unusually high clinical retention requirements may necessitate the use of bonded resin luting materials, which have shown the highest retentive strengths in laboratory studies. It is expected that the retentive ability of resin-modified luting cements will fall between those of resin composite luting agents and conventional glass-ionomer luting cements.

Pulpal biocompatibility

Pulpal sensitivity is a problem for both patients and clinicians which can arise unexpectedly after permanent cementation has been completed. Irreversible pulpal reactions require endodontic treatment with additional, unexpected expense and damage to the newly placed restoration. Such situations should be avoided, and biological considerations are of supreme importance in the provision of successful restorations. A varying incidence of pulpal necrosis is associated with the presence of crown-and-bridge units and has been documented at different time intervals after insertion. Incidence rates of approximately 2% in short-term studies[31,32] and up to 15% in long-term studies[33] have been reviewed.[34] Intermediate rates of 3% to 6% are typical.[35,36] Pulp necrosis was the second most prevalent reason for abutment failure (6%) after secondary caries (25%) in a small clinical evaluation of luting cements over 10 years.[35] Larger retrospective studies have documented an incidence rate of less than 3%.[1]

Postoperative sensitivity was linked to the use of glass-ionomer luting cements,[35,37] particularly in the early years of usage, but this has since been disputed. Smith and Ruse[38] attributed such sensitivity to the low initial pH of the freshly mixed cement and the prolonged setting time, particularly if mixed too thinly, to reach a "zinc-phosphate consistency." Its initial acidity was greater than that of a zinc polycarboxylate cement and the time to neutrality was much longer. Use of recommended powder-to-liquid proportions is therefore critical to avoid unduly prolonged setting. Glass-ionomer cements have pseudoplastic properties that allow adequate flow under pressure despite the more viscous mix from an optimal powder–liquid ratio.

No substantial differences have been found in monkey pulp response to cemented gold inlays using zinc-phosphate, conventional glass-ionomer, and bonded resin luting materials when mean remaining dentin thickness was 1 mm.[39] Severe pulpal reactions have been documented in primates when extensive crown preparations used conventional glass-ionomers with continuous-pressure full-crown seating and the residual dentin was 0.5 mm or less.[40] Stanley[41] recommended the application of calcium hydroxide for pulp protection in extensive and deep crown preparations.

A unique prospective comparison of zinc-phosphate and glass-ionomer luting cements,[31] reported in 1993, was specifically designed to evaluate the incidence of sensitivity under clinical conditions. This multicenter randomized trial involved 10 standardized clinicians and placement of over 100 crowns, with each cement, on vital teeth with at least one third of the crown surface area on dentin. No conditioning was performed prior to placement of the glass-ionomer, and a double application of cavity varnish was used before zinc phosphate insertion. Significantly more patient reports of sensitivity at cementation and sensitivity to cold 2 weeks after cementation occurred in the zinc-phosphate group (32% and 34%, respectively) than in the glass-ionomer group (19% in both cases). After 3 months there were no sensitivity differences between the two cements, and there was a low number (2%) of irreversible pulpal complications in both groups over the 3 months of the study. This clinical trial found no association between the use of glass-ionomer luting cement and increased incidence of pulpal sensitivity, which is in agreement with the results of other clinical studies.[42,43]

A retrospective analysis[32] of 1,435 cast restorations luted with a glass-ionomer cement in a general practice over a 5-year period also showed the material to be effective and to exhibit acceptable pulpal compatibility. Of the 1,184 vital teeth restored, only 2.4% subsequently required endodontic treatment. Postcementation sensitivity was observed in 3.1% of the vital teeth, but resolved spontaneously within 4 weeks. A higher incidence of irreversible pulpitis was observed when a hemostatic agent was used on the retraction cord and when dentin was etched with polyacrylic acid before cementation. All current proprietary hemostatic agents have been shown to have high acidity,[44] can remove the dentinal smear layer in areas of contact, and may potentiate any prolonged acidity from an acidic luting material. Removal of the smear layer with acid etching improves the bonding strength of glass ionomers in vitro,[28] but Pashley[45] has shown that this greatly increases dentin permeability, which could augment acidic effects on the pulp. An increase in pulpal response to glass-ionomers has been documented when acid etching has been used in vivo.[46] Acidic cements have self-etching properties that are effective in removing the smear layer and promoting close adaptation to the dentin surface.[47] Subsequent mechanical interlocking and specific chemical interactions provide excellent adaptation. Glass-ionomer restoratives produced less demineralization of the dentin surface than did glass-ionomer luting forms. Routine use of acid etchants thus may not be necessary for luting cements. The advantages and risks of routine dentin pretreatment must be considered carefully, because the increased bonding strength with glass-ionomer cements may be negated by an irreversible pulpal reaction.[48]

Prevention of postcementation pulpal pathology

Biologic factors are of critical importance in restorative dentistry, and each step in the delivery of restorations requires adequate pulp protection. Correct preoperative pulpal assessment, atraumatic tooth preparation in the presence of adequate water spray, avoidance of dehydration, optimal temporization procedures, and knowledgeable use of all ancillary restorative materials are prerequisites for maintaining pulp vitality. Glass-ionomer luting cements offer certain advantages over zinc-phosphate,

Box 8-2 Synergistic factors leading to adverse pulpal effects

- Large areas of freshly cut, deep vital dentin
- Young tooth with large pulp and permeable dentin
- Traumatic tooth preparation without coolant
- Iatrogenic tooth dessication
- Cement mixed too thinly
- Potentiation of acid effects by etchants
- Additional acidic effects from hemostatic agents
- Preexisting pulpal pathology

Box 8-3 Prevention of pulpal pathology

- Ensure adequate water coolant during tooth preparation
- Avoid tooth dessication and dull burs
- Provide optimal temporization coverage
- Avoid acid etching of vital dentin
- Use varnish or desensitizers when potential sensitivity is high
- Use a cool slab and ensure the product is mixed to optimal thickness (or use a preencapsulated product)
- Ensure that no salivary contamination occurs prior to final setting

but awareness of cement properties and synergistic factors that may potentiate any acidic effects ensure successful usage. Large areas of deep, freshly cut dentin, particularly in the young tooth, allows acid permeation to the pulp, especially if acid etching has been used. Pulpal effects are exaggerated if tooth preparation is traumatic, temporization is ineffective, or the cement is mixed too thinly. Synergistic factors for pulpal irritation are listed in Box 8-2.

Although it may minimize fluoride uptake and somewhat inhibit adhesiveness, the judicious use of cavity varnish or desensitization agents is recommended for extensive areas of deep, newly cut vital dentin or for areas with a high potential for sensitivity. To allow maximum fluoride exposure at the caries-prone marginal areas of the restoration, such pulpal protection agents may be avoided at the preparation perimeter. They are obviously not required on endodontically treated teeth or teeth with previous extensive restorations and/or maximal reparative secondary dentin. A copal varnish, a one-step resin desensitizer such as Gluma desensitizer, or a visible cavity varnish such as Hydroxyline (which contains suspended calcium hydroxide) are appropriate agents. Visibility is an advantage because it allows accurate spot placement. For all agents, the use of a disposable brush is recommended to ensure optimal usage in areas of perceived need, with application immediately prior to cementation. The subsequent reduced dentin permeability should minimize any acidic effects on the pulp when glass-ionomers are used for cementation and residual dentin thickness is minimal. Clinical steps to avoid pulpal damage and its sequelae are listed in Box 8-3.

Resistance to oral dissolution

An exposed margin of cement is inevitable with indirect restorations. Resistance to in vivo dissolution is necessary to maintain the marginal seal and to avoid crevice formation, which increases the potential for plaque retention and caries development. A correlation between gap size and cement degradation has been demonstrated,[49] and increased marginal precision provides optimal performance for any cement.

Many workers have investigated the solubility of cements in vitro by analysis of material loss under different physical and chemical conditions. Conventional glass-ionomer cements have shown less susceptibility to dissolution and erosion in dilute acids than have zinc-phosphate and zinc-polycarboxylate luting cements.[50,51] In vitro studies generally compare well with in vivo studies that have measured loss of cement from specimen holders worn intraorally within dentures[52,53] or orthodontic brackets.[54] Such simulated clinical studies have shown a loss of substance for zinc-phosphate cement as much as 40 times greater than that for glass-ionomers when the cements were set under optimal conditions and then immersed in specimen holders.[52,55] An intermittent erosion cycling test using immersion in buffered lactic acid at pH 4, alternating with distilled water at pH 5.5, showed glass-ionomer cements to be far less susceptible to erosion than zinc-phosphate and zinc-polycarboxylate cements.[56] All the materials showed significantly more erosion at 15 minutes set than at 1 hour, but the glass-ionomer, a freeze-dried form, was significantly more resistant than the other two materials. However, these results did not correlate with those of a clinical study of restorations performed by the same workers. It is likely that this contradiction is related to the glass-ionomer's early sensitivity to moisture which creates a defective layer of varying thickness at crown margins in vivo. Such a surface layer would be susceptible to toothbrush abrasion and dissolution.

All the reported solubility and erosion studies used fully set cement specimens. It has been shown[57,58] that early solubility, or sensitivity to moisture during setting, is a problem for conventional glass-ionomer luting cements, even up to 8 minutes after the start of mixing. It is therefore crucial to avoid salivary contamination of the setting cement at restoration margins to avoid a marginal area that is dissolution prone. Optimal cement properties are necessary at this critical marginal area. Use of varnish protection has been recommended, but this is difficult to achieve in subgingival locations (Fig 8-3). Susceptibility of the exposed cement margin depends on the properties achieved, the quality of the seal, and the differing oral conditions found at predominantly gingival locations. The presence of a material that contains and can release fluoride is considered advantageous. However, the clinical significance of the level and duration of fluoride release is still questionable, particularly for the small quantities involved in luting films. Whether the production of susceptible marginal cement is clinically common or the reduced dissolution and presence of fluoride content associated with glass-ionomer cements will reduce susceptibility to decay can only be assessed in clinical studies.

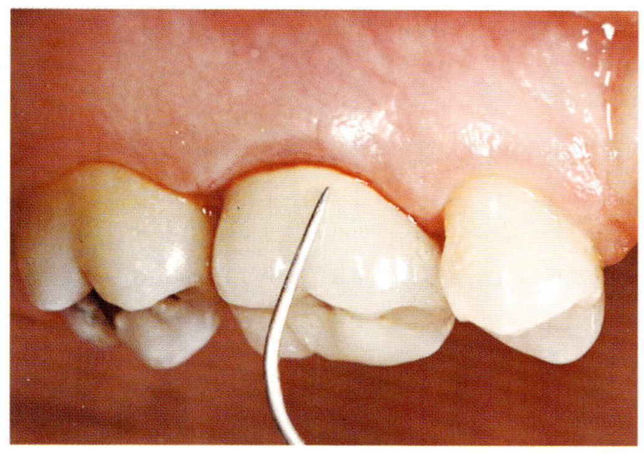

Fig 8-3 Newly placed crown immediately after removal of excess luting cement. This shows the difficulty of providing varnish protection to subgingival cement margins. Cement should be allowed to set as long as practicable to minimize surface contamination. Use of a retraction cord may be helpful.

Clinical evaluation of conventional glass-ionomer luting cements

Long-term clinical evaluations of glass-ionomer luting are sparse and those that are available involve a relatively small number of restorations, allowing little discernment between different cements. One of the longest studies involved 135 abutment teeth; used three different luting agents, two of which were glass-ionomers; and assessed the teeth after a period of 10 years.[35] Survival of abutments was 80% after 5 years and 71% after 10 years, with little overall difference between zinc phosphate and glass-ionomers. A 6% incidence of postoperative sensitivity and some continuing pulpal problems were more common with the glass-ionomers, but the authors concluded that the overall prognosis of abutment teeth was equally good with zinc phosphate or glass-ionomers. The development of secondary caries on retainers luted with both types of cement showed that the anticariogenic effects of the fluoride content in glass-ionomers is insufficient to prevent secondary decay under particularly unfavorable conditions.

A 4-year evaluation of 61 restorations performed by undergraduate dental students paradoxically showed few post-cementation problems and no cases of pulp pathology within this time frame with the three types of cement used (zinc-phosphate, zinc-polycarboxylate, and glass-ionomer).[48] Crowns retained with a glass-ionomer cement did, however, have a lower gingival index than those retained with zinc-phosphate or resin composite, which was attributed to the antimicrobial properties of glass-ionomers. Several studies have documented these antimicrobial effects,[59–61] which may be related to the presence of fluoride ions. Antimicrobial activity can influence plaque formation and may play a role in caries resistance. The small sample size did not allow definitive conclusions concerning cement superiority. However, the complete lack of pulpal problems was attributed to a longer than normal time interval between preparation and cementation.

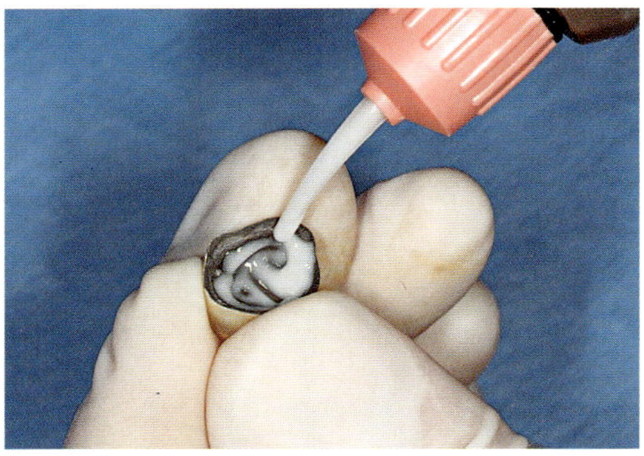

Fig 8-4 Use of a preencapsulated luting cement. Whether using conventional or resin-modified glass-ionomers, such a product ensures a consistent powder–liquid ratio and allows easy introduction into the interior of the crown.

A clinical study[62] evaluating all-ceramic crowns cemented with glass-ionomer cement documented a success rate of 98.4% at 3 years.[63] Only one crown fractured, for which inappropriate margin preparation was faulted. No cases of pulpal sensitivity were reported.

The use of glass-ionomers for luting purposes has gradually increased since their introduction. Reinhardt et al[64] reported that 75% of US dentists surveyed use glass-ionomer luting in their practices, and Christensen[65] stated that these cements were the most frequently used worldwide in the early 1990s. Correct usage, an optimal powder–liquid ratio, and avoidance of aggressive acid etching and tooth desiccation, combined with judicious use of desensitization agents, should provide predictable performance with these fluoride-releasing cements. McLean[66] encouraged the use of an encapsulated product (Fig 8-4) to control the powder–liquid ratio and suggested brushing the cement onto the crown and tooth to avoid excess hydrostatic pressure on the pulp. Sensitivity reports have declined substantially in recent years, probably due to manufacturing modifications and more knowledgeable handling by clinicians. Glass-ionomers are, however, still powder-liquid cements relying on optimum marginal accuracy and preparation retention design. Their improved solubility properties cannot overcome large marginal discrepancies, and the levels of adhesion attained cannot substantially increase clinical retention for short, unduly tapered crown preparations.

Resin-Modified Glass-Ionomer Luting Cements

Conventional glass-ionomer materials are generally accepted as the most durable of the dental cements. Their prolonged maturation time, however, allows early water sensitivity and they are also more susceptible to hydrolytic degradation than the more insoluble resin composite luting materials.[67] Over the last several years, modified glass-ionomer materials combining resin composite and glass-ionomer technologies have been introduced.

These materials are intended to increase conventional glass-ionomers' toughness and resistance to dissolution but preserve their clinical attributes of adhesion, fluoride content, and ease of use. In these hybrid materials, some of the water content of the glass-polyalkenoate system has been replaced by water-soluble polymers or polymerizable resins. This has resulted in cements with generally better physical and mechanical properties than those of conventional glass-ionomers,[68,69] but which are capable of comparable levels of fluoride release and similar in vitro artificial caries protection.[11] The resin-reinforced materials also show less early susceptibility to moisture.[13,58]

Resin-modified glass-ionomers represent one of the newest categories of dental materials and involve an interpenetrating cross-linking network of acid-base reaction and resin polymerization. The underlying chemistry is complex but the established presence of an acid-base reaction leading to the formation of a glass-ionomer polysalt matrix is essential to provide known glass-ionomer characteristics. The first resin-modified glass-ionomer material introduced commercially was a lining cement, Vitrebond, developed by Mitra.[70] This photo-cured hybrid glass-ionomer cement system retains a reactive fluoroaluminasilicate glass powder, but the liquid consists of an aqueous solution of a novel polyacrylic acid copolymer that contains pendant methacrylate groups, together with approximately 10% 2-hydroxyethylmethacrylate (HEMA). The acid-base reaction begins when the powder and liquid are mixed, but is relatively slow. Light activation starts the free radical resin polymerization reaction, which is relatively quick. Once polymerization has occurred and the material has hardened, there is a more limited acid-base reaction. Despite this, the end result is a strong liner with good adhesiveness to dentin and significant fluoride-releasing capability.[71]

Compositional approaches to hybridization

There have been different commercial approaches to the hybridization of resin and glass-ionomer technology. The three primary choices are discussed here.

Modification of the polyalkenoic acid to include photopolymerizable side groups

For this approach, the acid-base reaction is retained and the resin moiety is polymerized by light- and/or self-curing mechanisms to help the material attain optimal physical properties, depending on the access to light. Vitrebond fits this category, as does the tri-cured restorative material Vitremer with free radical self-curing and photo-curing capabilities. A purely chemically activated luting form of the latter material is available for luting purposes.

Addition of polymerizable monomer to the polyalkenoic acid

In this case, the polyalkenoic acid liquid component of conventional glass-ionomers is modified by adding a percentage of a polymerizable resin monomer that is compatible with water; HEMA is commonly used. Fuji Plus luting cement contains HEMA and tartaric acid and can be used with a 10:2 citric acid–ferric chloride etchant due to the more resinous character of this cement.

Substitution of the polyalkenoic acid with a polymerizable component

In this approach, the polyalkenoic acid component is totally replaced by new polymerizable resin monomers. Advance is an example of this type of product. A novel carboxylic acid monomer, water, and a diluent resin monomer make up the liquid that is mixed with the reactive glass to form the polyacid structure in situ.

Dyract-Cem on the other hand is a free radical polymerized luting material based on a strontium-aluminum glass and an anhydrous urethane dimethacrylate system containing an acidic monomer. After polymerization, diffusion of water into the set product is said to allow metal ion cross-linking. Such materials have been classified as polyacid-modified resin composites by McLean et al.[72] They behave more like composite materials than glass-ionomers and show lower levels of fluoride release.[73]

In other products, the liquid component is a conventional restorative resin monomer, such as bisphenol A–glycidyl methacrylate (Bis-GMA) in combination with triethyleneglycol dimethylamine (TEGDMA), that is polymerized by a free radical mechanism. No acid-base reaction is involved, and such materials are essentially resin composites containing aluminosilicate glasses and a preponderance of resin.

A range of chemistries is thus available, representing a spectrum from conventional glass-ionomer to resin-modified and polyacid-modified glass-ionomer to resin composite. Tooth attachment with predominantly resin-based materials requires the use of current resin bonding techniques, whereas glass-ionomer–type materials show some intrinsic adhesion to dentin. It has been shown that in Vitrebond the copolymer interacts chemically with dentin, indicating true glass-ionomer behavior.[74] Bonding is reduced, however, by a delay between application and photopolymerization. Bonding of the polyacid-modified material Dyract-Cem depends on the use of a resin primer. The resin-modified glass-ionomer Fuji Plus has been reported to provide high bonding strengths to enamel (18.4 MPa) and dentin (7.1 MPa) without the benefit of acid etchant or primer.[75] The Fuji system shows evidence of an ion exchange chemical bonding, as well as hybridization-type micromechanical attachment, when examined by transmission electron microscopy after polyacrylic acid etching.[76]

Classification and characterization of these new formulations are emerging gradually. Because two types of reactions are involved in true resin-modified glass-ionomers (free radical polymerization and an acid-base reaction) and because they proceed at the same time, there are problems in differentiating the contribution of each to the set product. Use of Fourier transform infrared spectroscopy (FTIR) has elucidated product differences for hybrid restorative materials and has confirmed the presence of an acid-base reaction in the Vitremer and Fuji II LC systems,[77] despite the difficulties of interpretation due to the presence of a free radical chemically cured reaction in Vitremer. The authors warn, however, that the influence of the retardation of the acid-base reaction on the performance of resin-modified glass-ionomer restorations over the long term is not known. They recommend the application of a protective resinous coating during the early setting stages to provide the time required for maturation of the glass-ionomer phase at the surface, thus minimizing the influence of salivary contamination. Others also have recommended the use of sealant barriers with resin-modified materials, even though these materials exhibit less early water sensitivity than do conventional glass-ionomers.[13]

Physical and mechanical properties

Resin-modified glass-ionomer cements show quite different mechanical and physical characteristics from those of conventional materials. Hybrid restorative materials show superior physical attributes to conventional glass-ionomers, but are inferior to conventional resin composites. Resin-modified glass-ionomer restoratives behave in a manner similar to conventional glass-ionomers, whereas polyacid-modified resin composites are more characteristic of microfilled resin composites in vitro.[78] These commercial products of varying compositions represent a continuum from conventional glass-ionomer to resin composite. Resin-modified glass-ionomers exceed conventional glass-ionomers in fracture strength and fatigue resistance under wet conditions in vitro.[78] They also show improved diametral tensile and flexural strengths, but a lower modulus of elasticity.[69] Limited research specific to luting forms of resin-reinforced materials is available. Data on film thickness has shown good crown seating for Vitremer luting cement (21.8 μm) compared to conventional glass-ionomers such as Fuji I (17.2 μm), but a substantially higher film thickness for the hybrid material Advance (106.6 μm).[79]

The new chemistry of these different approaches and the possibility of forming heterogeneous structures with hydrophilic and hydrophobic domains has raised questions about dimensional stability and the constancy of physical properties over time. Curing shrinkage is greater for resin-modified restoratives than for a hybrid resin composite or conventional glass-ionomer cement.[80] Peak initial strength is generally reached by 24 hours. Some researchers have reported stability in a wet environment,[68,69] but volumetric expansion also has been reported.[80] Because of significant expansion after water storage,[81–83] it has been suggested that resin-modified cements not be used for all-ceramic crowns or for post cementation, where such a property may prove deleterious. Indeed, fractures of a small number of all-ceramic crowns and even tooth roots have been reported.[84] Smith[6] concluded that resin-modified cements provide improved strength and fracture toughness and lower early moisture sensitivity, but cautioned that such improvements may be gained at the expense of increased dimensional change, loss of some intrinsic adhesion, and questionable long-term stability. Data specific to luting cements confirms the propensity to dimensional change due to imbibition. Fuji Plus showed double the net dimensional change over 1 week than that of a conventional glass-ionomer or a resin composite, with the greatest change occurring in the first 24 hours.[85]

Zinc-hosphate cement revealed a slight shrinkage effect. After a 2-week immersion, Fuji Plus, Vitremer, and Dyract-Cem all showed greater linear expansion than did a luting resin control.[86]

Pulpal biocompatibility

The initial pH is less acidic (around pH 4) for lining cements[87] compared with conventional glass-ionomers (pH 2), which may have implications for improved pulpal acceptance. Photo-cured resin-modified lining cements have elicited minimal pulpal response in Class V cavities in dogs[16] and in primates.[46] Limited information is available when they are used as luting cements. Proprietary products for luting have been commercially available for only a few years, but anecdotal reports are positive in the short term and manufacturers claim lower incidence of pulpal sensitivity problems. Clinical data is not available on these cements, but initial indications are positive for traditional luting purposes involving metal castings and crowns.

Improved adhesion has been shown with resin-modified glass-ionomer restoratives,[12,88] no doubt because of the addition of resin hybridization of the dentin surface due to HEMA penetration and to the known chemisorption of the polyacrylic acid moiety. The quicker setting reaction also provides higher early strength and water resistance which influence shear bond strengths. Restorative materials show higher bonding strengths to enamel than to dentin, but data on adhesion with resin-modified luting cements is more limited. The use of polyacrylic acid pretreatment of dentin has been shown to improve adhesion in some studies[88] but not in others.[89] The polyacrylic acids used produced etching patterns on enamel and completely removed the smear layer from dentin.[88] Fuji II LC showed greater adhesion to enamel and dentin than Vitremer. The bonding strength of Fuji Plus to bovine enamel was significantly improved with acid etching, but no differences were reported between treated and untreated dentin.[89]

Acid etchants that remove the smear layer should be used carefully (Fig 8-5). Tooth sensitivity after cementation of crowns is a common problem in dentistry. Although anecdotal reports suggest little problem with postoperative sensitivity using resin-modified luting cements, definitive information is lacking. In particular, teeth that are prepared for extracoronal restorations are at risk due to the large surface area of exposed dentinal tubules. Removal of the smear layer with acid etching may increase any subsequent chemical or physical effects. The application of resin desensitizers under conventional luting cements, on the other hand, is becoming fairly standard practice in North America and may be used judiciously under resin-modified cements. Sealing of dentin with resins has been shown to markedly decrease hypersensitivity.[90] Swift et al[91] found that the use of two such desensitizing resins (Gluma desensitizer and One-Step) had little or no effect on the retention of crowns luted with zinc-phosphate, glass-ionomer, or resin-modified glass-ionomer cements. It should be noted that in this in vitro study the retention of the resin-modified cement was essentially equivalent to that of the conventional glass-

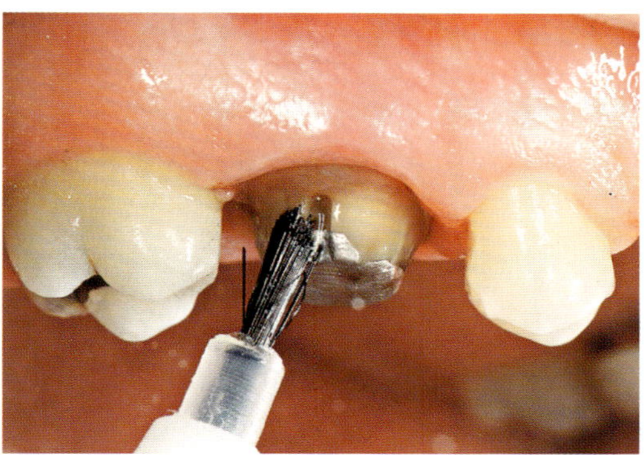

Fig 8-5 Pretreatment of the tooth. Prior to crown cementation, the prepared tooth should be cleaned thoroughly to remove all remnants of temporary cement, saliva, blood, or other debris. Acid etching is optional and should be used judiciously on the vital tooth.

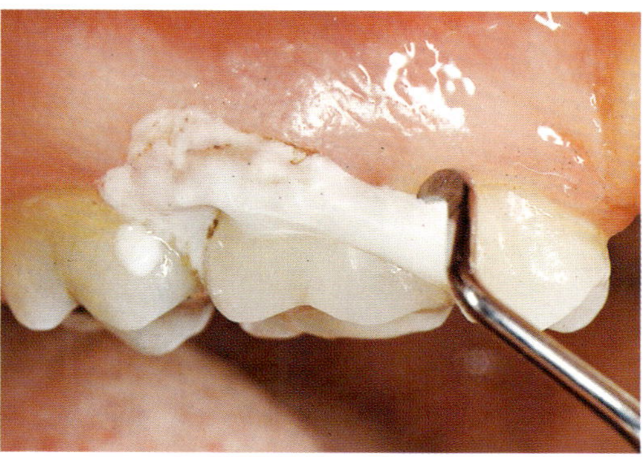

Fig 8-6 Initial removal of excess resin-modified glass-ionomer cement. Cleanup should begin in interdental areas when the cement has reached the first setting stage, while the restoration is maintained in place under pressure. If the cement is allowed to set completely, it is extremely tenacious and excess is difficult to remove.

onomer. The absence of reduced retention when the resin barrier was present between the glass-ionomer and dentin suggests that the physical properties of glass-ionomer materials have a greater effect than intrinsic tooth adhesion in determining the increased retention over zinc-phosphate cement that has been documented in many studies.

Clinical use

Clinical use of a resin-modified glass-ionomer is essentially similar to that of a conventional cement. Powder and liquid are dispensed according to the manufacturer's proportions and mixed on a glass slab. The cement consistency is somewhat thicker than that of zinc-phosphate but similar to that of a conventional glass-ionomer. The cement flow is optimal, allowing easy seating of castings and crowns. Setting time is more rapid than with conventional glass-ionomers, and the clinician must be alert for the first stages of set so excess cement can be removed while it is easily dislodged. Cleanup at this point is relatively easy (Fig 8-6), but delay allows further cement maturation and a hard set which, although clinically desirable in the exposed cement line, causes difficulty in removal for the clinician. A common clinical practice when cementing castings is to have the patient bite on a cotton roll or a soft wood stick. Although designed to ensure accurate seating, the inevitable tide of saliva engulfing the lingual margin unfortunately results in a weak and friable cement seal—as for any type of cement—and the practice is not recommended. Firm finger seating pressure and careful removal of excess resin-modified glass-ionomer luting cements provides successful cementation of inlays, onlays, and crowns (Fig 8-7).

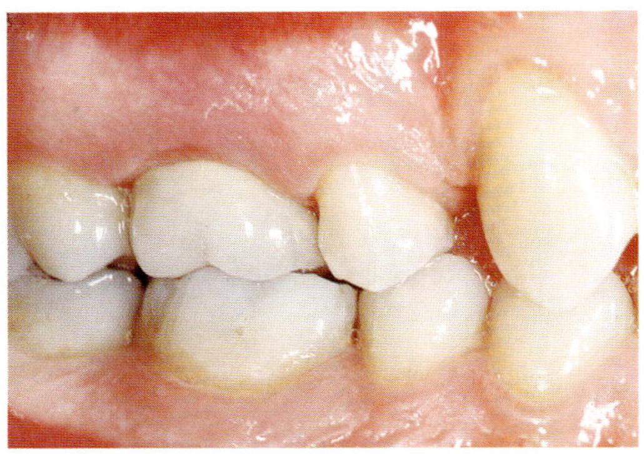

Fig 8-7 A crown successfully cemented with a resin-modified luting cement.

Further careful laboratory analyses and clinical data are necessary before resin-modified luting cements can be categorically accepted. It is relevant and interesting to note that Vitremer used in the challenging oral environment of post-radiation xerostomic patients has proved more robust than a conventional glass-ionomer restorative material (Ketac Fil), though not as sturdy as a resin composite.[92] Thus, it is possible that resin-modified luting forms provide a cementation material somewhere between resin composite and conventional glass-ionomer luting agents.

Summary

The characteristics and clinical advantages of glass-ionomer systems are well delineated. Conventional glass-ionomer luting cements are the most durable of the traditional cements available and provide easy clinical usage, good physical properties, inherent adhesive capability, fluoride release, and the potential for caries inhibition.

Clinical care in tooth preparation procedures, restoration quality, and marginal accuracy are likely to be more crucial for restoration longevity than the type of cement used. The choice and usage of cement should be based on sound biological and physical criteria for the particular clinical situation. Although glass-ionomer technology provides the potential for anticariogenic activity, it is unlikely this attribute can overcome particularly unfavorable clinical conditions.

Resin-modified glass-ionomer luting cements seem to combine the advantages of a glass-ionomer, including fluoride release, antibacterial activity, and the potential for caries inhibition, with improved physical properties from resin components. Initial acceptance from clinicians has been positive for routine cementation involving metal and metal-ceramic restorations, but it has been suggested that water sorption and associated expansion preclude usage with all-ceramic restorations and post cementation. More scientific information is required on these promising materials.

References

1. Schwartz NL, Whitsett LD, Berry TG, et al. Unserviceable crowns and fixed partial dentures: Life-span and causes for loss of serviceability. J Am Dent Assoc 1970;81:1395–1401.

2. Glantz P-O, Ryge G, Jendresen MD, Nilner K. Quality of extensive fixed prosthodontics after five years. J Prosthet Dent 1984;52:475–479.

3. Randow K, Glantz P-O, Zoger B. Technical failures and some related clinical complications in extensive fixed prosthodontics. Acta Odontol Scand 1986;44:241–255.

4. Swartz ML, Phillips RW, Clark HE. Long-term F release from glass-ionomer cements. J Dent Res 1984;63:158–160.

5. Lin A, McIntyre NS, Davidson RD. Studies on the adhesion of glass-ionomer cements to dentin. J Dent Res 1992;71:1636–1841.

6. Smith DC. Development of glass-ionomer cement systems. Biomaterials 1998;19:467–478.

7. Mount GJ. An Atlas of Glass-Ionomer Cements, 2d ed. London: Martin Dunitz Publisher, 1994.

8. McComb D, Sirisko R, Brown J. Comparison of physical properties of commercial glass-ionomer luting cements. J Can Dent Assoc 1984;9:699–701.

9. Mitchem JC, Gronas DG. Clinical evaluation of cement solubility. J Prosthet Dent 1978;40:453.

10. Groten M, Probster L. The influence of different cementation modes on the fracture resistance of feldspathic ceramic crowns. Int J Prosthodont 1997;10:169–177.

11. Nagamine M, Toshiyuki I, Yasuhiro T, Irie M, Staninec M, Inoue K. Effect of resin-modified glass-ionomer cements on secondary caries. Am J Dent 1997;10:173–178.

12. Miyazaki M, Iwasaki K, Soyamura T, Onose H, Moore BK. Resin-modified glass-ionomers: Dentin bond strength versus time. Oper Dent 1998;23:144–149.

13. Cho E, Kopel H, White SN. Moisture susceptibility of resin-modified glass-ionomer materials. Quintessence Int 1995;26:351–358.

14. Wilson AD. Resin-modified glass-ionomer cements. Int J Prosthodont 1990;3:425–429.

15. Sidhu S, Watson TF. Resin-modified glass-ionomer materials. A status report for the American Journal of Dentistry. Am J Dent 1995;8:59–67.

16. Gaitantzopoulou MD, Willis GP, Kafrawy AH. Pulp reactions to light-cured glass-ionomer cements. Am J Dent 1994;7:39–42.

17. Wilson AD, Crisp S, Lewis BG, McLean JW. Experimental luting agents based on glass-ionomer cements. Br Dent J 1977;142:117–122.

18. Wilson AD, McLean JW. Glass-Ionomer Cements. Chicago: Quintessence Publishing, 1988.

19. Øilo G. Luting cements: A review. Int Dent J 1991;41:81–88.

20. McLean JW, Wilson AD, Prosser HJ. Development and use of water hardening glass-ionomer cements. J Prosthet Dent 1984;52: 175–181.

21. Setchell DJ, Teo CK, Khun AT. The relative solubilities of four modern glass-ionomer cements. Br Dent J 1985;158:220–222.

22. Knibbs PJ, Plant CG, Shovelton DS. The performance of a zinc-polycarboxylate luting cement and a glass-ionomer luting cement in general dental practice. Br Dent J 1986;160:13–15.

23. McComb D. Retention of castings with glass-ionomer cement. J Prosthet Dent 1982;48: 285–288.

24. Dahl BL, Øilo G. Retentive properties of luting cements: An in-vitro investigation. Dent Mater 1986;2:17–20.

25. Omar R. A comparative study of the retentive capacity of dental cementing agents. J Prosthet Dent 1985;60:35–40.

26. Ayad MF, Rosenstiel SF, Salama M. Influence of tooth surface roughness and type of cement on retention of complete cast crowns. J Prosthet Dent 1997;77:116–121.

27. Gorodovsky S, Zidan O. Retentive strength, disintegration and marginal quality of luting cements. J Prosthet Dent 1992;68:269–274.

28. Powis DR, Folleras T, Merson SA, Wilson AD. Improved adhesion of glass-ionomer cement to dentin and enamel. J Dent Res 1982;61: 1416–1422.

29. Pashley DH, Michelich V, Kehl TJ. Dentin permeability. Effects of smear layer removal. J Prosthet Dent 1981;46:531–537.

30. Pashley DH. Smear layer. Physiological considerations. Oper Dent 1984;9(suppl):359–371.

31. Johnson GH, Powell LV, Derouen TA. Evaluation and control of post-cementation pulpal sensitivity: Zinc-phosphate and glass-ionomer luting cements. J Am Dent Assoc 1993;124:39–46.

32. Brackett WW, Metz JE. Performance of a glass-ionomer luting cement over 5 years in a general practice. J Prosthet Dent 1992;67:59–61.

33. Balmgvist S, Swartz B. Artificial crowns and fixed partial dentures 18–23 years after placement. Int J Prosthodont 1993;6:279–285.

34. Habsha E. The incidence of pulpal complications and loss of vitality subsequent to full crown restorations. Ont Dent 1998;75:19–24.

35. Jockstad A, Mjör IA. Ten years' clinical evaluation of three luting cements. J Dent 1997;24:309–315.

36. Jackson CR, Skidmore AE, Rice RT. Pulpal evaluation of teeth restored with fixed prostheses. J Prosthet Dent 1992;67:323–325.

37. American Dental Association. Council on Dental Materials, Instruments and Equipment. Reported sensitivity to glass-ionomer luting materials. J Am Dent Assoc 1984;109:476.

38. Smith D, Ruse ND. Acidity of glass-ionomer cements during setting and its relation to pulp sensitivity. J Am Dent Assoc 1986;112:654–657.

39. Inokoshi S, Fujitani M, Otsuki M, Sonoda H, Kitasako Y, Shimada Y, Tagami J. Monkey pulpal responses to conventional and adhesive luting cements. Oper Dent 1998;23:21–29.

40. Pameijer CH, Stanley HR, Ecker G. Biocompatibility of a glass-ionomer luting agent. Part II Crown cementation. Am J Dent 1991;4:134–142.

41. Stanley HR. Pulpal consideration of adhesive materials. Oper Dent 1992;5(suppl):151–164.

42. Norman RD, Wright JS. A comparison of glass-ionomer and zinc-phosphate cements via pulpal response. Compend Contin Educ Dent 1986;7: 41–47.

43. Kern M, Kleimeier B, Schaller H-G, Strub JR. Clinical comparison of postoperative sensitivity for a glass ionomer and a zinc-phosphate luting cement. J Prosthet Dent 1996;75:159–162.

44. Land MF, Rosenstiel SF, Sandrik JL. Disturbance of dentinal smear layer by acidic hemostatic agents. J Prosthet Dent 1994;72:4–7.

45. Pashley DH. Dentin-predentin complex and its permeability: Physiologic overview. J Dent Res 1985;64(special issue):613–620.

46. Felton DA, Cox CF, Odom M. Pulpal response of chemically cured and experimental light-cured glass-ionomer liners. J Prosthet Dent 1991; 65:704–712.

47. Shimada Y, Kondou Y, Inikoshi S, Tagami J, Antonucci JM. Demineralizing effect of dental cements on human dentin. J Dent Res 1998;77:680 [abstract 386].

48. Pameijer CH, Nilner K. Long-term clinical evaluation of three luting materials. Swed Dent J 1994;18:59–67.

49. Mesu FP. Degradation of luting cements measured in vitro. J Dent Res 1982;61:665–672.

50. Finger W. Evaluation of glass-ionomer luting cements. Scand J Dent Res 1983;91:143–149.

51. Walls AWG, McCabe JF, Murray JJ. An erosion test for dental cements. J Dent Res 1985; 64:1100–1104.

52. Pluim LJ, Arends J, Havinga P, Jongebloed WL, Stockroos I. Quantitative cement solubility experiments in vivo. J Oral Rehabil 1984; 11:171–179.

53. Mitchum JC, Gronas DG. Continued evaluation of the clinical solubility of luting cement. J Prosthet Dent 1981;45:289–290.

54. Earl MSA, Ibbetson RJ. The clinical disintegration of a glass ionomer cement. Br Dent J 1986;161:287–291.

55. Knibbs PJ, Walls AWG. A laboratory and clinical evaluation of three dental luting cements. J Oral Rehabil 1989;16:467–473.

56. Phillips RW, Swartz ML, Lund MS, Moore BK, Vickery J. In vivo disintegration of luting cements. J Am Dent Assoc 1987;114:489–492.

57. Oilo G. Early erosion of dental cements. Scand J Dent Res 1984;92:539–543.

58. Um CM, Oilo G. The effect of early water contact on glass-ionomer cements. Quintessence Int 1992;23:209–214.

59. McComb D, Ericson D. Antimicrobial action of new, proprietary lining cements. J Dent Res 1987;66:1025–1028.

60. Scherer W, Lippman N, Kaim J. Antimicrobial properties of glass-ionomer cements and other restorative materials. Oper Dent 1989;14:77–81.

61. DeSchepper EJ, White RR, von der Lehr W. Antibacterial effects of glass-ionomers. Am J Dent 1989;2:51–56.

62. Scotti R, Catapano S, D'Elia A. A clinical evaluation of In-Ceram crowns. Int J Prosthodont 1995;8:320–323.

63. Klaisner PJ, Brandau HE, Charbeneau GT. Glass ionomer cements in dental practice: A national survey on the use of glass-ionomer cements. Oper Dent 1989;18:56–60.

64. Reinhardt JW, Swift EJ Jr, Bolden AJ. A national survey on the use of glass-ionomer cements. Oper Dent 1993;18:56–60.

65. Christensen GJ. Why is glass ionomer cement so popular? J Am Dent Assoc 1994;125:1257–1258.

66. McLean JW. Clinical applications of glass-ionomer cements. Oper Dent 1992;5 (suppl):184–190.

67. Wilson AD, Groffman DM, Kuhn AT. The release of fluoride and other chemical species from a glass-ionomer cement. Biomaterials 1985;6:431–433.

68. Uno S, Finger WJ, Fritz U. Long-term mechanical characteristics of resin-modified glass-ionomer restorative materials. Dent Mater 1996;12:64–69.

69. Mitra SB, Kedrowski BL. Long-term mechanical properties of glass-ionomers. Dent Mater 1994;19:78–82.

70. Mitra SB. Adhesion to dentin and physical properties of a light-cured glass-ionomer liner/base. J Dent Res 1991;70:72–74.

71. Mitra SB. In-vitro fluoride release from a light-cured glass-ionomer liner/base. J Dent Res 1991;70:75–78.

72. McLean JW, Nicholson JW, Wilson AD. Proposed nomenclature for glass-ionomer dental cements and related materials. Quintessence Int 1994;25:587–589.

73. Marks LAM, Verbeek RMH. Water sensitivity of the fluoride release of modified glass-ionomers. J Dent Res 1998;77:939 [abstract 2463].

74. Titley KR, Smith DC, Chernecky R. SEM observations of the reactions of the components of a light-activated glass-polyalkenoate (ionomer) cement on bovine dentin. J Dent 1996;24:411–416.

75. Friedl K-H, Schmalz G, Hiller K-A, Geismeier R, Lang P. Bond strength of hybrid ionomer and compomer luting materials. J Dent Res 1998;77:814 [abstract 1463].

76. Van Meerbeek B, Yoshida Y, Lambrechts P, Vanherle G, Waakasa K, Nakayama Y. Mechanisms of bonding of a resin-modified glass-ionomer adhesive to dentin. J Dent Res 1998;77:911 [abstract 2236].

77. Kakaboura A, Eliades G, Palaghias G. An FTIR study on the setting mechanism of resin-modified glass-ionomer restoratives. Dent Mater 1996; 12:173–178.

78. Gladys S, Van Meerbeek B, Braem M, Lambrechts P, Vanherle G. Comparative physico-mechanical characterization of new hybrid restorative materials with conventional glass-ionomer and resin composite restorative materials. J Dent Res 1997;76:883–894.

79. Tan K, Lim CC, Chan YM. The effect of resin and resin-ionomer cements on crown seating. J Dent Res 1998;77:925 [abstract 2347].

80. Attin T, Buchalla W, Kielbassa AM, Hellwig E. Curing shrinkage and volumetric changes of resin-modified glass-ionomer restorative materials. Dent Mater 1995;11:359–362.

81. Feilzer AJ, Kakaboura AI, de Gee AJ, Davidson CL. The influence of water sorption on the development of setting shrinkage stress in traditional and resin-modified glass-ionomer cements. Dent Mater 1995;11:186–190.

82. Yap A, Lee CM. Water sorption and solubility of resin-modified polyalkenoate cements. J Oral Rehabil 1997;24:310–314.

83. Iwami Y, Yamamoto H, Sato W, Kawai K, Torii M, Ebusi S. Weight change of various light-cured restorative materials after water immersion. Oper Dent 1998;23:132–137.

84. Miller M (ed). Reality Now 68: 1 July, 1995 and 75: 4 March, 1996.

85. Ewoldsen E, Covey D. Effects of water storage on dimension of standardized luted interfaces. J Dent Res 1998;77:689 [abstract 462].

86. Salz U, Rumphorst A, Gianasmidis A, Rheinberger V. Comparative linear expansion study of various cements after water storage. J Dent Res 1998;77:689 [abstract 464].

87. Tam L, McComb D, Pulver F. Physical properties of proprietary light-cured lining materials. Oper Dent 1991;16:210–217.

88. Fritz UB, Finger WJ, Uno S. Resin-modified glass-ionomer cements: Bonding to enamel and dentin. Dent Mater 1996;12:161–166.

89. Yoshikawa T, Tosaki S, Hirota K. Effect of tooth treatment for bonding strength of resin-modified glass-ionomer. J Dent Res 1995;74(special issue):428 [abstract 222].

90. Watanabe T, Sano M, Itoh K, Wakumoto S. The effects of primers on the sensitivity of dentin. Dent Mater J 1991;7:148–150.

91. Swift EJ, Lloyd AH, Felton DA. The effect of resin desensitizing agents on crown retention. J Am Dent Assoc 1997;128:195–200.

92. Woods RE, McComb D, Lee L, Maxymiw WG. A clinical comparison of light-cured and conventional glass-ionomer cement restorations to bonded resin composite in the treatment of class V caries in xerostomic head and neck radiation patients. Unpublished data, 1998.

Chapter 9

Luting in Orthodontic Practice

Dorothy McComb

Orthodontic treatment with fixed appliances utilizes luting materials to effect a stable attachment of brackets and bands during tooth movement. A common clinical problem is demineralization, or caries, under or around the brackets or bands, particularly in caries-prone younger patients. Thorough oral hygiene is difficult with fixed appliances. Another frequent clinical problem is bracket or band detachment, which disrupts schedules, may delay treatment, and, if longstanding, can result in serious tooth decay. This chapter discusses usage of glass-ionomer materials in orthodontic therapy.

Band Cementation

Conventional glass-ionomer cements

Requirements for materials used in orthodontic band cementation are somewhat similar to those for luting crown-and-bridge units, except there is no need for low film thickness or long-term stability. An additional requirement is ease of cleanup at the completion of orthodontic therapy. The properties of conventional glass-ionomer cements, which include high strength, low solubility, fluoride release, and chemical adhesion, are just as advantageous for band cementation as for crown-and-bridge luting. Although zinc-phosphate has been the cement of choice for many years, the development of conventional glass-ionomer cements provided the potential for increased band retention—through superior tensile and compressive strength and adhesion to tooth structure—as well as the potential for decreased incidence of demineralization—through reduced cement solubility, antibacterial activity, initially high tooth fluoride uptake, and prolonged low levels of fluoride release. A series of clinical studies have clearly documented significantly superior retention rates for orthodontic molar bands cemented with glass-ionomers than for other conventional cements investigated.[1–5]

In a literature review of in vivo failure rates with zinc-phosphate–cemented bands by different workers, Stirrup[5] reported ranges of 6.5% to 23% failure in maxillary first molars and 20.1% to 31% failure in mandibular first molars over a range of treatment times. Fricker and McLachlan[1] compared glass-ionomer and zinc-phosphate band cementation over a 1-year treatment period and observed an 8.8% failure with zinc-phosphate and 0.6% with glass-ionomer.

A second 2-year follow-up study[2] with 198 patients confirmed the increased retention with glass-ionomer cement; bands cemented with zinc-phosphate loosened in 13.2% of teeth compared with only 2.3% for the glass-ionomer group. The authors reported enamel demineralization in 19 of the 198 patients, all in zinc-phosphate–banded teeth. Similar improved retention of bands cemented with glass-ionomer (1.9% failure over a mean treatment period of just under 2 years) was reported by Mizrahi[3] and no interjaw differences were observed. In another clinical comparison study[4] involving two sequential 9-month periods, 1,200 bands were cemented with zinc-phosphate and 500 with glass-ionomer. The number of recementations was reduced by more than 50% with the glass-ionomer, and more cement remained on the tooth after bands were removed at the end of treatment. Whereas 18 teeth showed demineralization in the zinc-phosphate group, none was observed in the glass-ionomer group. Greater cement loss, the presence of residual oral debris, and a higher incidence of demineralization confirmed the greater propensity of zinc-phosphate luting cements for leakage and solubility.

These results were confirmed decisively in a well-designed comparative survival study that used a split-mouth randomization technique to ensure no study design biases.[5] Band loss rates of 9.5% for an experimental conventional glass-ionomer luting cement and 28.9% for a standard zinc-phosphate cement were reported over a period of more than 600 days. The retentive superiority of the glass-ionomer over zinc-phosphate was clear and, 6 months into the trial, a decision was made that any further loose bands would be recemented with the "clearly superior glass-ionomer cement."

Thus, several clinical trials have shown conventional glass-ionomer materials to be more effective than zinc-phosphate cement in the retention of orthodontic molar bands, and many have reported decreased incidence of demineralization around band margins. Clinical comparison of different commercial brands of glass-ionomer cement[6] and the use of a 50% higher powder–liquid ratio[7] produced no significant improvement in retention rates.

A consistent characteristic of glass-ionomers in both in vitro and in vivo studies has been the site of cement failure; the cement has a propensity for remaining attached to tooth structure rather than to the metal band. This characteristic is felt to be favorable for increased tooth protection. In an in vitro study,[8] 100% of fracture sites between cement and stainless steel bands showed residual cement attached to enamel, which bears out other clinical research.

Resin-modified glass-ionomer cements

Newly developed resin-modified glass-ionomer cements, some introduced specifically for orthodontic use, are currently the subject of considerable interest. The promise of improved physical properties,[9] in particular their increased fracture toughness and resilience[10] and less sensitivity to moisture contamination,[11] and the preservation of adhesion and fluoride release, has suggested the use of these cements for orthodontic band cementation as well as bracket bonding. Other material developments have included polyacid-modified resin composites, similar in composition to compomers, and dual-cured resin-based adhesives that contain fluoroaluminosilicate glass, but the results of enamel bond strength studies for these materials have been less than satisfactory.[12–14] Such materials are essentially resin composites and their attachment to enamel requires acid etching as a preparatory step. Materials containing no acidic polymer provide no acid-base reaction, making the term "glass ionomer" inappropriate.[14]

Another 12-month clinical trial by Fricker[15] studying molar band cementation compared a true resin-modified, light-activated, dual-cured adhesive cement with both a fluoride-containing resin and a conventional glass-ionomer. Approximately 60 cemented bands per material type were used. A band failure rate of 2.9% was recorded for Fuji II LC, 8.1% for Bandlok, and 3.5% for Ketac-Cem, with no statistical difference between the three. The resin-modified glass-ionomer was used after enamel was etched with polyacrylic acid, but the dual-cured fluoridated resin was used without phosphoric acid enamel etching, per the manufacturer's instructions. No acid etching was used with the conventional glass-ionomer. Again, both types of glass-ionomers failed predominantly at the adhesive–metal interface, leaving residual cement on the enamel surface (Figs 9-1a and 9-1b). The fluoridated resin material failed at the interface between enamel and adhesive, showing more typical resin behavior when used without acid etching (Fig 9-1c). All the metal bands were roughened lightly on the inside with a diamond bur. It has been shown that this procedure can increase bond strength and reduce the clinical failure rate of first molar bands when a conventional glass-ionomer is used.[9,16] Further research will be necessary to evaluate whether resin-modified glass-ionomers, now available in self-curing luting forms, will provide any additional benefits over conventional glass-ionomers for orthodontic band cementation.

Bracket Bonding

Since the advent of enamel bonding, fixed appliance therapy has been possible with resin-bonded brackets, involving less tooth coverage, greatly improved esthetics, and easier patient cleansing. Despite this, demineralization, or white spot formation, around brackets (Fig 9-2) has been reported to occur within a month of placement.[17] Retention of resin-bonded brackets is predictable and reliable during therapy, but debonding procedures can be time-consuming and may cause damage to or loss of surface enamel. Indeed, the pursuit of even greater bond strengths to enamel in orthodontics has been challenged and a philosophy of optimized bond strengths has been encouraged.[18] The potential of glass-ionomer cements to provide adhesion, fluoride release, and easy cleanup has suggested their use for bracket bonding, despite their less desirable physical properties and lower bond strengths. However, the clinical reality is that conventional glass-ionomer cements show unacceptably high debonding rates, which precludes their usage.

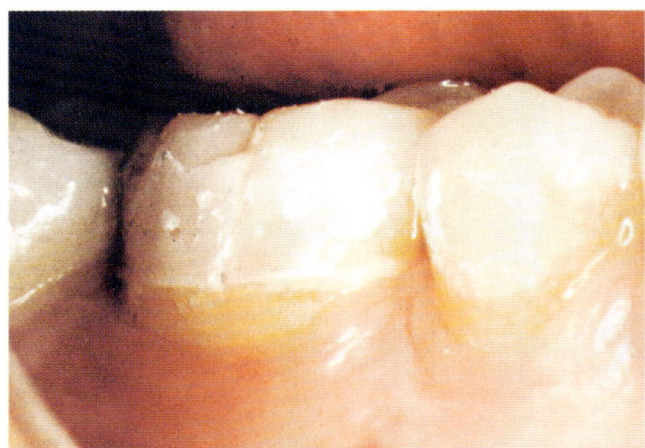

Fig 9-1a Conventional glass-ionomer cement after orthodontic band removal. Cement remains on the enamel surface. (From Fricker.[15] Reproduced with permission.)

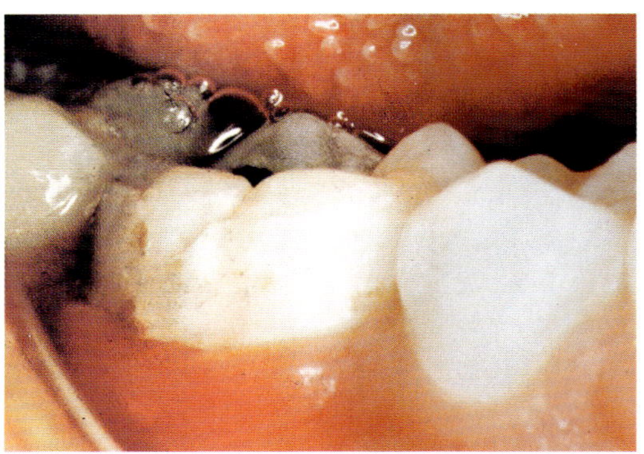

Fig 9-1b Resin-modified glass-ionomer cement after band removal. Cement remains on the enamel surface. (From Fricker.[15] Reproduced with permission.)

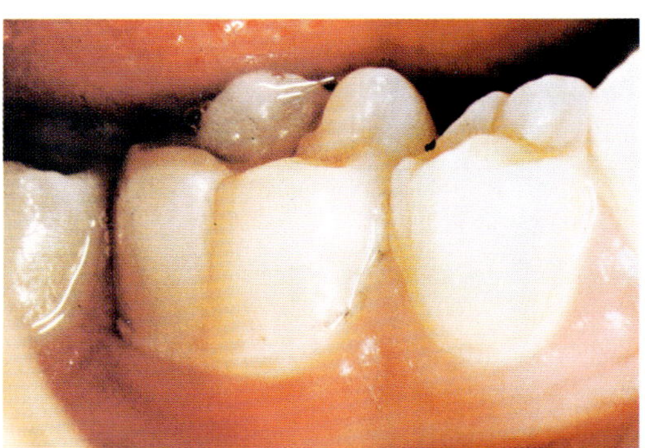

Fig 9-1c Cement with no adhesive properties after band removal. Minimal cement remains on the enamel surface. (From Fricker.[15] Reproduced with permission.)

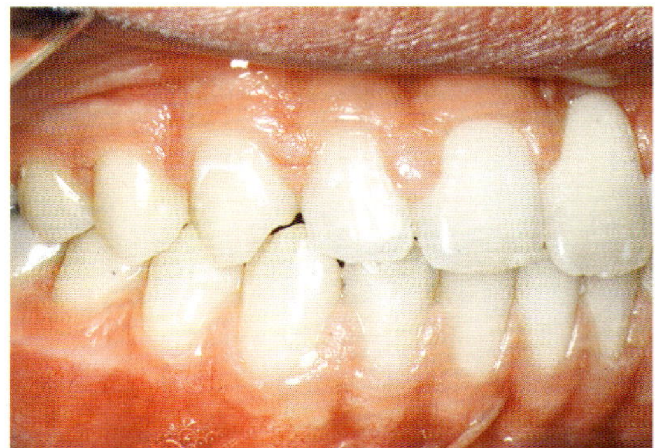

Fig 9-2 White spot formation due to localized demineralization during orthodontic treatment. Such areas may be minor, as here, or so prominent as to affect the esthetic result.

Conventional glass-ionomers

A 12-month clinical evaluation of a glass-ionomer cement for the direct bonding of orthodontic brackets was carried out by Fricker.[19] An unacceptable 20% rate of bracket debonding was reported, compared to 5% with resin composite. In a larger study comparing conventional glass-ionomer cement with an acrylic resin cement over an average treatment time of 653 days by Norevall et al[20] the frequency of failed brackets with glass-ionomer cement was 36% and 15% for the resin-based material. Meshed foil base brackets failed less often (22% with glass-ionomer and 7% with acrylic resin) than cut groove base brackets (50% with glass-ionomer and 23% with acrylic resin). The time required for debonding and cleanup at the end of orthodontic therapy was significantly shorter for glass-ionomer cement and reduced incidence of white spot formation was reported. Also, the vast majority of the glass-ionomer–bonded brackets failed cohesively, leaving cement on the enamel and bracket, showing that the physical strength properties of the cement are a major problem. Shear bond strengths for glass-ionomer cements are fairly low (3.6 to 5.8 MPa) depending on the stainless steel bracket retention design.[21] For resin-based orthodontic cements, shear bond strengths in the 17 to 18 MPa range are possible with stainless steel brackets and may be even higher (24 to 28 MPa) with ceramic brackets.[22]

It is therefore surprising that White[23] successfully used conventional glass-ionomer cement for bracket bonding and was able to achieve clinical results similar to those obtained with a resin adhesive. The newly set glass-ionomer cement was protected from moisture, salivary contamination was avoided, and only very light wires were inserted immediately after the bonding procedure. Silverman et al[24] later suggested that the success rate would be higher with conventional glass-ionomer cements if wires were not inserted at all during the bonding appointment, to allow the cement to achieve its maximum set and highest strength. There has even been some recent debate[18] on the merits of lower bond strengths to avoid iatrogenic enamel damage from the exceedingly high resin adhesive bonds to etched enamel.

It has been stated that a minimum of 10 MPa shear bond strength is necessary for successful clinical bonding, even though routine orthodontic forces on teeth are generally much lower.[25] Failure rates during therapy for conventional adhesive resin cements varied from 1.6% to 7% in most of the seven comparative clinical studies reviewed by Millett and McCabe.[26] Only one of the seven reported a higher (15%) failure with resin bonding[20] and only when grooved base brackets were used. Resin bracket bonding to dry, acid-etched enamel provides secure and predictable orthodontic bonding that cannot be reproduced with conventional glass-ionomer cements.

Millet and McCabe[26] have thoroughly reviewed both the in vitro and in vivo studies (80 references) on the topic of orthodontic bonding with glass-ionomer cement and have concluded that there is little support in the literature to suggest that conventional glass-ionomers are suitable for routine bracket bonding. The 37 laboratory studies on bond strength testing of orthodontic brackets failed to yield clear guidelines as to the best enamel pretreatment and cement proportioning but they confirmed the fracture pattern of adhesive failure between bracket and cement. Bond strengths were less than ideal and the presence of high standard deviations revealed the technique sensitivity of glass-ionomer usage for this purpose. Review of clinical studies of orthodontic brackets bonded with conventional glass-ionomer cements revealed a retention failure rate varying from 3.8% to 50.9%. The clinical disadvantages of unreliable bracket retention therefore outweigh the potential material advantages of these materials.

Resin-modified glass-ionomers

The development of modified glass-ionomers with the addition of resin moieties has rekindled interest in the use of alternative bonding materials with potential anticariogenic properties. Stronger, tougher, and more resilient than conventional glass-ionomer cements, these new materials offer both increased bond strength to tooth structure and fluoride-release capability. They have distinct possibilities for orthodontic bonding with the possibility of reduced incidence of demineralization. Many in vitro studies in the last few years have attempted to define the performance of resin-modified glass-ionomers in this role, with mixed results.[13,14,27–31] Shear bond strength studies used a range of early resin-modified glass-ionomer materials, some developed as lining materials and some as restoratives. Part of the problem was the lack of information about the chemistry of many of these materials and confusion with resins containing fluoroaluminosilicate glass filler without any acid-base polyalkenoate reaction.

In vitro shear bond strength studies for orthodontic purposes in recent years therefore reflect an eclectic mix of commercial materials, and the results must be assessed carefully. Disappointing results were obtained with a compomer restorative[27] and a resin-modified glass-ionomer restorative[31] and lining.[27]

However, in vitro results with true resin-modified cements developed for orthodontic use have shown considerable promise for bonding brackets.[13,14,28,30] In one study, Fuji Ortho resin-modified cement, optimized specifically for orthodontic purposes, showed elevated bond strength, increased viscosity to prevent drift on the tooth, and a modified chemical-curing reaction.[30] Adhesive cement remained firmly attached to enamel after testing. Using metal brackets, Subenberger et al[13] obtained shear bond strengths of 28.17 MPa with Fuji Ortho LC and 23.90 MPa with Photac-Bond, which approached the control resin bond strengths of 33 MPa. The resin-modified glass-ionomer cements were used with polyacrylic acid etching, as were two materials better described as polyacid-modified resins. The two latter materials gave much lower bond strengths. Similar materials were used in the same manner with ceramic brackets and yielded essentially similar results.[14] The one marked difference was the comparatively low shear bond strength of Concise resin to ceramic brackets with micromechanical retention, which was exceeded by that of Fuji Ortho LC.

In a comparison of different tooth conditions for enamel bonding with Fuji

Ortho LC, Jobalia et al[28] demonstrated that this resin-modified glass-ionomer cement approached and even exceeded the strength observed for resin adhesives. They reported that a moist enamel surface after 10% polyacrylic acid etching gave optimal performance.

Newer generation resin-modified glass-ionomers appear to show markedly superior clinical retention than that of conventional glass-ionomers in orthodontic bracket bonding. Of the 11 clinical reports reviewed by Millett and McCabe[26] and involving glass-ionomer bonding, two of the latest involved the use of a resin-modified cement. Whereas Fricker[19] found a 20% failure rate with the conventional cement Fuji I, he obtained a vastly reduced (3%) failure rate with the dual-cured material Fuji II LC.[32] In both studies a 10-second polyacrylic acid pretreatment of enamel was performed and a Begg light-wire technique used. Of particular note is the fact that Fricker[32] reported no significant difference between the failure rate of brackets bonded with the resin-modified glass-ionomer and that of brackets bonded with a resin composite (1.6%). Using a tri-cured resin-modified glass-ionomer involving an acid-base reaction, resin photopolymerization, and oxidation-reduction resin self-curing (Fuji Ortho LC), Silverman et al[24] also reported a low failure rate of bracket debonding, in this case using an edgewise technique, over a period of approximately 8 months.

Resin-modified glass-ionomer orthodontic cements are available in photopolymerized and self-curing versions. The manufacturers' directions state that the materials can be used either with or without acid etching for 10 to 20 seconds using 10% polyacrylic acid. Most of the clinical studies report using a pretreatment step. In all cases, a pumice-cleaned surface is necessary and a desiccated or overly dry enamel surface is to be avoided (Figs 9-3a and 9-3b). The photopolymerized version requires 40 seconds of light curing for each bracket (Fig 9-4). Light-gauge wires can be placed immediately after photopolymerization, but clinicians should allow at least 7 to 10 minutes after the last bracket cementation with the self-curing material (Fig 9-5).

Prevention of Demineralization

Orthodontic treatment increases mouth plaque, levels of *Mutans streptococci*,[33] and the risk of caries development.[34] Recent studies have shown that 50% to 75% of all orthodontic patients develop some demineralization on labial surfaces, on at least one tooth, during fixed appliance treatment.[35–37] Overall incidence of white spot formation during orthodontic therapy is 11% to 12%, with little difference after either bonding or zinc-phosphate banding.[35] It has been shown that development of demineralization is a significant clinical problem present on teeth even 5 years after orthodontic therapy.[36]

Several authors have reported less enamel demineralization under orthodontic bands or brackets retained with conventional glass-ionomer cements in vivo.[2,4,9,38–41] Using photographic records, as well as visual examination, Marcusson et al[40] found demineralization after debonding on 24% of surfaces bonded with Ketac-Cem and 40.5% of surfaces bonded with resin. Before

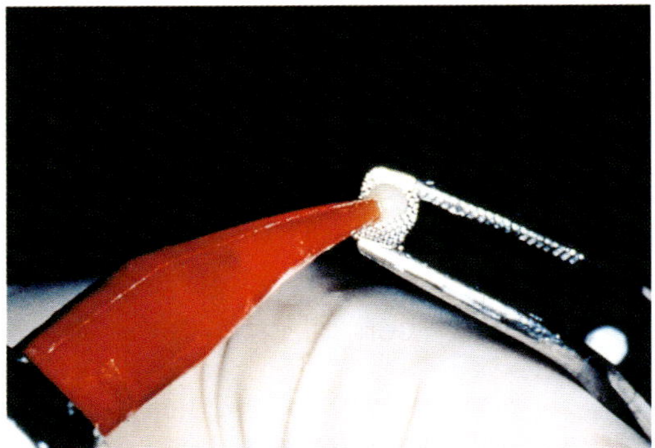

Fig 9-3a The mixed powder-liquid photopolymerized resin-modified glass-ionomer being placed on the bracket using a syringe. (Courtesy Dr Scott Dillingham.)

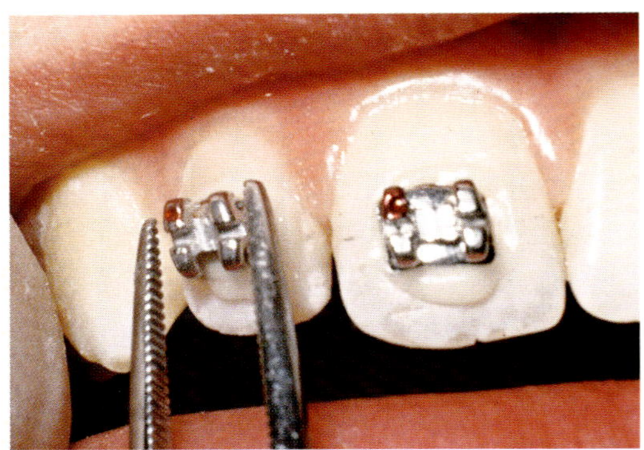

Fig 9-3b The cement-loaded bracket positioned on a pumice-cleaned, acid-etched, moist enamel surface. Acid etching of enamel with 10% polyacrylic acid for 10 to 20 seconds is recommended. (Courtesy Dr Scott Dillingham.)

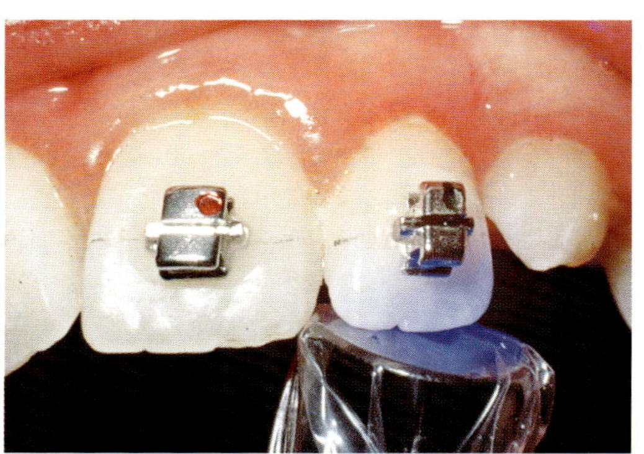

Fig 9-4 Light curing of the brackets. When using photopolymerized material, each bracket is light cured for 40 seconds, with care taken not to disturb the cement but to ensure light application to all exposed surfaces of cement. (Courtesy Dr Scott Dillingham.)

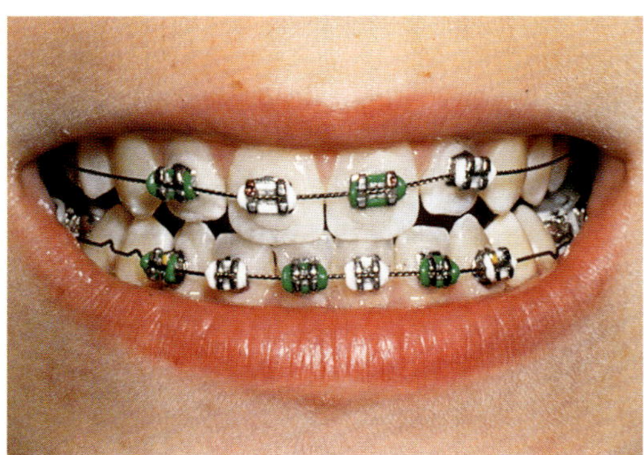

Fig 9-5 Patient with full bracketing bonded with a photopolymerized resin-modified glass-ionomer orthodontic cement. (Courtesy Dr Scott Dillingham.)

treatment, 8.1% (Ketac-Cem) and 6.3% (resin) of the examined surfaces were classified as having white spots, and mean treatment time was 22 months. One year later, white spot incidence was reduced for both bonding agents. At 2 years, the incidence of demineralized surfaces was less for glass-ionomer (16%) compared with resin (29%), but for both groups white spots were significantly more frequent than before orthodontic treatment. In an in vivo caries model[39] with specially designed bands to create a serious cariogenic challenge, no visual white spots were seen after 4 weeks. Microradiographic data of the extracted teeth, however, showed a significant reduction in early lesion development under a glass-ionomer cement.

Thus, investigations have shown that fluoride released from glass-ionomer cements contributes substantially to reducing demineralization but cannot provide complete caries protection. An alternative material approach, the addition of fluoride to resin composite bonding agents, has been shown to have little effect on the incidence of demineralization in some studies,[42,43] but therapeutic effects in others.[44,45] Where caries reduction was recorded, it was suggested that the effect was most likely due to a localized concentration of fluoride rather than to an elevation of fluoride levels in saliva.[45] The presence of glass-ionomer restorations has been shown to increase the amount of fluoride in saliva,[46] but no information involving luting use is available.

The percentage of *Mutans streptococci* in plaque adjacent to orthodontic brackets cemented with a glass-ionomer cement has been shown to be less than that adjacent to brackets retained with resin over a period of just less than 10 months.[41] Although the results in this small clinical trial using 11 patients were not significantly different, further microbiological research is indicated. The authors suggested that in patients with relatively high pretreatment salivary levels of *Mutans streptococci*, and especially those who harbor *S sobrinus*, the use of glass-ionomer cement for bonding may prevent incipient caries formation because lesions formed adjacent only to resin-retained brackets in subjects with *S sobrinus.*

Less demineralization and white spot formation also was reported when resin-modified glass-ionomer cements were used for orthodontic bonding during a 4-week trial period in vivo.[47] Results with a polyacid-modified resin, however, showed no significant difference from those with a conventional bonding resin. Using a tri-cured resin-modified glass-ionomer material specifically designed for orthodontic bonding, Silverman et al[24] reported no visual demineralization over approximately 8 months.

The clinical evidence for glass-ionomers' potential to provide protection from demineralization is still sparse, and white spot occurrence is not eliminated by their use. The in vitro studies, although providing evidence of substantial reduction in demineralization adjacent to glass-ionomer materials, still do not show complete caries protection. Use of a glass-ionomer for band or bracket cementation therefore does not preclude the need for well-fitting bands and careful monitoring for retention, nor the need for good patient oral hygiene and other caries prevention treatment modalities throughout orthodontic therapy. The potential for appropriate orthodontic resin-modified glass-ionomer bracket bonding materials to provide reduced demineralization, fewer cleanup problems, and predictable retention is promising. Carefully designed, longer term studies with more patients will be necessary to prove these advantages.

Summary

Conventional glass-ionomers show proven benefit over zinc phosphate cement for orthodontic band cementation. Clinical retention rates are significantly higher and the incidence of demineralization around the bands is reported to be lower. Handling properties are good; the cement shows a greater tendency to attach to enamel surfaces, which is considered protective if the band should loosen; and cleanup is relatively easy. Whether resin-modified glass-ionomer cements will provide additional advantages for orthodontic band cementation remains to be assessed, but results to date show similar efficacy. With regard to orthodontic bracket bonding, clinical studies provide little support for the routine use of conventional glass-ionomer luting cement due to unacceptably high debonding rates. Newly formulated resin-reinforced glass-ionomer orthodontic cements, however, show considerable potential to provide predictable bonding without the debonding difficulties associated with resin-bonded brackets, shorter cleanup time, and the possibility of fewer demineralization problems.

References

1. Fricker JP, McLachlan MD. Clinical studies of glass-ionomer cements—part 1, a twelve-month clinical study comparing zinc-phosphate cement to glass ionomer. Aust Orthod J 1985;9:179–180.

2. Fricker JP, McLachlan MD. Clinical studies of glass-ionomer cements—part 2, a two-year clinical study comparing glass-ionomer cement with zinc phosphate cement. Aust Orthod J 1987;10:12–14.

3. Mizrahi E. Glass ionomer cements in orthodontics—an update. Am J Orthod Dentofacial Orthop 1988;93:305–307.

4. Maijer R, Smith DC. A comparison between zinc-phosphate and glass-ionomer cement in orthodontics. Am J Orthod Dentofacial Orthop 1988;93:273–279.

5. Stirrup DR. A comparative clinical trial of a glass-ionomer and a zinc-phosphate cement for securing orthodontic bands. Br J Orthod 1991;18:15–20.

6. Fricker JP. A 12-month clinical study comparing four glass-ionomer cements for the cementation of orthodontic molar bands. Aust Orthod J 1989;11:10–13.

7. Fricker JP. A clinical comparison of different powder:liquid ratios of two glass-ionomer cements on the retention of orthodontic molar bands. Aust Orthod J 1989;11:89–92.

8. Norris DS, McInnes-Ledoux P, Schwanginger B, Weinberg R. Retention of orthodontic bands with new fluoride-releasing cements. Am J Orthod 1986;89:206–211.

9. Seeholzer HW, Dasch W. Bonding with a glass-ionomer cement. J Clin Orthod 1986;22:165–169.

10. Momoi Y, Hirosaki K, Kohno A, McCabe JF. Flexural properties of resin-modified "hybrid" glass-ionomers in comparison with conventional acid-base glass ionomers. Dent Mater J 1995;14:109–119.

11. Mongolnam P, Tyas MT. Light-cured lining materials: A laboratory study. Dent Mater 1994;10:196–202.

12. Phijaisanit P, Tyas MT. Comparison of the shear bond strength of a so-called "dual-cured glass-ionomer cement" and a conventional resin

composite used in orthodontic bonding. Aust J Orthod 1997;15:23–29.

13. Subenberger U, Cacciafesta V, Jost-Brinkman PG. Shear bond strengths of brackets bonded with light-cured glass-ionomers. Eur J Orthod 1996; 18:543 [abstract 101].

14. Cacciafesta V, Subenberger U, Jost-Brinkman PG. Shear bond strengths of ceramic brackets bonded with light-cured glass-ionomers. Eur J Orthod 1996;18:512 [abstract 17].

15. Fricker JP. A 12 month clinical comparison of resin-modified light-activated adhesives for the cementation of orthodontic molar bands Am J Orthod Dentofacial Orthop 1997;112:239–243.

16. Millett DT, McCabe JF, Bennett TG, Carter NE, Gordon PH. The effect of sandblasting on the retention of first molar orthodontic bands cemented with glass-ionomer cement. Br J Orthod 1995;22:161–169.

17. O'Reilly MM, Featherstone JDB. Demineralization and remineralization around orthodontic appliances: An in vivo study. Am J Orthod Dentofacial Orthop 1987;92:33–60.

18. Kusy RP. When is stronger better? [letter to the editor]. Am J Orthod Dentofacial Orthop 1994;106:17A.

19. Fricker JP. A 12-month clinical evaluation of a glass-polyalkenoate cement for direct bonding of orthodontic brackets. Am J Orthod Dentofacial Orthop 1992;101:381–384.

20. Norevall L-I, Marcusson A, Persson M. A clinical evaluation of glass-ionomer cement as an orthodontic bonding adhesive compared with an acrylic resin. Eur J Orthod 1996;18:373–384.

21. Voss A, Hickel R, Molkner S. In vivo bonding of orthodontic brackets with glass-ionomer cement. Angle Orthod 1993;63:149–153.

22. Joseph VP, Roussouw E. The shear bond strength of stainless steel and ceramic brackets used with chemical and light-activated composite resins. Am J Orthod Dentofacial Orthop 1990; 97:121–125.

23. White LW. Glass-ionomer cement. J Clin Orthod 1986;20:387–391.

24. Silverman E, Cohen M, Demke RS, Silverman M. A new light-cured glass-ionomer cement that bonds brackets to teeth without etching in the presence of saliva. Am J Orthod Dentofacial Orthop 1995;108:231–236.

25. McCourt JW, Cooley RL, Barnwell S. Bond strength of light-cured fluoride-releasing base-liners as orthodontic bracket adhesives. Am J Orthod Dentofacial Orthop 1991;100:47–52.

26. Millett DT, McCabe J. Orthodontic bonding with glass-ionomer cement—a review. Eur J Orthod 1996;18:385–399.

27. Cook PA, Luther F, Youngson CC. An in vitro study of the bond strength of light-cured glass-ionomer cement in the bonding of orthodontic brackets. Eur J Orthod 1996;18:199–204.

28. Jobalia SB, Valente RM, de Rijk W, BeGole EA, Evans CA. Bond strength of visible light-cured glass-ionomer orthodontic cement. Am J Orthod Dentofacial Orthop 1997;112:205–208.

29. Ashcroft DB, Staley RN, Jakobsen MA. Fluoride release and shear bond strengths of three light-cured glass-ionomer cements. Am J Orthod Dentofacial Orthop 1997;111:260–265.

30. Komori A, Ishikawa H. Evaluation of a resin-reinforced glass ionomer cement for use as an orthodontic bonding agent. Angle Orthod 1997;67:189–196.

31. Ewoldsen N, Beatty MW, Erickson L, Feely D. Effects of enamel conditioning on bond strength with a restorative light-cured glass-ionomer. J Clin Orthod 1996;29:621–624.

32. Fricker JP. A 12 month clinical evaluation of a light activated glass-polyalkenoate (ionomer) cement for the direct bonding of orthodontic brackets. Am J Orthod Dentofacial Orthop 1994;105:502–505.

33. Hallgren A, Oliveby A, Twetman S. Caries associated microflora in plaque from orthodontic appliances retained with glass-ionomer cement. Scand J Dent Res 1992;100:140–143.

34. Øgaard B, Rölla G, Arends J. Orthodontic appliances and enamel demineralization, part 1: Lesion development. Am J Orthod Dentofacial Orthop 1988;94:68–73.

35. Gorelick L, Geiger AM, Gwinnett AJ. Incidence of white spot formation after bonding and banding. Am J Orthod 1982;81:93–98.

36. Øgaard B. Prevalence of white spot lesions in 19-year-olds: A study on untreated and orthodontically treated persons 5 years after treatment. Am J Orthod Dentofacial Orthop 1989;96:423–427.

37. Banks PA, Richmond S. Enamel sealants: A clinical evaluation of their value during fixed appliance therapy. Eur J Orthod 1994;16:19–25.

38. Kvam E, Broch J, Nissen-Meyer IH. Comparison between a zinc-phosphate cement and a glass-ionomer cement for cementation of orthodontic bands. Eur J Orthod 1983;5:307–313.

39. Rezk-Lega F, Øgaard B, Arends J. An in-vivo study on the merits of two glass-ionomers for the cementation of orthodontic bands. Am J Orthod Dentofacial Orthop 1991;99:162–167.

40. Marcusson A, Norevall LI, Persson M. White spot reduction when using glass-ionomer cement for bonding in orthodontics: A longitudinal and comparative study. Eur J Orthod 1997;19:233–242.

41. Ortendahl T, Thilander B, Svanberg M. *Mutans streptococci* and incipient caries adjacent to glass-ionomer cement or resin-based composite in orthodontics. Am J Orthod Dentofacial Orthop 1997;112:271.

42. Mitchell L. An investigation into the effect of a fluoride releasing adhesive on the prevalence of enamel surface changes associated with directly bonded orthodontic attachments. Br J Orthod 1992;19:207–214.

43. Banks PA, Burn A, O'Brien K. A clinical evaluation of the effectiveness of including fluoride into an orthodontic bonding adhesive. Eur J Orthod 1997;19:391–395.

44. Sonis AL, Snell W. An evaluation of a fluoride-releasing visible light-activated bonding system for orthodontic bracket placement. Am J Orthod Dentofacial Orthop 1989;95:306–311.

45. Øgaard B, Arends J, Helseth H, Dijkman G, van der Kuiji M. Fluoride level in saliva after bonding orthodontic brackets with a fluoride containing adhesive. Am J Orthod Dentofacial Orthop 1997;111:199–202.

46. Hatibovic-Kofman S, Koch G. Fluoride release from glass-ionomer in vivo and in vitro. Swed Dent J 1991;15:253–258.

47. Chung CK, Millett DT, Creanor SL. Cariostatic ability of resin-modified glass-ionomer cements for orthodontic bonding. Eur J Orthod 1996;18:513 [abstract 21].

Chapter 10

Application of Glass-Ionomer Cements in Endodontics

Shimon Friedman

Glass-ionomer cements have been used in endodontics for sealing root canals orthogradely and retrogradely, for sealing and restoring the pulp chamber, for repairing perforations, and, rarely, for treating vertically fractured teeth. These applications, which evolved in the 1980s and 1990s, share their rationale with the more common application of glass-ionomer cement as a restorative material and a luting cement. Thus, glass-ionomer cement is used in endodontics for its capacity to bond to dentin, its good biocompatibility, and its fluoride release. The first property is expected to enhance the seal and reinforce the tooth, the second to minimize the irritation of the periradicular tissues, and the third to impart an antimicrobial effect to combat root canal infection.

This chapter reviews the most recent data regarding the various applications of glass-ionomer cements in endodontics. Basic information on the properties of glass-ionomer cement is given in earlier chapters in this text.

Root Canal Sealing

The outcome of root canal treatment critically depends on the elimination of existing root canal infection and the long-term prevention of reinfection.[1] In many cases, the root canal cannot be disinfected predictably using conventional intracanal procedures.[2,3] There may be an advantage, therefore, in filling the canal with materials that can eliminate or curtail the residual microorganisms.[4] Such materials also may resist the ingress of microorganisms and prevent reinfection.

The root canal, being normally free of salivary or blood contamination, is an ideal environment for the placement of glass-ionomer cement. The concept of using this cement as a root canal sealer was first introduced by Pitt Ford.[5] Using a commercially available restorative material in conjunction with silver cones, he observed that the material set too quickly to allow application in conjunction with condensed gutta-percha. To extend the working time, Stewart[6] mixed together two formulations of glass-ionomer cement, then added barium sulfate to in-

Figs 10-1a and 10-1b Radiographs of a mandibular first molar treated with a glass-ionomer cement sealer and single gutta-percha cones.

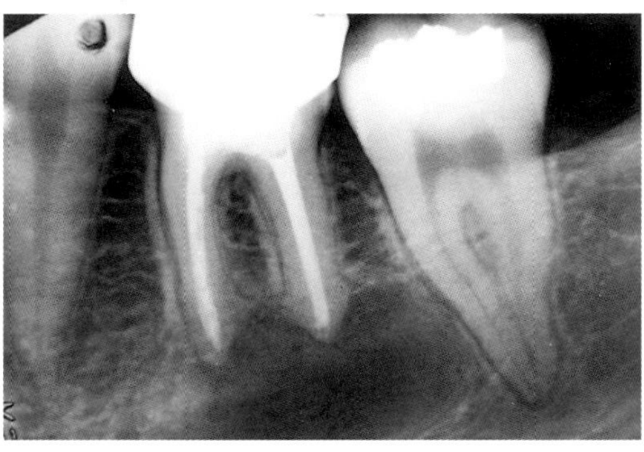

Fig 10-1a Immediate postoperative view shows an extensive periapical pathosis.

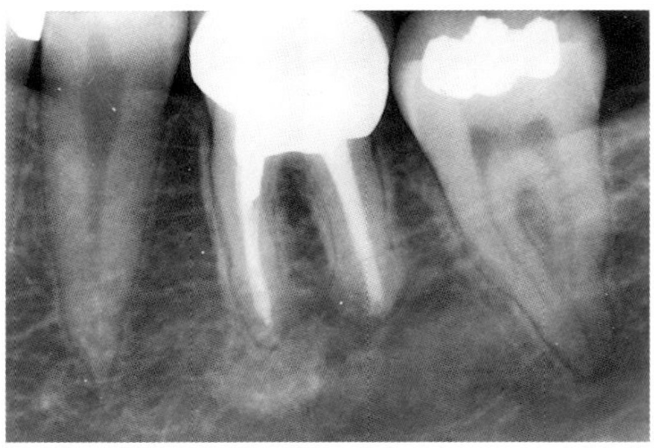

Fig 10-1b Three-year follow-up shows complete healing of the lesion, along with development of condensing osteitis at the mesial root tip.

crease the radiopacity. Ray and Seltzer[7] filled root canals entirely with a modified glass-ionomer cement and concluded that it was easy to use, was adequately radiopaque, and adapted closely to the canal wall. This material was later introduced commercially (Ketac-Endo), and to date it is the sole glass-ionomer cement available specifically as a root canal sealer. Similarly, Saunders et al[8] used a resin-based glass-ionomer cement (Vitrebond) as a root canal sealer in conjunction with gutta-percha and found it adapted closely to the canal wall. In addition, Trope and Ray[9] reported that roots filled with a glass-ionomer cement had an increased resistance to vertical fracture. All these early reports formed the basis for the use of glass-ionomer cement as a root canal sealer in endodontic therapy (Fig 10-1).

Retreatability and removal

Any material used for root canal filling has to allow retreatment of the canal.[10] For this reason, the glass-ionomer cement sealer is placed in conjunction with a gutta-percha core. Retreatment is facilitated by dissolving the gutta-percha and using ultrasonic vibration in the canal to disperse the cement.[11–13] In a series of in vitro studies, glass-ionomer cement was slower to retreat than conventional sealers; however, it could be removed effectively without an excessive amount of residue attached to the canal walls (Fig 10-2).[11–13] Partial removal of the root filling, for preparation of a post space, also is somewhat slower in canals filled with glass-ionomer cement than in those filled with other sealers.[14]

Sealing efficacy

Since the introduction of glass-ionomer cement as a root canal sealer, its sealing efficacy has been the subject of many in vitro studies employing different methodologies. The results of these studies are diverse and inconclusive, and their clinical relevance questionable.[15,16] In a few studies, the seal provided by the glass-ionomer cement was poor[17–21]; however, in the majority it was comparable to the seal provided by conventional sealers[22–33] or better.[34] The seal may be improved by using the cement in conjunction with condensed gutta-percha rather than with a single gutta-percha cone,[34,35] but this suggestion has been disputed.[21,32,33] As with all other root canal sealers, the seal appears to be conversely related to the thickness of the sealer layer.[26,28,30,36] Possibly, when applied in bulk, the shrinkage of the glass-ionomer cement undermines the seal of the root canal space.[17]

Recently, Friedman et al[37] introduced an animal model designed to assess the resistance of root fillings to bacterial ingress from an inoculated pulp chamber. Such evaluation closely simulates clinical conditions and is considered more relevant than evaluations in vitro. When tested with this model, an experimental glass-ionomer cement sealer performed better than a conventional sealer of a zinc-oxide–eugenol type.[38]

Antimicrobial efficacy

The antimicrobial activity of glass-ionomer cement is believed to result from the release of fluoride. The uptake of fluoride by the root canal dentin has been studied by Saunders et al.[8] Using a resin-based glass-ionomer cement as a sealer, these researchers observed a variable degree of increase in fluoride in the dentin after periods of 2, 4, and 12 weeks.

Several studies have addressed the potential antimicrobial efficacy of glass-ionomer cement sealers. In the agar diffusion test, two glass-ionomer cements demonstrated a strong antimicrobial effect when freshly mixed[39,40] and after 48 hours.[41] In this short time frame, the antimicrobial efficacy of these cements was better than that of several conventional sealers.[39–41] In a direct contact test, the short-term antimicrobial efficacy of a glass-ionomer cement was comparable to that of a zinc-oxide–eugenol sealer; however, within 1 week it diminished considerably.[40] In another study, an experimental glass-ionomer cement sealer failed to suppress the growth of microorganisms on its surface.[42] In a model designed to assess the antimicrobial effect of materials within the dentinal tubules of bovine teeth, a glass-ionomer cement sealer had no effect within the first 24 hours.[4] After 7 days, however, some antimicrobial effect was evident, although considerably less than that of other sealers.[4]

Adhesion

The adhesion of glass-ionomer cement sealer to the canal wall dentin has not been thoroughly investigated. Initial reports demonstrated close adaptation.[7,8] Apparently, the interface of the sealer and the canal wall is influenced by the various endodontic irrigants and medicaments used prior to root filling. However, the nature of this influence is the subject of controversy. When the smear layer was

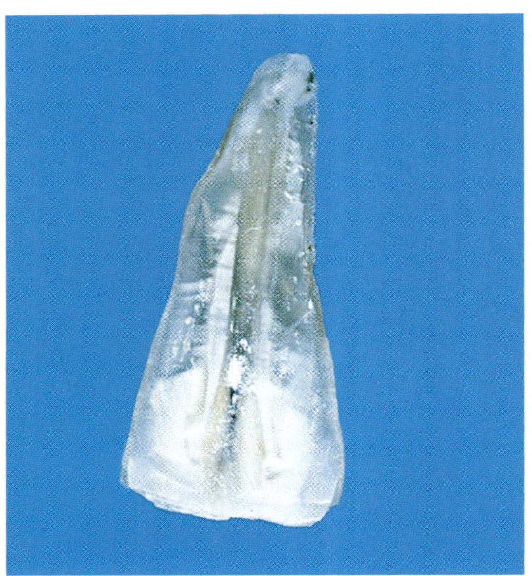

Fig 10-2 Photomicrograph of a split root after retreatment. The root canal was originally filled with glass-ionomer cement and a gutta-percha cone. Little residue of the root filling materials remains attached to the canal wall.

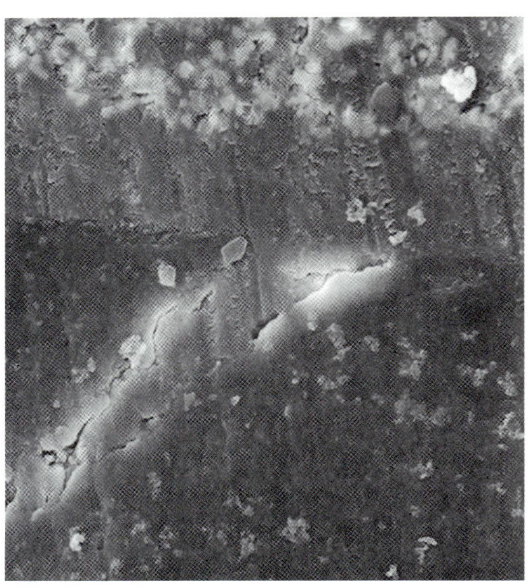

Fig 10-3 Scanning electron micrograph of the interface between a glass-ionomer cement sealer *(top)* and bovine dentin *(bottom)* conditioned with sodium hypochlorite. A hybrid layer is evident at the interface between the sealer and the dentin. (Courtesy of Lalh et al[46] and the Journal of Endodontics.)

removed, tags of the glass-ionomer cement were observed penetrating into the dentinal tubules,[8] but to a lesser degree than with other sealers.[27] Penetration of the filling material into the tubules is believed to improve the seal. Indeed, canals sealed with glass-ionomer cement after removal of the smear layer, demonstrated less leakage in vitro than those in which the smear layer was not removed.[24,29,32] However, in other studies, removal of the smear layer did not appear to affect the seal.[25,43,44] In fact, one study reported the seal was better with the smear layer present.[27]

A recent investigation assessed the bond strength of two glass-ionomer cement sealers to bovine dentin conditioned with the common endodontic irrigants.[45,46] The bond was weakest when the dentin was rinsed with 17% ethylenediaminetetraacetic acid (EDTA) to remove the smear layer.[45] When the dentin was rinsed only with sodium hypochlorite, a hybrid layer was observed in the cement–dentin interface, which may have contributed to the strength of the bond[46] (Fig 10-3).

Biocompatibility

Although it is widely accepted that glass-ionomer cement is biocompatible, several studies specifically assessed the biocompatibility of glass-ionomer cement sealers. In a comprehensive evaluation, Jonck et

Figs 10-4a to 10-4c Radiographs of maxillary incisors treated with a glass-ionomer cement sealer and single gutta-percha cones.

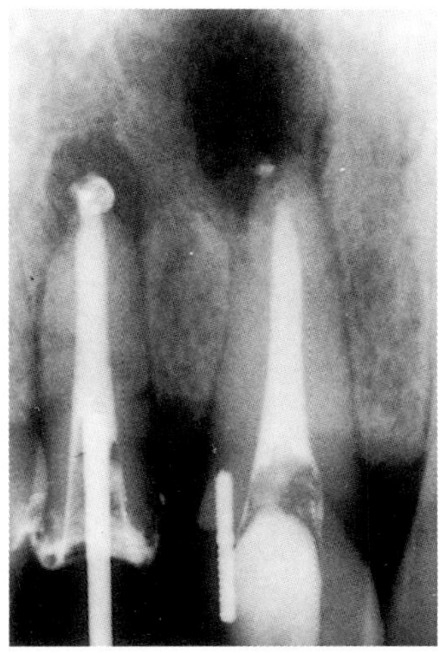

Fig 10-4a Immediate postoperative view shows periapical pathoses and extrusion of small amounts of the sealer.

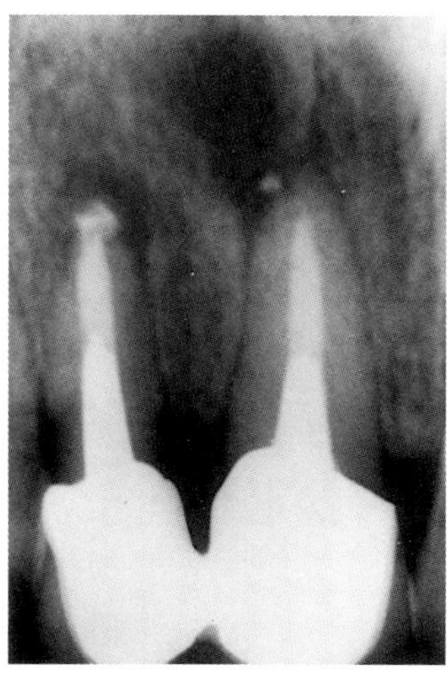

Fig 10-4b Six-month follow-up shows incomplete healing of the lesions without absorption of the extruded sealer.

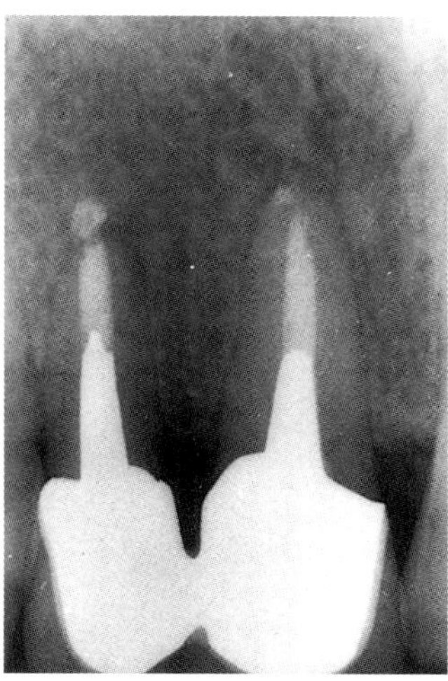

Fig 10-4c Three-year follow-up shows complete healing of both lesions, but still no absorption of the extruded sealer.

al[47,48] demonstrated excellent bone tolerance of experimental glass-ionomer cements, including a root canal sealer and a bone cement used in orthopedic surgery. The biocompatibility of the glass-ionomer sealer also was confirmed in the subcutaneous connective tissue.[49]

Clinical efficacy

To date, only one clinical study has been reported on the outcome of endodontic therapy using a glass-ionomer cement sealer.[50] The results of this study were influenced by the nature of the cases treated, many of which had been complicated by a variety of factors known to lower the prognosis of treatment, and by the criteria used for assessment of the outcomes.[50] Nevertheless, the reported rates of 78% success and only 6% failure are well within the range of those reported in many other studies in which conventional sealers were used.[1,50] One of the observations in the clinical study was that the glass-ionomer cement persisted in the tissues when extruded periapically (Fig 10-4), in contrast to other sealers which are normally absorbed within a relatively short period of time.[51] The persistence of the glass-ionomer sealer in the periradicular tissues confirms its very low tissue solubility, as well as its biocompatibility in the osseous environment.[47,48]

Figs 10-5a to 10-5c Radiographs of a maxillary lateral incisor with a glass-ionomer cement retrograde filling.

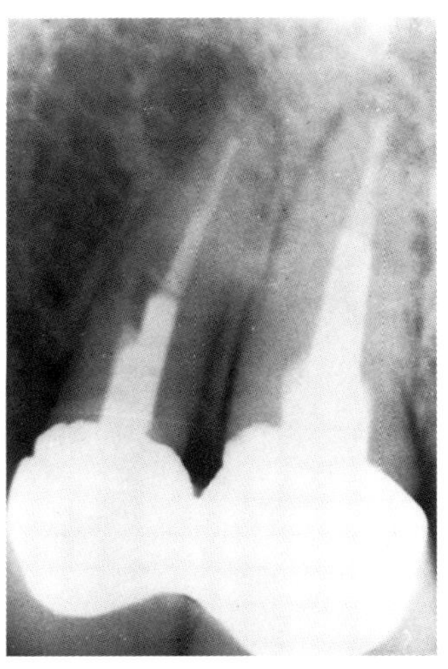

Fig 10-5a Preoperative view shows a periapical pathosis due to root canal infection. Retreatment was considered unfeasible because of the restoration and suspected perforation.

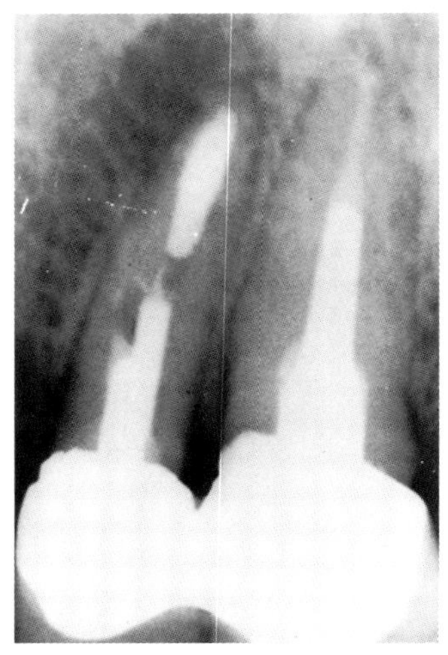

Fig 10-5b Immediate postoperative view shows the retrograde filling and extent of the periapical bone cavity.

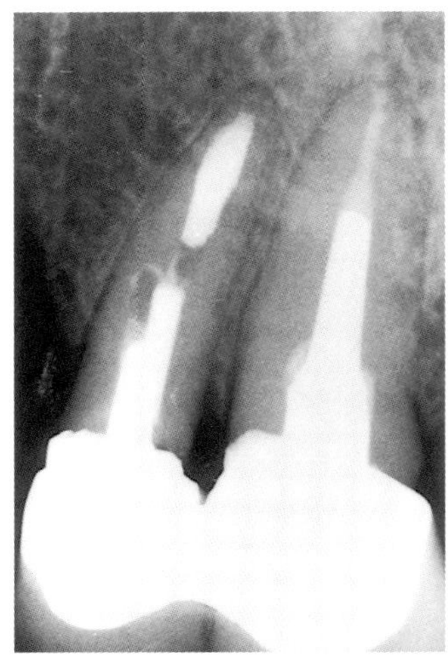

Fig 10-5c Three-year follow-up shows complete healing of the lesion and confirms that the retrograde filling effectively sealed the infected root canal.

Retrograde Root Canal Filling

A retrograde filling is placed to provide an apical seal in teeth with infected canals that cannot be accessed or negotiated coronally. Because the canal remains infected, the quality of the retrograde seal determines the outcome of the treatment (Fig 10-5). In this application, short working and setting times are not an impediment; in fact, they may be an advantage. Therefore, glass-ionomer cements used routinely for restorative applications were considered for retrograde filling long before a specific glass-ionomer sealer was developed. Consequently, studies have evaluated conventional glass-ionomer cements, as well as resin-based and silver-containing formulations. The main obstacle in the clinical application of glass-ionomers as retrograde filling materials is the difficulty of controlling the dryness of the surgical working field. On the other hand, in contrast to conventional cavity-retained retrograde fillings, the bonding of the glass-ionomer cement to the root dentin allows its application as a bonded cap over the resected root surface to improve the seal (Fig 10-6).

Figs 10-6a to 10-6c Radiographs of a mandibular first molar treated with a glass-ionomer cement apical cap.

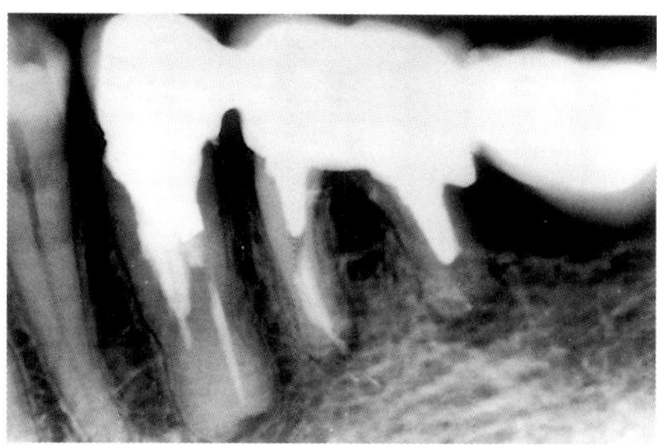

Fig 10-6a Preoperative view shows a periapical pathosis at the distal root due to root canal infection. Retreatment was considered unfeasible because of the extensive restoration.

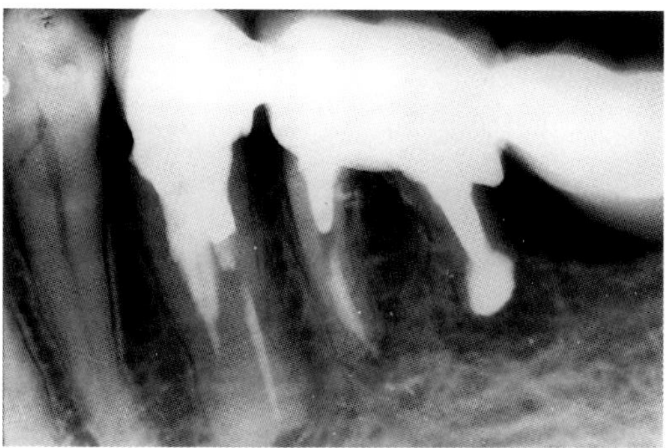

Fig 10-6b Immediate postoperative view shows the apical cap and extent of the periapical bone cavity.

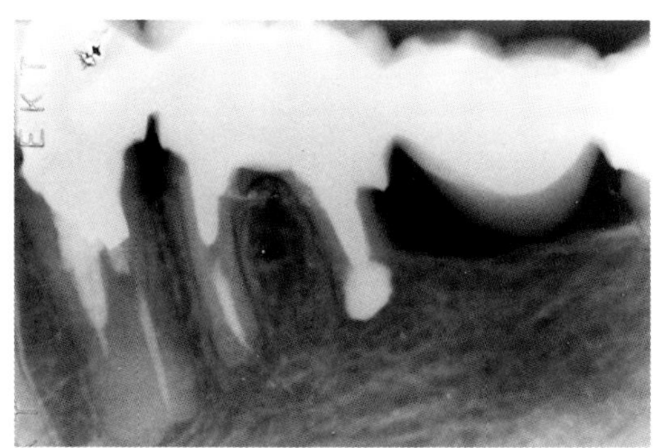

Fig 10-6c Four-month follow-up shows complete healing of the lesion, which confirms that the apical cap effectively sealed the infected root canal.

Sealing efficacy

Many in vitro studies have compared various formulations of glass-ionomer cement, with and without varnish, to other retrograde filling materials, mainly amalgam (Fig 10-7).[52] Contradictions among these studies and the limitations of their methodologies do not warrant a clear conclusion; however, the overall performance of glass-ionomer cement in earlier leakage studies was better than that of other materials, with the exception of resin composite.[52]

Several of the later studies also demonstrated minimal leakage with glass-ionomer retrograde fillings,[53–58] particularly when it was applied in conjunction with

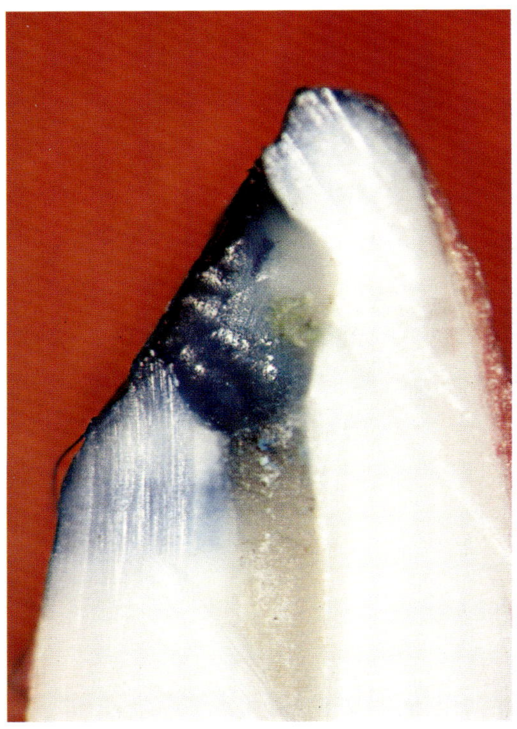

Fig 10-7 Photomicrograph of a split root of a canine tooth tested for apical dye leakage. The root canal was originally sealed with an amalgam retrograde filling for a period of 6 months. The filling was dislodged to demonstrate the amount of dye penetration.

varnish.[59,60] Other studies failed to demonstrate a better seal with glass-ionomers,[61–64] or even observed a poorer seal than that achieved with other materials.[65,66] When the different formulations of glass-ionomer cement were compared with each other, the resin-modified material demonstrated a better seal than the conventional cement, and both were better than a silver-containing material.[67]

Biocompatibility

When glass-ionomer cement is used as a retrograde filling, it is expected to come into direct contact with the healing alveolar bone, as opposed to when it is used as a restorative that interacts with the dentin, pulp, and gingiva. As healing takes place after apical surgery, deposition of mineralized tissue is expected to occur over the resected root surface and the retrograde filling.[68,69] Accordingly, several studies have focused on the interaction between glass-ionomer cements and bone. From bone implantation studies, it appears that the different types of glass-ionomer cement are well tolerated by bone.[47,48,70–73] However, the interpretation and correlation of results obtained in such studies is problematic.[74] The more clinically relevant usage studies, in which functioning retrograde fillings interact with the surrounding tissues, also have confirmed the compatibility of glass-ionomer cement with bone.[75–78] Due to this compatibility, bone

Figs 10-8a and 10-8b Radiographs of mandibular premolars of a dog with infected root canals, 6 months after retrograde filling with glass-ionomer cement. Some roots demonstrate periapical lesions, suggesting that the fillings failed to seal the infected root canals.

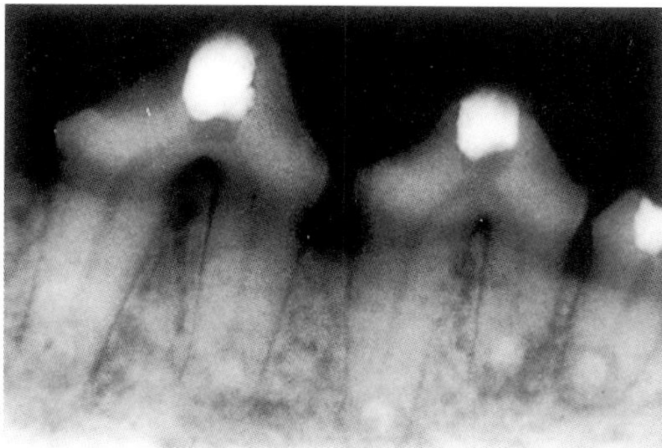

Fig 10-8a Right quadrant.

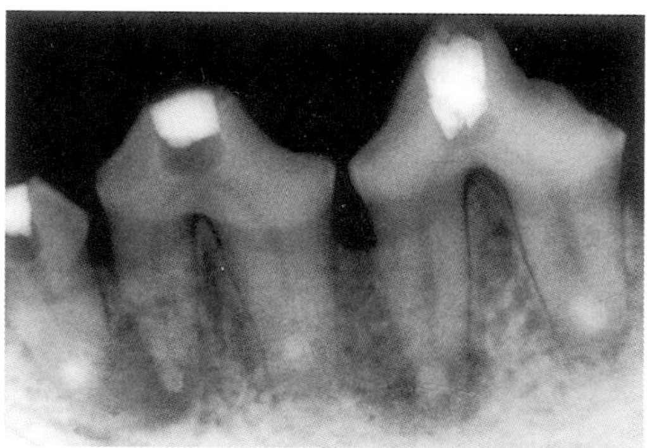

Fig 10-8b Left quadrant.

can grow directly over the glass ionomer, without an interface of connective or inflammatory tissue.[47,48,73]

Clinical efficacy

Zetterqvist et al[79] and later Jesslén et al[80] assessed the long-term outcome of apicoectomy relying on retrograde filling with glass-ionomer cement or amalgam. Using clinical and radiographic criteria to assess healing, these researchers demonstrated comparable results for the two materials. Thus, glass-ionomer cement proved to be an acceptable retrograde filling material, and it did not appear to be affected by the wet environment of surgery.[80]

Assessment of the clinical efficacy of a retrograde filling material in a clinical study is difficult due to multiple factors that may influence the outcome of the treatment. To minimize the variables, Friedman et al[81] assessed the efficacy of retrograde filling materials in an animal model. The root canals, deliberately infected to induce periapical pathosis, were sealed by retrograde fillings and periapical healing was examined several months later (Fig 10-8). The reported performance of glass-ionomer cement in studies based on this model has been comparable to that of amalgam,[81–83] but somewhat poorer than that of zinc oxide–eugenol cements.[82] These results contrast the failure of glass-ionomer cement to seal infected canals in an earlier study.[84]

Figs 10-9a and 10-9b Radiographs of a mandibular first molar with a perforation in the distal root repaired with glass-ionomer cement. (Courtesy of Fuss and Trope[85] and Endodontics and Dental Traumatology.)

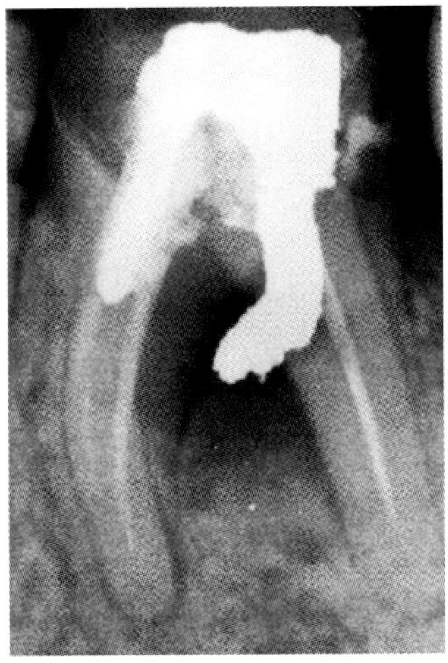

Fig 10-9a Preoperative view shows amalgam originally used to seal the perforation extruded into the furcation area, and extensive bone loss in the area.

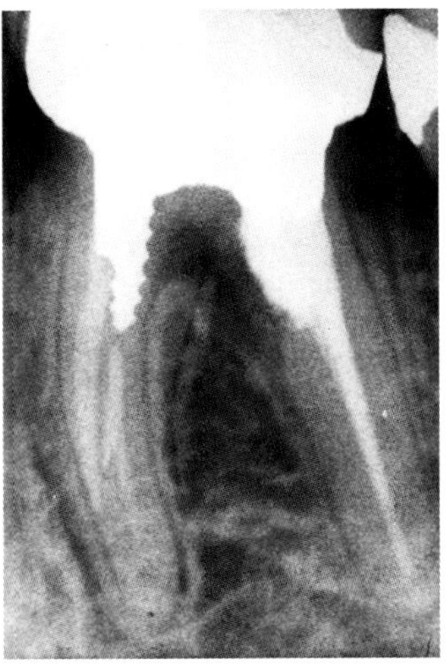

Fig 10-9b Thirty-month follow-up after perforation repair and root canal retreatment shows complete healing of the bone in the furcation.

Perforation Repair

The prognosis of perforation repair depends primarily on the ability to eliminate the pathway of the periradicular infection.[85] Secondary factors include the healing potential of the periradicular tissues, which is related to the duration of the perforation, its size and location, and the tissue compatibility of the repair material.[85] Thus, the material used for perforation repair should possess good sealing, antimicrobial, and biocompatibility properties. The prevalence of perforations in endodontically treated teeth is under 10%.[85] Because a variety of materials have been used for the repair of perforations, only limited information is available on the suitability and efficacy of glass-ionomer cements applied in this capacity.

Although of limited clinical relevance, several in vitro leakage studies have tested the seal of repaired perforations. With the exception of one study,[86] they support the suitability of glass-ionomer cement for this application.[87–92] Another in vitro study demonstrated the potential of a glass-ionomer root canal sealer to stimulate osteoblastic activity in cell culture.[93] In a well-documented case report, Goon and Lundergan[94] demonstrated the successful repair of a perforation with a glass-ionomer sealer after previous treatment attempts with gutta-percha and guided tissue regeneration had failed. Additional cases of successful perforation repair with glass-ionomer cement were reported by Fuss and Trope[85] (Fig 10-9). From the reported cases it appears that glass-ionomer cement is well suited for perforation repair in a variety of clinical situations.[85,95]

Glass-ionomer cement also can be applied over dentin in near-perforation situations to prevent potential infection of the periradicular tissues. In these situations, the glass-ionomer cement substitutes for the lost dentin (Fig 10-10).

Treatment of Vertical Fractures

Repair attempts of vertically fractured teeth are rare. The pathogenic mechanism of vertical fractures is through the propagation of intraoral microorganisms and the resulting bone loss along the fracture line.[96] Accordingly, treatment attempts should be directed toward the elimination of the fracture line as a pathway for microbial propagation, while maintaining a biocompatible environment for reattachment of the periradicular tissues. For teeth that are completely fractured, bonding the tooth segments together is an additional requirement.

The ability of glass-ionomers to bond split teeth is less than that of bonding agents and cyanoacrylate cement.[97] However, due to its good biocompatibility, glass-ionomer cement has been considered the material of choice for filling the canals of treated fractured teeth,[98] filling the fracture line,[99] and repairing completely fractured teeth.[100]

Stewart[101] filled canals temporarily with calcium hydroxide to combat microorganisms and induce repair of the fracture line by deposition of cementum. After initial healing, the canals were filled with glass-ionomer cement.[98] In the few cases treated in this manner, the teeth were retained for 2 to 10 years.[98,102] Another approach to treatment involves a surgical intervention, during which the fracture line is filled. The few clinical cases reported on incompletely fractured teeth treated in this manner demonstrated a poor outcome for this procedure. At best, the teeth were retained for several months, even when treatment was combined with guided tissue regeneration.[99]

The author is aware of only one report regarding the repair of a completely fractured tooth with glass-ionomer cement, in which the fracture extended to the furcation but not along the roots.[100] This tooth was still functioning 1 year after treatment. In addition, the author has treated two teeth with incomplete root fractures by means of extraction, filling of the fracture line with glass-ionomer cement, and replantation. Both these teeth are still functioning, at 2 and 4 years after treatment (Fig 10-11).

Coronal Sealing After Root Canal Treatment

Even after completion of endodontic treatment, teeth are at risk of reinfection via ingress of microorganisms from the access cavity into the filled canals.[37,38,103,104] The ability of the coronal restoration to prevent bacterial ingress is therefore one of the factors that influence the outcome of treatment.[1] The restorative applications of glass-ionomer cement in general are reviewed in several chapters of this book. There are, however, specific considerations for the application of glass-ionomer cement in conjunction

Figs 10-10a to 10-10d Radiographs of a mandibular first molar with a near-perforation at the pulp chamber floor treated with glass-ionomer cement.

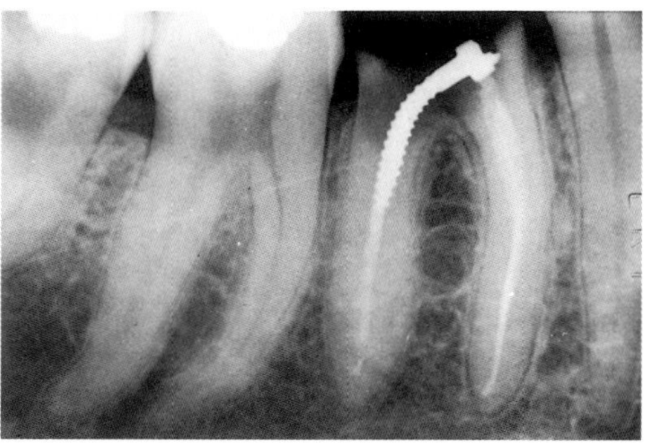

Fig 10-10a Preoperative view shows extension of a carious lesion to the pulp chamber.

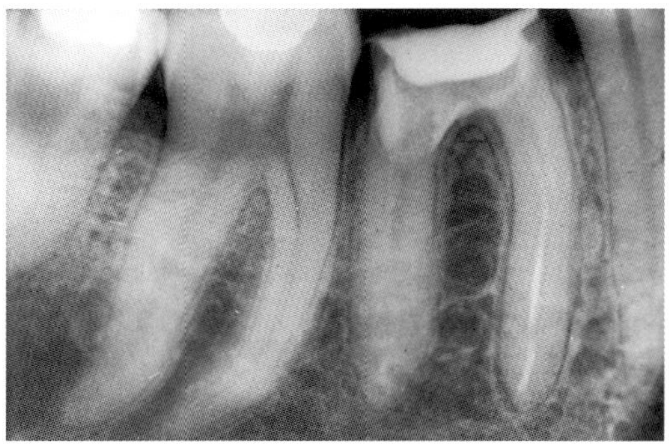

Fig 10-10b Intraoperative view shows application of a resin-modified glass-ionomer cement over the floor and walls of the pulp chamber, after excavation of caries, to protect the bone in the furcation from infection.

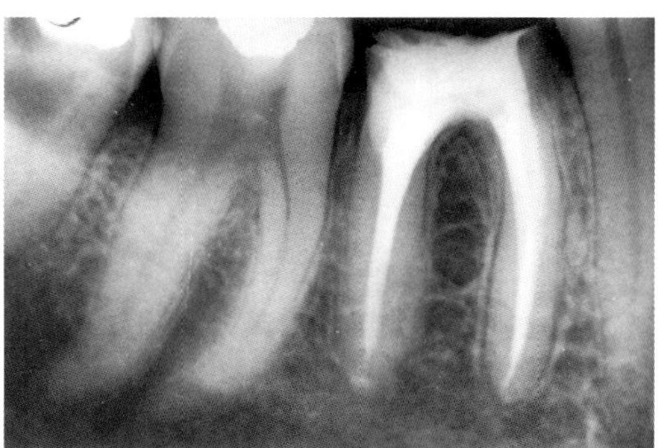

Fig 10-10c Immediate postoperative view shows completion of retreatment and root filling with a glass-ionomer cement sealer and single gutta-percha cones.

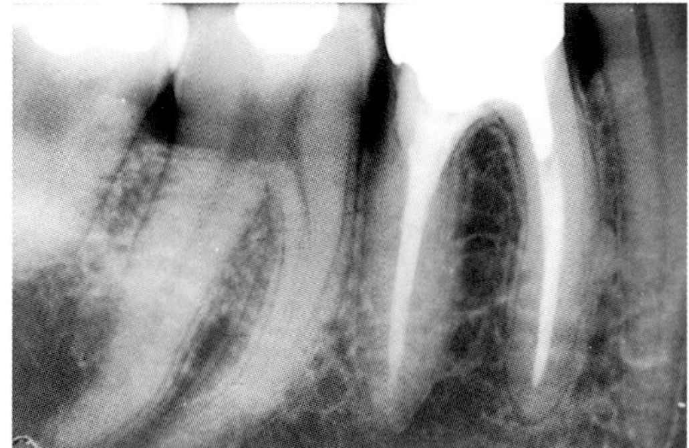

Fig 10-10d Seven-year follow-up shows the post-and-core restoration applied over the cement layer in the pulp chamber. The glass-ionomer serves as a dentin substitute. Periapical and furcation tissues are intact.

Figs 10-11a to 10-11c Radiographs of a vertically fractured maxillary premolar repaired with glass-ionomer cement prior to replantation.

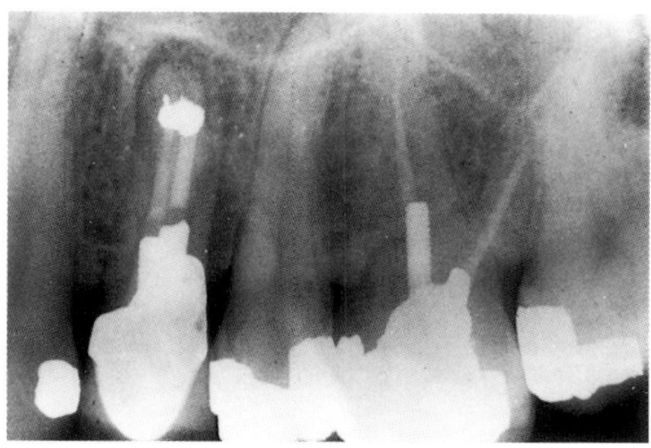

Fig 10-11a Preoperative view shows periapical and distal pathoses. The tooth had retrograde root canal fillings placed 2 years previously. Distal probing revealed a 9-mm periodontal pocket.

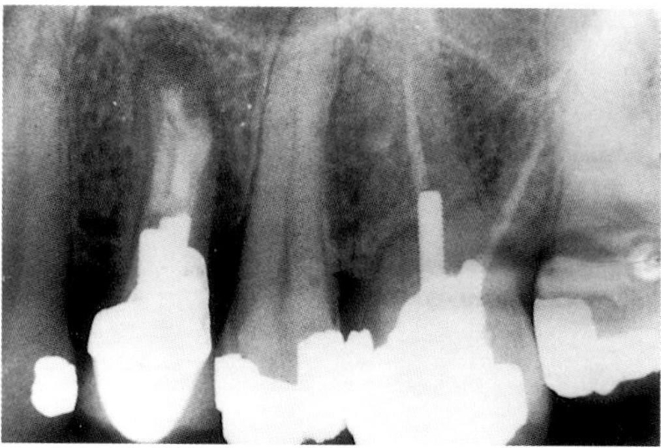

Fig 10-11b Immediate postoperative view. The tooth was extracted, the retrograde cavities refilled, and the vertical fracture line on the distal aspect of the root filled. All fillings were glass-ionomer cement.

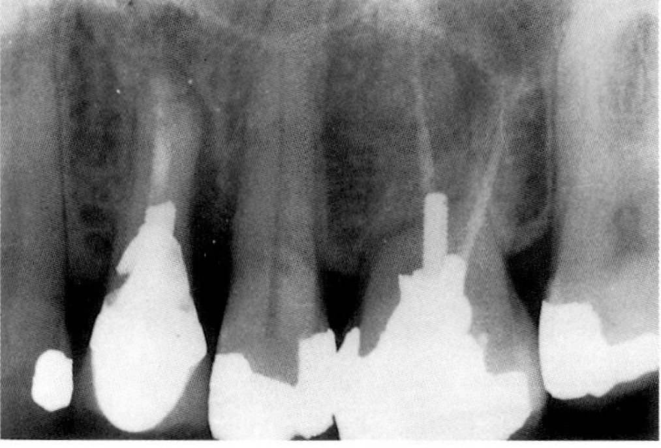

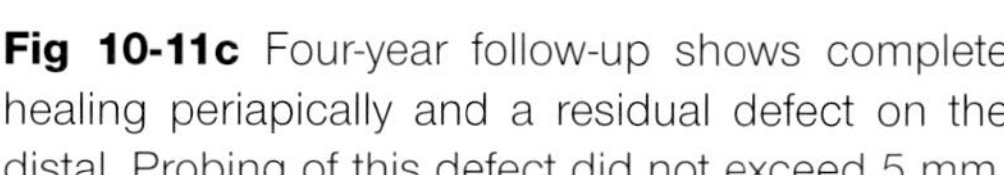

Fig 10-11c Four-year follow-up shows complete healing periapically and a residual defect on the distal. Probing of this defect did not exceed 5 mm.

with the restoration of endodontically treated teeth.

To prevent bacterial ingress into the filled canals, the canal orifices and the floor of the pulp chamber in multirooted teeth can be sealed with a restorative material.[105,106] Again, materials with good sealing properties are best suited for this application; accordingly, they are assessed by means of leakage studies in vitro. In one such study, glass-ionomer cement was found to be inferior to other materials.[105] However, a barrier of resin-modified glass-ionomer cement was effective against microbial ingress into the canals.[106]

Summary

Glass-ionomer cements have been used in endodontics for a variety of applications. Overall, they appear to be well suited for these uses, in which bone and soft tissue compatibility, sealing efficacy, and antimicrobial activity are more critical than tensile strength. Although the results of the numerous in vitro studies of glass-ionomer cement may appear diverse and inconclusive and the antimicrobial activity of glass-ionomer cement may not be optimal, clinical reports and well-designed animal studies have demonstrated acceptable clinical performance of this material in endodontic therapy.

References

1. Friedman S. Treatment outcome and prognosis of endodontic therapy. In: Ørstavik D, Pitt Ford TR (eds). Essential Endodontology. Oxford: Blackwell Science, 1998.

2. Sjögren U, Figdor D, Persson S, Sundqvist G. Influence of infection at the time of root filling on the outcome of endodontic treatment of teeth with apical periodontitis. Int Endod J 1997;30:297–306.

3. Sundqvist G, Figdor D, Persson S, Sjögren U. Microbiologic analysis of teeth with failed endodontic treatment and the outcome of conservative re-treatment. Oral Surg 1998; 85:86–93.

4. Heling I, Chandler NP. The antimicrobial effect within dentinal tubules of four root canal sealers. J Endod 1996;22:257–259.

5. Pitt Ford TR. The leakage of root fillings using glass-ionomer cement and other materials. Br Dent J 1979;146:273–278.

6. Stewart GG. Clinical application of glass-ionomer cements in endodontics: Case reports. Int Endod J 1990;23:172–178.

7. Ray HL, Seltzer S. A new glass ionomer root canal sealer. J Endod 1991;17:598–603.

8. Saunders WP, Saunders EM, Stephens E, Herd D. The use of glass-ionomer as a root canal sealer—a pilot study. Int Endod J 1992;25:238–244.

9. Trope M, Ray HL. Resistance to fracture of endodontically treated roots. Oral Surg 1992; 73:99–102.

10. Nguyen TN. Obturation of the root canal system. In: Cohen S, Burns RC (eds). Pathways of the Pulp. St. Louis: Mosby Year Book, 1991;193–195.

11. Friedman S, Moshonov J, Trope M. Efficacy of removing glass-ionomer cement, zinc oxide eugenol and epoxy resin sealers from retreated root canals. Oral Surg 1992;73:609–612.

12. Friedman S, Moshonov J, Trope M. Residue of gutta-percha and a glass-ionomer cement sealer following root canal retreatment. Int Endod J 1993;26:169–172.

13. Moshonov J, Trope M, Friedman S. Retreatment efficacy 3 months after obturation using glass-ionomer cement, zinc oxide-eugenol, and epoxy resin sealers. J Endod 1994;20:90–92.

14. Raiden G, Posleman I, Peralta G, Olguin A, Lagarrigue G. Dowel space preparation in root canals filled with glass-ionomer cement. J Endod 1998;24:197–198.

15. Wu M-K, Wesselink PR. Endodontic leakage studies reconsidered. Part 1. Methodology, application and relevance. Int Endod J 1993; 26:37–43.

16. Al-Ghamdi A, Wennberg A. Testing of sealing ability of endodontic filling materials. Endod Dent Traumatol 1994;10:249–255.

17. De Gee AJ, Wu M-K, Wesselink PR. Sealing properties of Ketac-Endo glass-ionomer cement and AH26 root canal sealers. Int Endod J 1994;27:239–244.

18. Smith MA, Steiman HR. An in vitro evaluation of microleakage of two new and two old root canal sealers. J Endod 1994;20:18–21.

19. Ahlberg KMF, Assavanop P, Tay WM. A comparison of the apical dye penetration patterns shown by methylene blue and India ink in root-filled teeth. Int Endod J 1995;28:30–34.

20. Horning TG, Kessler LTC Jr. A comparison of three different root canal sealers when used to obturate a moisture-contaminated root canal system. J Endod 1995;21:354–357.

21. Rohde TR, Bramwell JD, Hutter JW, Roahen JO. An in vitro evaluation of microleakage of a new root canal sealer. J Endod 1996;22:365–368.

22. Oguntebi BR, Shen C. Effect of different sealers on thermoplasticized gutta-percha root canal obturations. J Endod 1992;18;363–366.

23. Brown RC, Jackson R, Skidmore AE. An evaluation of apical leakage of glass-ionomer root canal sealer. J Endod 1994;20:288–291.

24. Holland R, Sakashita MS, Murata SS, Junior ED. Effect of dentine surface treatment on leakage of root fillings with a glass-ionomer sealer. Int Endod J 1995;28:190–193.

25. Goldberg F, Artaza LP, De Silvio A. Apical sealing ability of a new glass-ionomer root canal sealer. J Endod 1995;21:498–500.

26. Georgopoulou MK, Wu M-K, Nikolaou A, Phil M, Wesselink PR. Effect of thickness on the sealing ability of some root canal sealers. Oral Surg Oral Med Oral Pathol Oral Radiol Endod 1995;80:338–344.

27. Sen BH, Psikin B, Baran N. The effect of tubular penetration of root canal sealers on dye microleakage. Int Endod J 1996;29:23–28.

28. Wu M-K, De Gee AJ, Wesselink PR. Leakage of AH26 and Ketac-Endo used with injected warm gutta-percha. J Endod 1997;23:331–334.

29. Taylor JK, Jeansonne BG, Lemon RR. Coronal leakage: Effects of smear layer, obturation technique, and sealer. J Endod 1997;23:508–512.

30. Kontakiotis EG, Wu M-K, Wesselink PR. Effect of sealer thickness on long-term sealing ability: A 2-year follow-up study. Int Endod J 1997;30:307–312.

31. Malone KH, Donnelly JC. An in vitro evaluation of coronal microleakage in obturated root canals without coronal restorations. J Endod 1997; 23:35–38.

32. Raiden GZ, Olguin A, Peralta G, Posleman I, Lagarrigue G. Apical leakage in canals filled with glass-ionomer sealer and gutta-percha after dentin conditioning. Endod Dent Traumatol 1997; 13:289–291.

33. Dalat DM, Önal B. Apical leakage of a new glass-ionomer root canal sealer. J Endod 1998; 24:161–163.

34. Koch K, Min PS, Stewart GG. Comparison of apical leakage between Ketac-Endo sealer and grossman sealer. Oral Surg Oral Med Oral Pathol 1994;78:784–787.

35. Lee CQ, Harandi L, Cobb CM. Evaluation of glass-ionomer as an endodontic sealant: An in vitro study. J Endod 1997;23:209–212.

36. Wu M-K, De Gee AJ, Wesselink PR. Leakage of four root canal sealers at different thicknesses. Int Endod J 1994;27:304–308.

37. Friedman S, Torneck CD, Komorowski R, Ouzounian Z, Syrtash P, Kaufman A. In vivo model for assessing the functional efficacy of endodontic filling materials and techniques. J Endod 1997;23:557–561.

38. Friedman S, Komorowski R, Maillet W, Nguyen HQ, Klimaite R, Torneck CD. Resistance of coronally induced bacterial ingress by an experimental glass-ionomer cement root canal sealer in vivo. J Endod (in press).

39. Coogan MM, Creaven PJ. Antibacterial properties of eight dental cements. Int Endod J 1993;26:355–361.

40. Shalhav M, Fuss Z, Weiss EI. In vitro antibacterial activity of a glass-ionomer endodontic sealer. J Endod 1997;23:616–619.

41. Abdulkader A, Duguid R, Saunders EM. The antimicrobial activity of endodontic sealers to anaerobic bacteria. Int Endod J 1996;29:280–283.

42. Patel V, Santerre JP, Friedman S. Suppression of adherent *E. faecalis* by an experimental root canal sealer. J Endod 1998;24:289 [abstract 73].

43. Saunders WP, Saunders EM. Influence of smear layer on the coronal leakage of thermafil and laterally condensed gutta-percha root fillings with a glass ionomer sealer. J Endod 1994;20:155–158.

44. Tidswell HE, Saunders EM, Saunders WP. Assessment of coronal leakage in teeth root filled with gutta-percha and a glass-ionomer root canal sealer. Int Endod J 1994;27:208–212.

45. Lalh M, Titley K, Torneck CD, Friedman S. Smear layer affects the adhesion of glass-ionomer cement sealers to bovine dentin. J Endod 1998;24:275 [abstract 16].

46. Lalh M, Titley K, Torneck CD, Friedman S. SEM study of the interface of glass-ionomer cement sealers and conditioned bovine dentin. J Endod 1998;24:300 [abstract 42].

47. Jonck LM, Grobbelaar CJ, Strating H. Biologlass ionomer cemental evaluation of glass-ionomer cement (Ketac-O) as an interface material in total joint replacement. A screening test. Clin Mater 1989;4:201–224.

48. Jonck LM, Grobbelaar CJ, Strating H. The biocompatibility of glass-ionomer cement in joint replacement: Bulk testing. Clin Mater 1989; 4:85–107.

49. Kolokuris I, Beltes P, Economides N, Vlemmas I. Experimental study of the biocompatibility of a new glass-ionomer root canal sealer (Ketac-Endo). J Endod 1996;22:395–398.

50. Friedman S, Löst C, Zarrabian M, Trope M. Evaluation of success and failure after endodontic therapy using a glass-ionomer cement sealer. J Endod 1995;21:384–390.

51. Augsburger RA, Peters DD. Radiographic evaluation of extruded obturation materials. J Endod 1990;16:492–497.

52. Friedman S. Retrograde approaches in endodontic therapy. Endod Dent Traumatol 1991;7:97–107.

53. Pissiotis E, Sapounas G, Spangberg LSW. Silver glass-ionomer cement as a retrograde filling material: A study in vitro. J Endod 1991; 17:225–229.

54. Alhadainy HA, Elsaed HY, Elbaghdady YM. An electrochemical study of the sealing ability of different retrofilling materials. J Endod 1993; 19:508–511.

55. Pretorius S, Van Heerden WFP. The use of tricure glass-ionomer cement as an apical sealant after apicoectomy. J Dent Assoc S Afr 1995; 50:367–370.

56. Hosoya N, Lautenschlager EP, Greener EH. A study of the apical microleakage of a gallium alloy as a retrograde filling material. J Endod 1995; 21:456–458.

57. Chong BS, Pitt Ford TR, Watson TF, Wilson RF. Sealing ability of potential retrograde root filling materials. Endod Dent Traumatol 1995;11: 264–269.

58. Gerhards F, Wagner W. Sealing ability of five different retrograde filling materials. J Endod 1996;22:463–466.

59. Aktener BO, Pehlivan Y. Sealing ability of cermet ionomer cement as a retrograde filling material. Int Endod J 1993;26:137–141.

60. Özata F, Erdilek N, Tezel H. A comparative sealability study of different retrofilling materials. Int Endod J 1993;26:241–245.

61. Olson AK, MacPherson MG, Hartwell GR, Weller RN, Kulild JC. An in vitro evaluation of injectable thermoplasticized gutta-percha, glass-ionomer, and amalgam when used as retrofilling materials. J Endod 1990;16:361–364.

62. Friedman S, Rotstein I, Koren L, Trope M. Dye leakage in retrofilled dog teeth and its correlation with radiographic healing. J Endod 1991;17: 392–395.

63. Roth S. A laboratory study of glass-ionomer cement as a retrograde root-filling material. Aust Dent J 1991;36:384–390.

64. Danin J, Linder L, Ramsköld L, Sund M-L, Strömberg T, Telme I, Torstenson B. A study in vitro of threaded titanium pins used for retrograde obturation of root canals. Int Endod J 1994;27:257–262.

65. Danin J, Linder L, Sund M-L, Strömberg T, Torstenson B, Zetterqvist L. Quantitative radioactive analysis of microleakage of four different retrograde fillings. Int Endod J 1992;25:183–188.

66. Biggs JT, Benenati FW, Powell SE. Ten-year in vitro assessment of the surface status of three retrofilling materials. J Endod 1995;21:521–527.

67. Rosales JI, Vallecillo M, Osorio R, Bravo M, Toledano M. An in vitro comparison of micro-leakage in three glass-ionomer cements used as retrograde filling materials. Int Dent J 1996;46; 15–21.

68. Craig KR, Harrison JW. Wound healing following demineralization of resected root ends in periradicular surgery. J Endod 1993;19:339–347.

69. Torabinejad M, Hong CU, Lee SJ, Monsef M, Pitt Ford TR. Investigation of mineral trioxide aggregate for root-end filling in dogs. J Endod 1995;21:603–608.

70. Zmener O. Tissue response to a glass ionomer used as an endodontic cement. A preliminary study in dogs. Oral Surg 1983;56:198–205.

71. Lehtinen R. Tissue reaction to glass ionomer cement and dental amalgam in the rat. Proc Finn Dent Soc 1986;82:144–147.

72. Blackman R, Gross M, Seltzer S. An evaluation of the biocompatibility of a glass-ionomer-silver cement in rat connective tissue. J Endod 1989;15:76–79.

73. DeGrood ME, Oguntebi BR, Cunningham CJ, Pink R. A comparison of tissue reactions to Ketac-Fil and amalgam. J Endod 1995;21:65–69.

74. Mjör IA. A comparison of in vivo and in vitro methods for toxicity testing of dental materials. Int Endod J 1980;13:139–142.

75. Callis P, Santini A. Tissue response to retrograde root fillings in the ferret canine: A comparison of a glass-ionomer cement and gutta-percha with sealer. Oral Surg Oral Med Oral Pathol 1987;64:475–479.

76. Zetterqvist L, Anneroth G, Nordenram A. Glass ionomer cement as retrograde filling material. An experimental investigation in monkeys. Int J Oral Maxillofac Surg 1987;16:459–464.

77. Chong BS, Pitt Ford TR, Kariyawasam SP. Tissue response to potential root-end filling materials in infected root canals. Int Endod J 1997;30:102–114.

78. Chong BS, Pitt Ford TR, Kariyawasam SP. Short-term tissue response to potential root-end filling materials in infected root canals. Int Endod J 1997;30:240–249.

79. Zetterqvist L, Hall G, Holmlund A. Apicectomy: A clinical comparison of amalgam and glass-ionomer cement as apical sealant. Oral Surg Oral Med Oral Pathol 1991;71:489–491.

80. Jesslén P, Zetterqvist L, Heimdahl A. Long-term results of amalgam versus glass-ionomer cement as apical sealant after apicectomy. Oral Surg Oral Med Oral Pathol Oral Radiol Endod 1995;79:101–103.

81. Friedman S, Rotstein I, Mahamid A. In vivo efficacy of various retrofills and of carbon dioxide laser in apical surgery. Endod Dent Traumatol 1991;7:19–25.

82. Trope M, Löst C, Schmitz H-J, Friedman S. Healing of apical periodontitis in dogs after apicoectomy and retrofilling with various filling materials. Oral Surg Oral Med Oral Pathol Oral Radiol Endod 1996;81:221–228.

83. Chong BS, Pitt Ford TR, Wilson RF. Radiologic assessment of the effects of potential root-end filling materials on healing after endodontic surgery. Endod Dent Traumatol 1997;13:176–179.

84. Pitt Ford TR, Roberts GJ. Tissue response to glass-ionomer retrograde root fillings. Int Endod J 1990;23:233–238.

85. Fuss Z, Trope M. Root perforations: Classification and treatment choices based on prognostic factors. Endod Dent Traumatol 1996;12:255–264.

86. Moloney LG, Feik SA, Ellender G. Sealing ability of three materials used to repair lateral root perforations. J Endod 1993;19:59–62.

87. Alhadainy HA, Himel VT. Evaluation of the sealing ability of amalgam, Cavit, and glass-ionomer cement in the repair of furcation perforations. Oral Surg Oral Med Oral Pathol 1993;75:362–366.

88. Alhadainy HA, Himel VT. An in vitro evaluation of Plaster of Paris barriers used under amalgam and glass-ionomer to repair furcation perforations. J Endod 1994;20:449–452.

89. Himel VT, Alhadainy HA. Effect of dentin preparation and acid etching on the sealing ability of glass-ionomer and composite resin when used to repair furcation perforations over Plaster of Paris barriers. J Endod 1995;21:142–145.

90. Mannocci F, Vichi A, Ferrari M. Sealing ability of several restorative materials used for repair of lateral root perforations. J Endod 1997; 23:639–641.

91. Chan JYM, Hutter JW, Mork TO, Nicoll BK. An in vitro study of furcation perforation repair using calcium phosphate cement. J Endod 1997; 9:588–592.

92. Alhadainy HA, Abdalla AI. Artificial floor technique used for the repair of furcation perforations: A microleakage study. J Endod 1998;24:33–35.

93. Snyder WR, Hoover J, Khoury R, Farach-Carson MC. Effect of agents used in perforation repair on osteoblastic cells. J Endod 1997; 23:158–161.

94. Goon WWY, Lundergan WP. Redemption of a perforated furcation with a multidisciplinary treatment approach. J Endod 1995;21:576–579.

95. Lemon RR. Nonsurgical repair of perforation defects—internal matrix concept. Dent Clin North Am 1992;36:439–457.

96. Walton RE, Michelich RJ, Smith GN. The histopathogenesis of vertical root fractures. J Endod 1984;10:48–56.

97. Friedman S, Moshonov M, Trope M. Resistance to vertical fracture of roots, previously fractured and bonded with glass-ionomer cement, composite resin and cyanoacrylate cement. Endod Dent Traumatol 1993;9:101–105.

98. Stewart GG. The detection and treatment of vertical root fractures. J Endod 1988;14:47–53.

99. Selden HS. Repair of incomplete vertical root fractures in endodontically treated teeth—in vivo trials. J Endod 1996;22:426–429.

100. Trope M, Rosenberg ES. Multidisciplinary approach to the repair of vertically fractured teeth. J Endod 1992;18:460–463.

101. Stewart GG. Calcium hydroxide induced root healing. J Am Dent Assoc 1975;90:793–800.

102. Barkhordar RA. Treatment of vertical root fracture: A case report. Quintessence Int 1991;22:707–709.

103. Saunders WP, Saunders EM. Coronal leakage as a cause of failure in root canal therapy: A review. Endod Dent Traumatol 1994;10:105–108.

104. Saunders WP, Saunders EM. The root filling and restoration continuum—prevention of long-term endodontic failures. Alpha Omegan 1997; 90:40–46.

105. Beckham BM, Anderson RW, Morris CF. An evaluation of three materials as barriers to coronal microleakage in endodontically treated teeth. J Endod 1993;19:388–391.

106. Chailertvanitkul P, Saunders WP, Saunders EM. An evaluation of microbial coronal leakage in the restored pulp chamber of root-canal treated multirooted teeth. Int Endod J 1997;30:318–322.

Chapter 11

Glass-Ionomers and Compomers in Pediatric Dentistry

Reinhard Hickel and Juergen Manhart

The controversy (especially in Germany and Sweden) over dental amalgam and its alleged adverse health effects due to the release of mercury, governmental restrictions on its use, and the still growing demand of patients for esthetic dentistry have led to an increased use of alternative filling materials. In Germany, the federal health authorities (BGA and BfArM) ruled in 1992[1] that amalgam fillings should no longer be placed in children under 6 years of age, for reasons of potential prophylactic health care. However, the guidelines of these authorities contradict numerous German and international professional dental organizations on several issues and are not verified by independent scientific investigations.

During recent years, other restorative materials such as casting alloys, glass-ionomer cements, and resin composites also have received criticism due to their alleged side effects. In general, many of these allegations have been made without any documented scientific evidence. Like all other drugs, a certain risk of potential side effects, or residual risk, can never be excluded. However, based on current knowledge, it must be emphasized that none of the recommended restorative materials, including amalgam, resin composites, compomers, and glass-ionomer cements, presents an irresponsible risk for the patient, who is the focus of all dental practitioners and material researchers. Except for allergic and lichenous reactions, none of the supposed side effects has been clinically diagnosed.[2,3]

The Letter of Consensus issued on July 1, 1997, by the German Federal Ministry of Health, together with BfArM, the German Dental Association (BZÄK/KZBV), the German Scientific Dental Association (DGZMK), and the German Association for Operative Dentistry (DGZ), states clearly that the stipulation of a general ranking of restorative materials is not justified based on current knowledge.[4] In all cases, the decision about which restorative material is selected and used has to consider the clinical situation of the individual patient. Benefits and drawbacks of all possible restorative materials must be estimated, and the informed patient needs to be involved in the treatment decision.

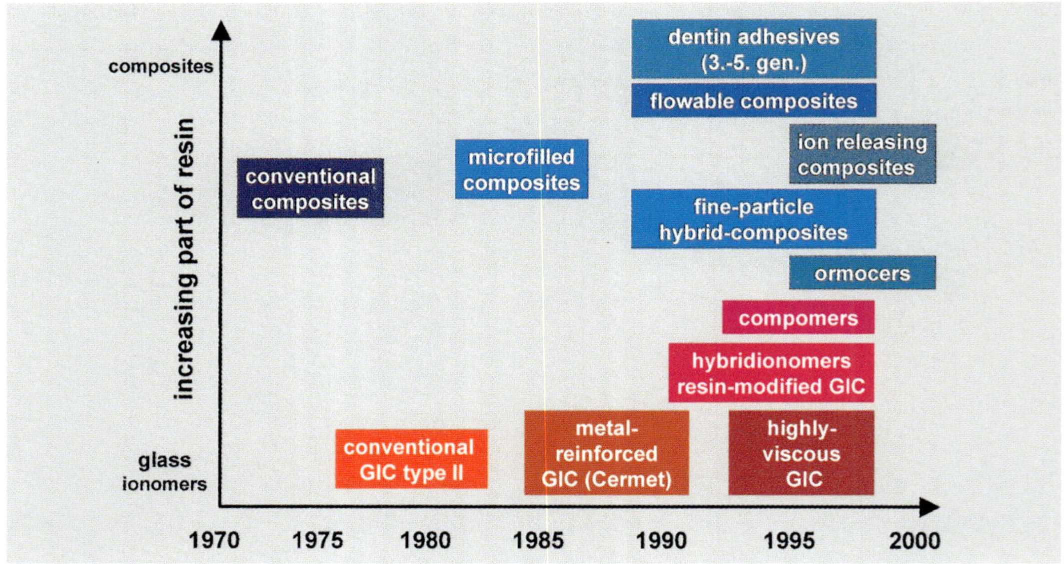

Fig 11-1 Historical development of different types of filling materials.

Glass-Ionomer and Resin Composite Restoratives

During the last two decades, many new filling materials and material groups have been developed. The number of available restoratives has increased dramatically, especially during the last 5 years (Fig 11-1). The great variety of products originally made it difficult to classify the materials and caused uncertainty for dentists in identifying proper usage.

To create a clearly structured classification for tooth-colored plastic restorative materials, Hickel[5] suggested assigning the materials to classes corresponding to their water content or a possible acid-base reaction during setting. Consequently, two main groups were recognized—glass-ionomer cements and resin composites—with subdivisions in each. Today, tooth-colored direct restorative materials are subdivided into the following groups: conventional and highly viscous glass-ionomer cements; resin-modified glass-ionomer cements, or hybrid ionomers; polyacid-modified resins and compomers; and (hybrid and microfilled) resin composites, including dentin adhesive systems (Table 11-1). Numerous products are available in each of these subgroups (Table 11-2).

Conventional glass-ionomer cements

Conventional glass-ionomer materials represent the oldest category of glass-ionomers. They were developed during the late 1960s by Wilson and Kent.[6] The first commercial product, called ASPA, was

Table 11-1 Classification of plastic direct filling materials based on glass ionomers and resin composites

Glass-Ionomer Cements (water based)	Resin Composites (no water added)
Conventional	Hybrid composite
Metal-reinforced (cermet)	Microfilled composite
Highly viscous	Ormocers
Resin-modified (hybrid ionomer)	Compomer

Table 11-2 Survey of commercially available products in the different material classes (1997)

Manufacturer	Conventional GIC	Metal-reinforced GIC	Highly viscous GIC	Hybrid ionomer	PAMR	Compomers
3M				Vitremer		F 2000
Degussa						(Xeno)
DenMat					Geristore	
Dentsply	Chem-Fil II Superior					Dyract, Dyract AP
DMG	Alpha Fil			Ionosit FilP/L		Luxat
Espe	Ketac-Fil, Chelon-Fil	Ketac Silver, Chelon Silver	Ketac Molar	Photac Fil Quick		Hytac
GC	Fuji II	Miracle Mix	Fuji IX GP	Fuji II LC Improved		
Kerr						Elan
Shofu	Glass Ionomer Type II	Hi-Dense	Hi-Fi, Hi-Dense			
Vivadent	Vivaglass Fil					Compoglass F
Voco	Aqua Ionofil	Argion Molar	Ionofil Molar			

GIC = glass-ionomer; PAMR = polyacid-modified resins.

introduced in 1972, and early materials required multiple improvements before gaining popularity in the 1980s. Changes were made in the glass particles, as well as in the composition of the polyacrylic acids. An essential improvement was the acceleration of the setting process, resulting in reduced moisture sensitivity during the critical initial reaction period.

The primary focus of this chapter is on restorative materials, but glass-ionomers also are used for the final cementation of stainless steel crowns in deciduous molars, as bases or liners, and in the sealing of pits and fissures.

Metal-reinforced glass-ionomer cements

This type of cement is commonly referred to as *cermet*, derived from the abbreviation of *cer*amic and *met*al, or metal-modified glass-ionomer cement. Cermets were developed in the mid-1980s based on conventional glass-ionomers.[7–9] Through high temperature sintering of silver particles to fusing glass powder, the wear resistance and flexural strength of the glass-ionomer cement was improved.[8–12]

Previous to this development, efforts had been made to improve the properties of conventional cements by mixing alloy powder with the glass-ionomer powder; the resulting product was called Miracle Mix.[13,14] Metal-reinforced glass-ionomers show excellent radiopacity.[15] However, they are not tooth-colored due to the addition of the metal particles. In some cases, discoloration of restored teeth by oxidized silver particles has been reported.[16] The bond strength to hard tooth tissues and the fluoride release of these materials are lower than those of conventional glass-ionomers.[12,17–24]

Cermets are only available with silver particles (eg, Ketac-Silver, Chelon-Silver); versions with gold particles are not commercially available because of the high costs. Cermets fell short of McLean's high expectations[7] as an alternative material to amalgam and exhibited frequent fractures in Class II cavities, as do conventional glass-ionomer cements (Table 11-3).

Highly viscous glass-ionomer cements

Due to the possibility of reduced secondary caries by fluoride release and to the comparative ease of use of conventional glass-ionomers, further developments have been made for posterior restorations in primary and permanent dentition. These highly viscous glass-ionomer cements are currently used in developing countries, in particular within the scope of atraumatic restorative treatment (ART) supported by the World Health Organization.[33] The objective was to design a restorative material that could be used without modern technical devices such as light-curing units, amalgamators, and micromotors that require electricity. Furthermore, a material with a high level of fluoride release was required because caries removal with hand instruments (eg, spoon excavators and enamel hatchets) is often incomplete, increasing the risk of recurrent caries or the development of new caries due to imperfect cavity margins.

Table 11-3 Failure (fracture) rates of glass-ionomer and cermet restorations in Class II cavities

Author(s)	Dentition	Period	Failure Rates (%)
Hickel et al[25] (1988)	Permanent	3 years	67
Lidums et al[26] (1993)	Permanent	2 years	43
Wilkie et al[27] (1993)	Permanent	2 years	55
Krämer et al[28] (1994)	Permanent	8 years	59
Hickel[29,30] (1989, 1990)	Deciduous	3 years	41
Hung and Richardson[31] (1990)	Deciduous	1 year	40
Qvist et al[32] (1997)	Deciduous	3 years	50

The highly viscous glass-ionomer cements have been well accepted, especially in improved encapsulated versions (eg, Fuji IX GP, Ketac-Molar). Due to their opacity, they have esthetic disadvantages when used for cervical fillings or Class III cavities. Predominant indications are fillings in deciduous molars and temporary restorations in permanent posterior teeth.

The formulations of conventional, metal-reinforced, and highly viscous glass-ionomer cements have no additional functional polymerizable monomers. These cements are therefore advantageous for patients who are allergic to components of resin composites. Based on reports from Scandinavia, increasing rates of allergic reactions (eg, to monomers) may be important for the future of these materials.[34]

Resin-modified glass-ionomer cements

In the late 1970s and early 1980s, the spread of light polymerization units began with the introduction of photopolymerizable resin composites. These materials became popular within a short time because of their handling and storage advantages. Light-curable glass-ionomers were developed in the mid-1980s, and are better described as hybrid ionomers or resin-modified glass-ionomers. The setting reaction of these materials has a light-curing mechanism in addition to the acid-base reaction of the glass-ionomer. The initial setting is by light-mediated polymerization of methacrylate monomers, while the slow acid-base reaction allows the bulk of the cement to mature to its final strength.

Table 11-4 Abrasion and wear resistance of different classes of restorative materials using two wear simulation devices*

	Material Loss	
Type of Material	Munich Oral Environment	ACTA Machine
Compomers	110–260 µm	30–60 µm
Hybrid ionomers	> 1,000 µm	40–150 µm
Highly viscous GICs	280–380 µm	28–50 µm
Metal-reinforced GICs	450–500 µm	30–85 µm
Conventional GICs	800–900 µm	30–150 µm

GIC = glass-ionomer cement.

* Data obtained from Hickel,[3] Kunzelmann,[35] and authors' unpublished material. Values were collected at 20,000 cycles for the Munich Oral Environment and at 200,000 for the ACTA machine. Abrasion values for the same materials are different for both simulators due to different wear phenomena.

Most of the mechanical properties of hybrid ionomers (eg, flexural strength) are improved by the addition of the polymerizable monomers. The fluoride release rate of the resin-modified materials is similar to that of conventional glass-ionomers; for patients with high levels of caries activity, both groups of materials may exhibit equivalent benefits. In spite of the resin content, wear resistance is low in most hybrid ionomers (Table 11-4).

Due to the usefulness of light polymerization, many dentists changed from conventional to resin-modified glass-ionomers. Besides their ease of handling, they also offer reduced susceptibility to crazing and cracking as a result of desiccation. In deep cavities, light-cured materials can be completely polymerized only in thin increments (1.5 to 2 mm). Even in those areas of the mouth with limited access, the tip of the polymerization unit has to be placed as close to the restorative material as possible to obtain sufficient light intensity for the initial setting process.

Polyacid-modified resins and compomers

The term *polyacid-modified resins* was suggested by McLean et al.[36] Unlike conventional and resin-modified glass ionomers, polyacid-modified resins and compomers have no or insignificant acid-base reaction during their setting process (see Table 11-1). Due to water sorption of the filling during clinical service, a negligible acid-base reaction can occur. Polyacid-modified resins are closely related chemically to compomers, which are sometimes integrated into this group. However, compomers have only one component, whereas polyacid-modified resins are mixed with a precise powder–liquid ratio. Since the introduction of compomers, which offer easier handling, the importance of mixable polyacid-modified resins has significantly decreased.

The term *compomer* is derived from *compo*site and glass-iono*mer*. This class of restorative materials combines some of the chemical and mechanical properties of resin composites with others of glass-ionomer cements. Compomers were introduced in the European market in 1993. Today, several products from different manufacturers are available (see Table 11-2). Compomers are similar to resin composites in their chemical structure. However, they include reactive, ion-leachable glass particles and polymerizable acidic monomers. In contrast to glass-ionomers, compomers contain no water in their formulations and are one-component materials, with the exception of dual-curing compomers for cementation, which do not need mixing. An acid-base reaction, which is typical in the setting of glass-ionomer cements, does not occur during the setting process of compomers. However, similar to glass-ionomers, compomers release fluoride.[37]

With regard to their mechanical properties, particularly tensile and flexural strength and wear resistance, compomers are superior to glass-ionomers but less effective than resin composites.[3,5,38] Prior to the application of compomer, the enamel and dentin need to be primed by a bonding agent (acid etched) to obtain optimum adhesion and bond strength to hard tooth tissues. Glass-ionomer cements bond chemically to the tooth structure, partially by chelation of the calcium in the apatite of enamel and dentin with the carboxyl groups of their polyacids. In contrast, compomer bonding to tooth structure is primarily mediated by micromechanical retention (resin tags and resin-dentin-interdiffusion zone hybrid layer), as with resin composites.

Concerning esthetics and finishing/polishing procedures, compomers are superior to conventional and even resin-modified glass-ionomer cements (Table 11-5), although considerable differences may be found among individual products in all groups. They match almost perfectly with the surrounding tooth structure, unlike glass-ionomers, which sometimes look chalky and opaque.

Indications for Use

Until a few years ago, amalgam was the worldwide material of choice for the restoration of deciduous molars. However, a partial change has occurred due to the controversy over amalgam's possible side effects. Although Christensen et al[39] found that 73% of fillings were still amalgam, compared to glass ionomers (15%) and composite resins (10%), Widstrom and Forss[40] reported that in Finland amalgam fillings are inserted in only 29% of all adult patients and 15% of children and adolescents; glass-ionomer cements were used in 91% of restorations of primary teeth and in 47% of permanent teeth for patients up to 16 years of age. This frequency of glass-ionomer fillings is remarkably high in comparison to other countries and depends greatly on the size

Table 11-5 Direct comparison of characteristics of conventional glass-ionomers, resin-modified glass-ionomers, and compomers

Characteristic	Conventional Glass-Ionomers	Resin-Modified Glass-Ionomers	Compomers
Handling properties/ preparation of the material	Powder-liquid system, aqueous based; hand-mixing versions or precapsulated systems	Powder-liquid system, water-monomer based; hand-mixing versions or precapsulated systems	One-component material, no water; no mixing necessary
Working time	1–2 min	Several minutes (setting initiated by light curing)	Unlimited (light cured)
Setting mechanism	Acid-base reaction (4–8 min); second phase within the next 24 h	Light curing (40 s); radical polymerization and acid-base reaction	Light curing only (40 s); incremental technique imperative for deep cavities
Moisture sensitivity after placement	High, especially during first setting stage (protective varnish required)	Moderate to low	None
Final polish	Fair	Good	Excellent
Adhesion to tooth structure	Self-adhesive, chemical bond to enamel and dentin	Self-adhesive; primer necessary for certain products	Acid etching and primer necessary
Strength	High compressive strength, low flexural strength	High compressive strength, medium flexural strength	High compressive strength, high flexural strength
Wear resistance	Low (highly viscous cements: moderate to acceptable)	Poor	Moderate to good
Marginal quality	Acceptable	Acceptable to good	Good to excellent
Fluoride release	Very high	Moderate to very high	Moderate to high
Esthetics/translucency	Good (highly viscous cements: moderate due to high opacity)	Good to excellent	Excellent
Typical problems	Crazing and cracking; appearance sometimes too opaque; susceptible to fractures in Class II restorations	Tendency to discolor during clinical service	Tendency toward marginal discoloration due to gap formation and material swelling; usually removable
Indication, if allergies to resin composites	Yes	No; allergological examination recommended	No; allergological examination recommended

Table 11-6 Indications for classes of restorative materials in different locations and cavity sizes

	Cavity Class in Primary Teeth				
	I	II	III	IV	V
Resin composites	++	++	++	+++	++
Compomer	+++	+++	+++	++	+++
Resin-modified glass-ionomers	++	++	++	–	+++
Highly viscous glass-ionomers	+++	+	+	–	++
Conventional glass-ionomers	++	(+)	+	–	+++

+++ = highly indicated; ++ = indicated; + = indicated with limitations; – = not indicated.
Note: Bond strength of dentin adhesive systems is usually higher to freshly cut dentin than to sclerotic dentin.

and the location of the restorations. As shown in Table 11-3, conventional glass-ionomers and cermets fracture more frequently in Class II cavities due to the comparatively low flexural strength of these materials. Oldenburg et al[41] reported 18% failure for Class II composite restorations in deciduous teeth, only 4% in Class I, and none in Class V lesions.

Therefore, indications for the different types of glass-ionomer cements and compomers are to some extent dependent on the type and size of the cavity (Table 11-6). Due to a greater supply of better alternatives, conventional glass-ionomers are today mainly used in Class V and Class III cavities, especially for patients exhibiting high caries activity. These materials also are employed for lesions in sclerotic dentin. Highly viscous glass-ionomer cements are esthetically inferior to all other types of materials described due to their high opacity. Except for the ART, they are applied only in deciduous molars and as temporary restorations in permanent posterior teeth.

Indications for resin-modified glass-ionomers correspond closely to those of conventional glass-ionomers; that is, primary indications are the restoration of cervical defects. They also are recommended for Class III cavities as well as for fillings in deciduous teeth.

Further developments, improvements, and clinical trials are needed to extend the indications for compomers to permanent restorations in Class I and Class II cavities in permanent dentition.

One important advantage of glass-ionomer cements is the release of fluoride. Hicks et al[42] showed less formation of secondary caries around glass-ionomer restorations in vitro. Svanberg et al[43] reported less plaque formation on glass ionomers than on amalgam or resin composites. Caries-inhibiting effects also were described in a 5-year in vivo study,[44] and for pit and fissure sealants.[45] In contrast, two articles about the reasons for replacement of failed restorations reported a high rate of secondary caries with glass-ionomer cements.[46,47]

Considerably less fluoride is released from compomers than from resin-modified or conventional glass-ionomers. However, improvements have been made in this area and are still ongoing. For example, amine fluoride has been added to the new primer systems and the percentage of fluoride-containing filler particles in compomers has been increased.

Clinical Procedures

Morphologic considerations of primary teeth

The technique of cavity preparation in primary dentition differs in part from that in permanent teeth. Several anatomic differences of primary teeth must be considered. Primary teeth have a thinner enamel (about 1 mm thick throughout the entire crown) than permanent teeth, and the distance occlusally and particularly mesiodistally from the tooth surface to the pulp chamber is smaller (only 2 to 3 mm). This knowledge of the relative thickness of enamel and dentin is important in cavity preparation to avoid accidental pulp exposure. The pulp horns in primary teeth, especially the mesiobuccal pulp horn of the first deciduous molars, are high and prominent. Pulp chambers are proportionately larger; thus, there is comparatively less tooth structure protecting the pulp in primary teeth. The occlusal surface of primary molars is narrow, and the buccal and lingual surfaces diverge strongly toward the root, making the crowns rounded and bulbous. The distinct constriction at the neck of primary molars demands special care during preparation of the gingival seat of a proximal box. In contrast to permanent teeth, the orientation of the enamel rods of the gingival third of the crowns is directed toward the occlusal surfaces.

The mineral content of the enamel of primary teeth is lower than that of permanent dentition. Primary teeth show about 10 times more pores (1 to 5 vol%).[48] In many cases, the enamel surface is characterized by a prismless outer layer, which is normally 30 to 50 μm thick but may be up to 100 μm.[49,50] Due to this prismless layer, it was frequently postulated that adhesive composite restorations were not possible in deciduous teeth. However, when the enamel margins are beveled, prismatic structures are exposed, allowing adhesive bonded fillings even in primary teeth. The etching time was originally controversial. In the past, 60-second etching of the enamel with 37% phosphoric acid was used for permanent teeth, and from 120 to 240 seconds was allowed for primary teeth. However, from 30 to 60 seconds, depending on the fluoride content of the enamel for deciduous teeth, is now considered sufficient to expose a proper microretentive etching pattern.[51,52]

Use of rubber dam

With few exceptions, the use of rubber dam in restorative pediatric dentistry is strongly recommended, regardless of the filling material. The isolation of the operating field presents many advantages, such as keeping spray from the dental handpiece, distasteful medicaments, disinfectants, monomers, and etching gel away from the tongue, throat, and soft tissues. It also saves time through elimination of spitting and rinsing by the patient, resulting in rare defensive reactions from the child. Tongue and lips are retracted and somewhat protected from rotating instruments. Many procedures in pediatric dentistry are performed more quickly and are less stressful when rubber dam is applied. This more than compensates for the short time required to place it.

Preparation and restoration

The formerly justified claims of "extension for prevention" have changed to "prevention of extension," thanks to highly improved preparation instruments and restorative materials and more sophisticated application techniques. Furthermore, high standards of oral hygiene and the availability of efficient mechanical devices and chemical agents for tooth cleaning and plaque removal are now available. Broader knowledge about the importance of proper dietary habits also has been achieved.

When employing adhesive restoratives, in contrast to amalgam fillings, unsupported but nonfriable enamel overhangs can be preserved and the cavity size can be kept as small as possible. The size of the cavity is mainly influenced by the extent of decay rather than by macroretentive considerations. Adhesive techniques result in the maximum preservation of tooth tissue, with positive effects on the strength and fracture resistance of the restored tooth and filling.

After preparation of the primary outline form of the cavity and caries excavation, the margins are finished by smoothing with very fine diamond burs (25-μm grain size). Unlike cavities in anterior teeth, Class I and Class II cavities in primary teeth do not require specific beveling of the margins. This only enlarges the occlusal surface of the restoration unnecessarily. Internal and external line and point angles should be well rounded to permit better adaptation of the restorative material and to lower stress concentration in the restoration and tooth, reducing the potential for fractures.

Cervical lesions in deciduous dentition are rare and, in most cases, completely limited to the enamel. If conventional glass-ionomer cements are used for restoring these cavities, butt joint margins are generally recommended to avoid fracture of thin marginal areas of the fillings. On the other hand, if compomers or resin-modified ionomers are employed, the margins can be prepared using a butt joint relationship between the tooth and the restorative material or by beveling.

With regard to compomers, there is still ongoing controversy about the necessity and usefulness of additional acid etching of the enamel margins. Acid etching results in a significantly higher bond strength of compomers to enamel.[53,54] If the coronal margin in mixed Class V cavities is beveled and etched, the marginal quality is improved and there is less microleakage of compomer restorations in this area.[55] However, in most cases, the gingival margin shows more marginal gaps in primed dentin due to the better and more durable adhesion and higher bond strength achieved with etched and primed enamel. An ideal solution for this problem is still pending.

In occlusal cavities of permanent molars, etching of the enamel improves the marginal quality, but no studies on primary teeth are available. At the present time, treatment in routine dental practice mainly occurs without additional etching because ease of use and time saved is a major benefit in the treatment of children. All available studies have been carried out in compliance with this procedure.

In contrast to amalgam and resin composite restorations without the use of dentin adhesives, the application of a base or liner in deciduous teeth is not imperative for any of the restorative materials mentioned. Usually, due to limited cavity size, it is only recommended in deep cavities.

Acid etching of the tooth structures prior to filling should always be handled in compliance with the manufacturer's instructions. Many glass-ionomers require etching of the dentin (eg, with 10% polyacrylic acid) to remove the smear layer, thus improving the adhesion (Figs 11-2a to 11-2d). Compomers must always be applied with the corresponding primer system.

When restoring Class II cavities, a matrix and wedges are placed prior to filling. The use of metal matrix bands, which are more reliable in producing physiologically contoured proximal contact areas than plastic matrices, is approved for all materials. Precontoured clear plastic matrices are available for Class V defects.

Conventional glass-ionomer cements can be bulk packed into the cavities with a hand instrument or injected from a capsule. Encapsulated versions of glass-ionomers are advantageous because they optimize the mixing process, have an ideal premeasured powder–liquid ratio, and facilitate placement into the cavity by direct injection. It is important to pay attention to the working time. If exceeded, it compromises the adhesive bond to tooth structure (accomplished by a chelation reaction between positively charged calcium ions present on the dentin and enamel surface, and setting by cross-linking chains of polyacrylic acids of the glass-ionomer cements that contain negatively charged carboxyl groups).

Due to their moisture sensitivity, the surface of glass-ionomer cements should be protected immediately at placement and during the initial setting stages. This can be accomplished with a special varnish (eg, Ketac Glaze) or a light-cured bonding agent to avoid desiccation or water uptake. Additional water sorption causes a dissolution in the matrix and yields a weaker cement with higher solubility. Dehydration results in crazing and cracking of the cement surface. Resin-modified glass-ionomers are less sensitive to moisture; however, their desiccation also results in a cracked and crazed surface. Therefore, these materials also should receive surface protection.

Although the resin-modified materials are dual-cured due to the acid-base reaction, attention should be given to sufficient light polymerization. This is also

Figs 11-2a to 11-2d Placement of a glass-ionomer filling (Ketac-Molar) in a permanent molar.

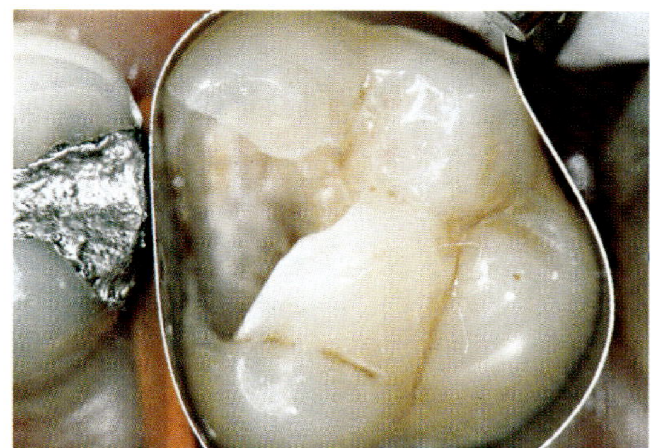

Fig 11-2a Tooth 26 shows a mesio-occlusal cavity after caries removal.

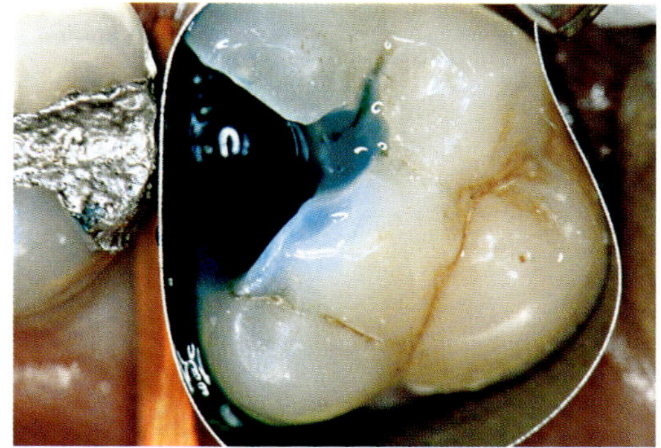

Fig 11-2b After protecting deep dentinal areas with a $Ca(OH)_2$ liner, the tooth tissues are conditioned with polyacrylic acid.

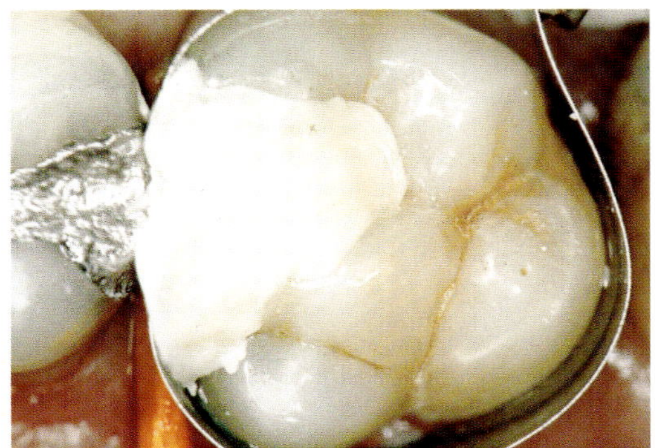

Fig 11-2c A highly viscous glass-ionomer filling is placed into the cavity as a bulk.

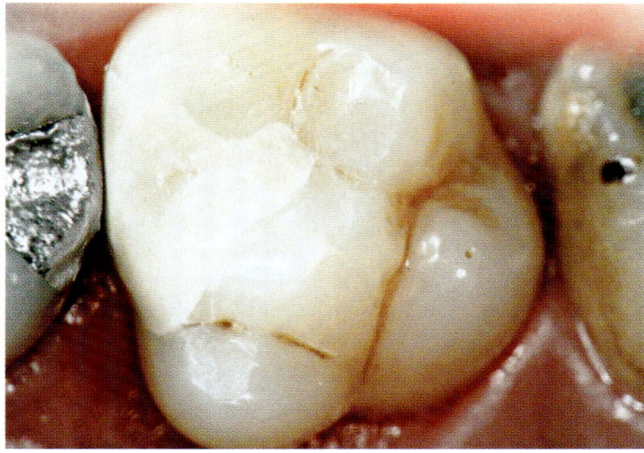

Fig 11-2d The polished restoration shows proper proximal contact to the mesial amalgam filling.

Figs 11-3a to 11-3k Placement of a compomer filling (Dyract-AP) in a primary molar.

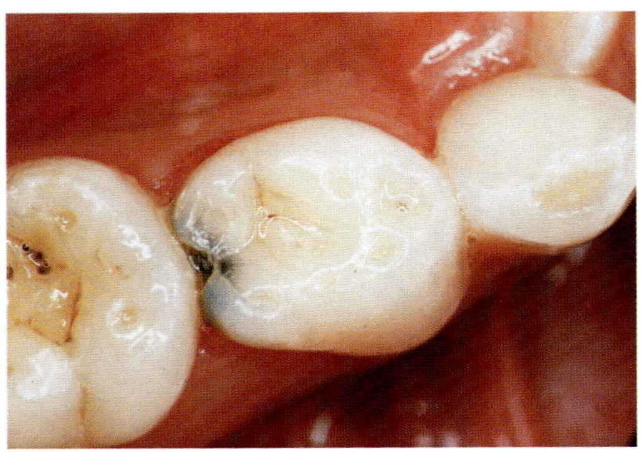

Fig 11-3a Tooth 84 exhibits caries on the distal proximal surface, causing pain. The second deciduous molar shows slightly occlusal caries.

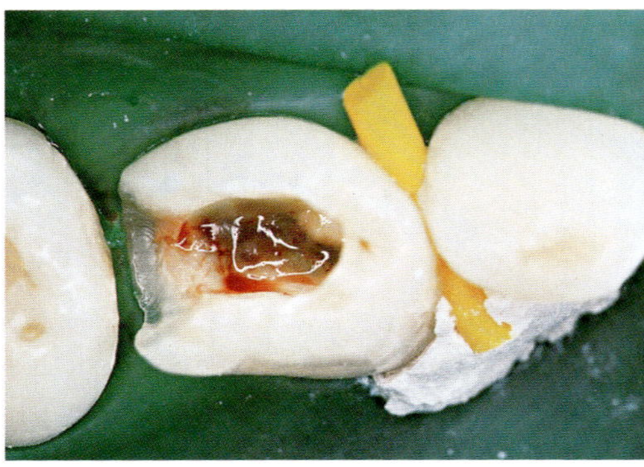

Fig 11-3b The extension of the caries in tooth 84 made it necessary to amputate the coronal part of the pulp (pulpotomy).

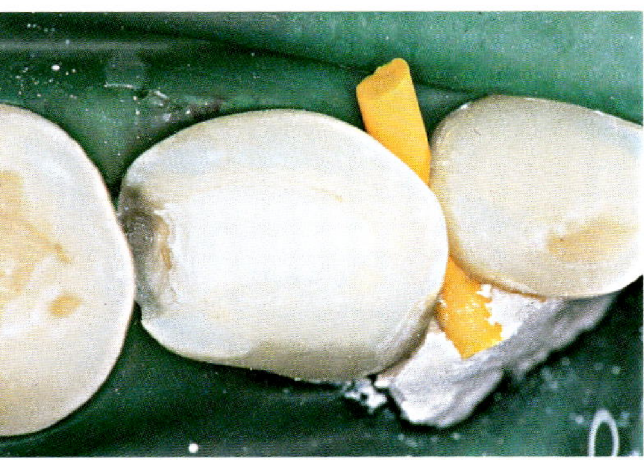

Fig 11-3c A formocreosolized zinc oxide–eugenol base is applied.

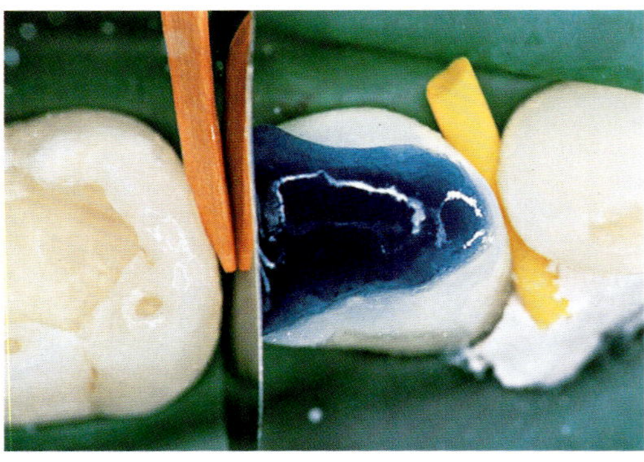

Fig 11-3d Enamel and dentin are etched with 37% phosphoric acid. The adjacent tooth is protected with a metal matrix.

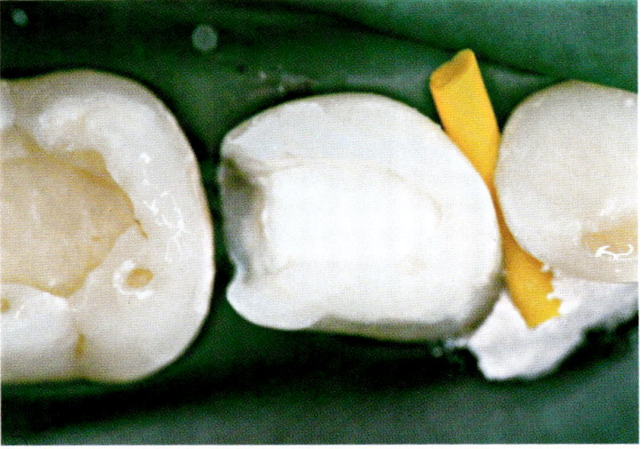

Fig 11-3e The enamel of the cavity finish lines appears dull and frosty white, signaling a successful pretreatment process yielding a microretentive etch pattern.

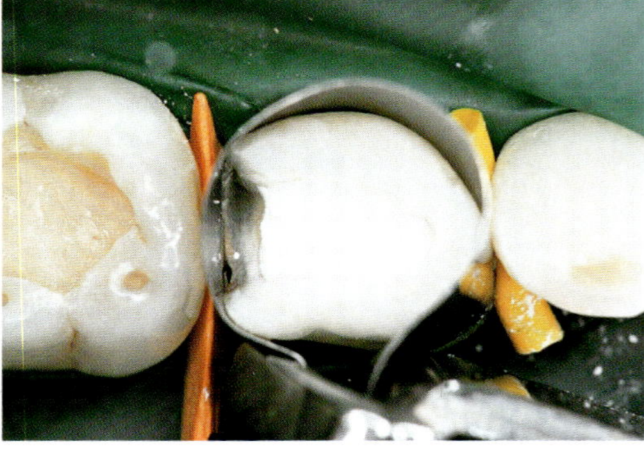

Fig 11-3f A metal matrix band ensures a proper proximal contour.

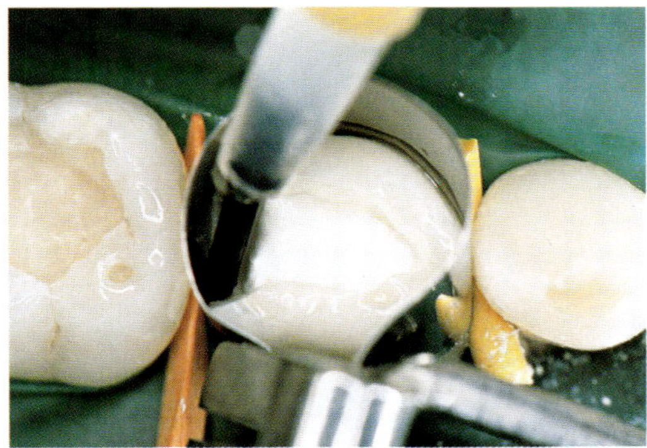

Fig 11-3g The dentin adhesive (Prime & Bond 2.1) is applied.

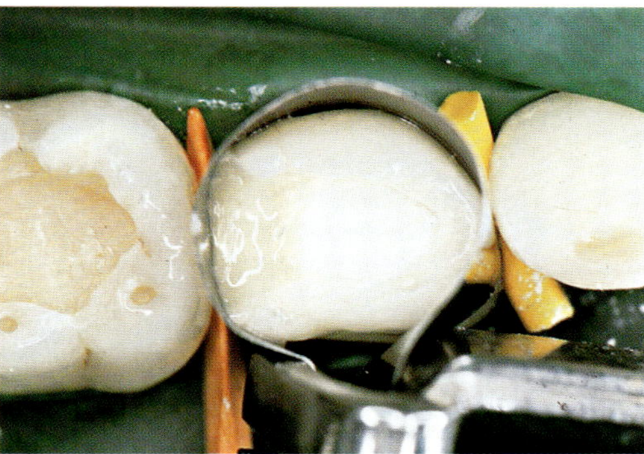

Fig 11-3h The restorative material is placed incrementally. The first layer fills the gingival part of the proximal box. Each increment is light cured separately for 40 seconds.

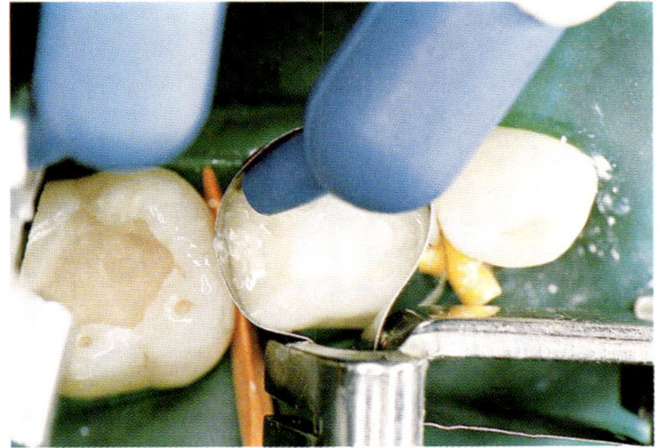

Fig 11-3i The next increment is applied directly in the cavity from the compule.

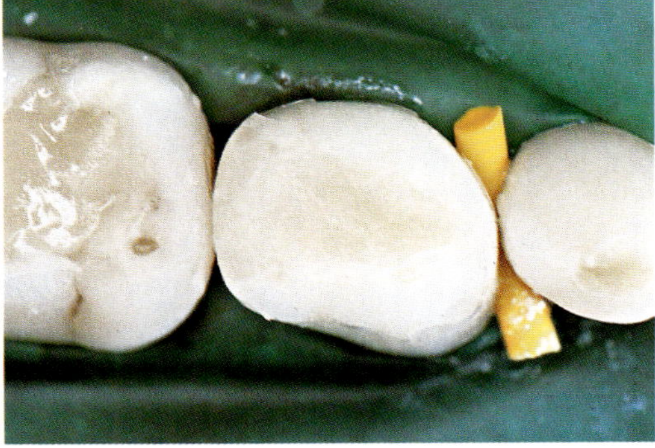

Fig 11-3j The teeth are completely filled with the restorative material.

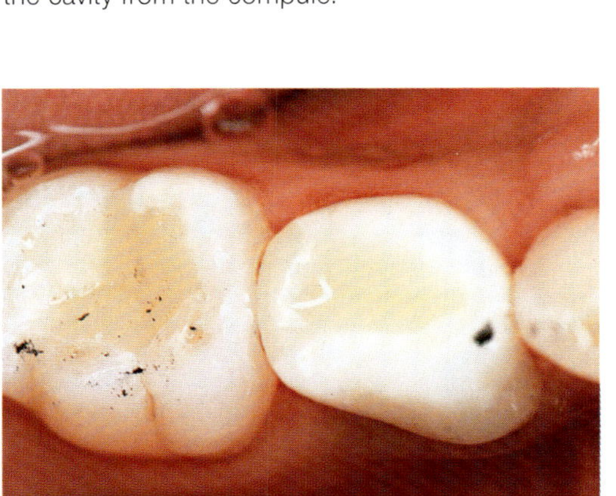

Fig 11-3k After removal of excess material, finishing, and polishing, the occlusion is checked for prematurities. Tooth 84 exhibits a physiological distoproximal contact, and both restorations on both teeth show anatomically correct occlusal surfaces.

imperative for compomers, which have to be applied incrementally in deep cavities, with each increment light cured individually for 40 seconds. This ensures proper polymerization with maximum material properties and significantly reduces shrinkage. Undercuring leads to a weakened restoration that is susceptible to failure during clinical service. The placement time for compomers is similar to that for amalgam (Figs 11-3a to 11-3k).

Finishing and polishing

The process of contouring, finishing, and polishing resin-modified glass-ionomers, polyacid-modified resins, and compomers is basically equivalent to that for resin composite restorations. The anatomy of the occlusal surface should be shaped as much as possible with the appropriate hand instruments prior to polymerization. Flash material can be removed easily while the compomer is still in a plastic condition. However, care must be taken not to compromise the marginal quality by removing excess material from the boundaries of the filling. Finishing and polishing can be initiated immediately after polymerization. The margins of the restoration are smoothed with fine-grit finishing diamond burs, and the occlusal anatomy is improved. Occlusal contacts and lateral movement paths are controlled and refined, if needed. Polishing is done with flexible aluminum oxide disks, abrasive silicon points, disks, and cups provided by different manufacturers. A final high-gloss appearance can be achieved with fine and extra-fine composite polishing pastes applied with mandrel-mounted foam polishing cups.

For conventional glass-ionomers, the following finishing and polishing procedure has proven successful. Depending on the product, approximately 5 minutes after placement of the glass-ionomer into the cavity, the matrix is removed and the excess cement at the margins is trimmed without water spray using hand instruments. It is important that all carving is done from the restoration toward the hard tooth tissue and not in reverse, to avoid ditching of the cement at the margins. After removal of the flash, the surface of the glass-ionomer restoration is coated with a protective varnish/bonding agent to avoid dehydration and water sorption. Occlusion is checked for proper contact, if applicable. Further finishing and polishing should be done during the next appointment, ideally at least 24 hours later when the cement has reached its full maturity. Sufficient water cooling during rotary instrumentation is imperative. If the glass-ionomer cement becomes heated because of dry instrumentation, cracking and crazing in the cement will occur due to desiccation. Ultrafine finishing diamonds (15-μm grain size) are used for contouring and finishing. Final polishing is accomplished with fine and ultrafine flexible abrasive aluminum oxide disks.[56–58] Sufficient cooling with water spray is necessary throughout the entire process.

Clinical Results in Primary Dentition

In comparison to restorations in permanent dentition, the longevity of those in primary teeth is significantly different for all materials. This makes the assessment of these fillings as a separate group meaningful.[30] Qvist et al[59,60] and others[61,62] found an average longevity of less than 2 years for amalgam fillings in children 4 years old and under, and only 1 year or less for composite restorations in this age group. According to Holland et al,[62] failure of amalgam fillings occurs more frequently in deciduous teeth, especially in small children, due to moisture contamination of the cavities during condensation. The age of the children at the time of placement is therefore a major factor in restoration longevity.[62–64]

In contrast to studies of permanent dentition, no separate investigations of glass-ionomer fillings in Class III and Class V lesions in primary dentition are known. For this reason, only Class I and II restorations in deciduous molars are discussed in the rest of this section.

Studies of primary molars with resin composite and amalgam restorations have presented different results. Barr-Agholme et al[63] reported significantly better results for composite restorations (88% satisfactory) after 2 years compared to amalgam (68%), while Östlund et al[64] found better results for amalgam fillings (92% acceptable) than for composites (84%) or glass ionomers (40%) after 3 years of service. Varpio[65] revealed less favorable results with earlier resin composites, which had less than 60% success after 3 years and only about 35% acceptability after 4 to 6 years. Oldenburg et al[41] found a success rate of 89% after 4 years for composite restorations, but reported great discrepancies between different types of restorations. Longevity data for all groups of glass-ionomers and compomers are summarized in Table 11-7.

Conventional and metal-reinforced glass-ionomer cements

During the last 10 to 20 years, glass-ionomer cements have been employed to an increasing degree as a restorative material in the primary dentition.[66–70,86–93] Walls et al[66] showed that after 2 years of clinical service the performance of glass-ionomer cements in posterior teeth was similar to that of amalgam fillings. But, after 5 years, amalgam had a median survival time of 3.5 years, which was superior to that of conventional glass-ionomers (2.8 years).[71] Qvist et al[32] compared amalgam and conventional glass-ionomer cements after 3 years and found a significantly higher failure rate with glass-ionomers, especially in Class II cavities.

Cermet restorations revealed a comparable success rate to amalgam fillings in small children. In older children and larger cavities, especially in Class II restorations, amalgam was superior.[70] Compared to amalgam, encapsulated glass-ionomers offered the advantage of a shorter application time.

Table 11-7 Longevity studies of restorations in primary molars with glass-ionomer cements and compomers according to class of restoration

Author(s)	Period (y)	Black Class (*n*)	Restorative Materials	*n*	Success Rate	Remarks
Walls et al[66]	2	II (102) I (14)	Ketac-Fil Amalgam	65 51	64% 60%	No significant difference, GICs showed worse anatomical form
Engelsmann et al[67]	4 (2.5–6)	I/II	Ketac-Fil Amalgam	128 60	64% 68%	Class II GIC had significantly (76%) more failures than amalgam (53%)
Hickel[29]	2	II (56) I (50)	Ketac-Silver	106	II: 84% I: 90%	Retentive cavity is necessary, Class II restorations often fracture more
Stratmann et al[68]	1	II	Ketac-Silver	40	93%	Rubber dam necessary
Forsten et al[69]	1	II	Ketac-Fil Ketac-Silver	100 99	84% 77%	No significant difference for cavity designs
Hickel and Voß[70]	3	II (132) I (83)	Ketac-Silver Amalgam	125 90	II:59% I:75% II:66% I:79%	Class II fillings showed worse results than Class I, in particular for GICs
Hung and Richardson[31]	1	II	Ketac-Silver Amalgam	40 33	60% 100%	Cermet had fractures in 16 fillings; not recommended for Class II lesions
Welbury et al[71]	5	II (222) I (16)	Ketac-Fil Amalgam	119 119	67% 80%	Cavities for GIC fillings could be smaller
Ostlund et al[64]	3	II	Chem-Fil Occlusin Amalgam	25 25 25	40% 84% 92%	Conventional Class II cavities, only second molars
Frencken et al[33]	1	I II	Chem-Fil	116 138	79% 55%	ART used in Thailand; minimal intervention
Andersson-Wenckert et al[72]	3	II	GIC GIC small cavities	56	68% 75%	Microcavity without occlusal extension
Croll and Helpin[73]	1–1.5	II	Vitremer	250	100%	Minor wear, no fractures
Espelid and Tveit[74]	1	II	Ketac-Silver Vitremer	32 32	97% 100%	1 cermet with secondary caries; Vitremer had better marginal adaptation

Author(s)	Period (y)	Black Class *(n)*	Restorative Materials	*n*	Success Rate	Remarks
Kilpatrick et al[75]	2.5	II	Ketac-Fil Ketac-Silver	46 46	77% 59%	Cermet had significantly worse results and marginal openings
Qvist et al[76]	1	II/I	Ketac-Fil Photac-Fil	46 46	77% 59%	Resin-modified GIC showed higher longevity; no difference in cariostatic effects
Reeka et al[77]	0.5–2	I (186) II (80)	Dyract (−1 y) Dyract (>1 y)	180 86	97% 95%	Marginal staining in 20%, but only 1 case with marginal caries
Donly and Kanellis[78]	2	II	3M-EXM155 Amalgam	20 20	90% 85%	Experimental GIC performed at least as well as amalgam
Kimura et al[79]	1	II	Fuji II LC	25	88%	12% fractures and loss of fillings
Peters et al[80]	1	II (80) I (11)	Dyract	91	97%	High wear rates (x = 190 µm) (33% more than 200 µm)
Roeters et al[81]	2	II/I	Dyract	76	95%	Only 2 fractures
Peters et al[82]	3	II/I	Dyract	37	91%	Shift in anatomical form; 9% caries
Krämer et al[28]	1	I/II	Hi-Dense Ketac-Molar (0.5 y)	47 13	94% 100%	Both materials had 50% marginal fractures or ditching
Frankenberger et al[83]	2	I/II	Hi-Dense Ketac-Silver	52 73	72% 72%	K-M-estimator after 2.3 years; no difference, in Class II both materials showed higher fracture rates
Qvist et al[32]	3	II/I	Ketac-Fil Amalgam	515 543	63% 82%	In Class II restorations, GIC had 50% fractures
Vulicevic et al[84]	1	II/I	Dyract Luxat	30 30	100% 100%	No differences
Kitty and Wie[85]	1	I/II	Dyract Prisma TPH	60 60	98% 98%	Compomer was only worse for marginal discoloration and wear resistance

GIC = glass-ionomer cement.

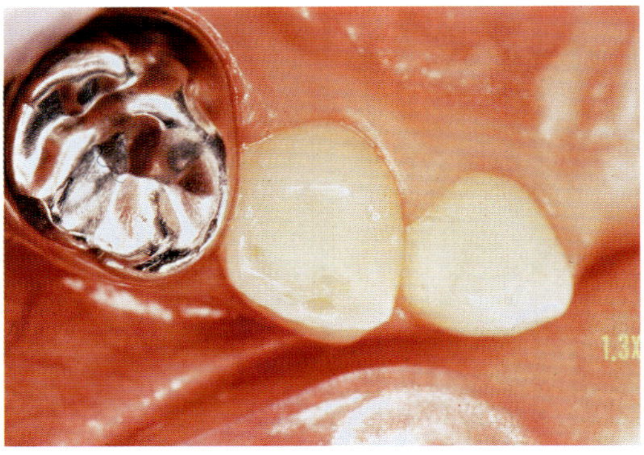

Fig 11-4 Successful Class I restoration with a compomer (Dyract) in tooth 64 after 18 months of clinical service. Tooth 65 is restored with a stainless steel crown.

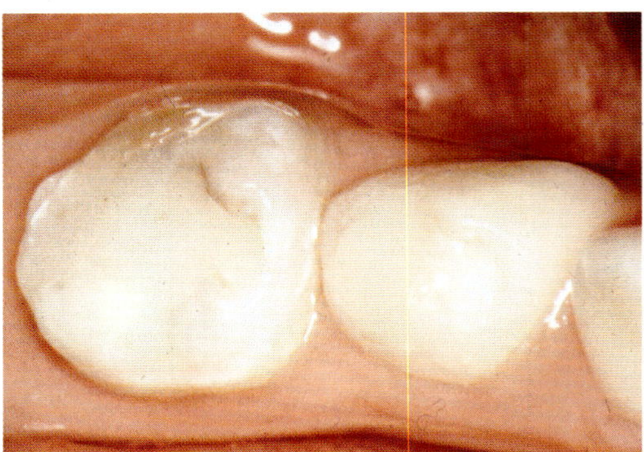

Fig 11-5 Class I Dyract filling in tooth 84 after 24 months. The restoration in tooth 85 (Dyract) showed marginal staining due to a swelling of the material. This discoloration was removed by polishing.

Highly viscous glass-ionomer cements

Due to the relative newness of highly viscous glass-ionomers, only a few clinical studies using these materials in primary molars have been published. Frankenberger et al[83] reported a 72% success rate for Hi-Dense with an observation period up to 2 years, showing no statistically significant difference compared to the results using Ketac-Silver. As in previous studies of conventional glass-ionomers and cermets (see Table 11-3), Hi-Dense revealed more fractures in Class II cavities than in Class I lesions. This result was to be expected because of the low flexural strength of the resin-free glass-ionomer cements compared to resin-modified materials and compomers.

Resin-modified glass-ionomer cements

Few published studies are available for the hybrid ionomers. Kimura et al[79] showed a success rate of 80% for Fuji II LC after only 1 year. Qvist et al[76] compared conventional glass-ionomers with resin-modified cements and found a higher success rate for the latter, with the same anticariogenic effect for both materials. The resin-modified material Vitremer showed a better marginal adaptation than cermet, as observed by Espelid and Tveit.[74] Donly et al[78] reported equivalent results for resin-modified cement and amalgam. Croll and Helpin[73] analyzed more than 250 Vitremer Class II restorations after 12 to 18 months and observed no fractures, no marginal stain, no recurrent caries, and only minor wear.

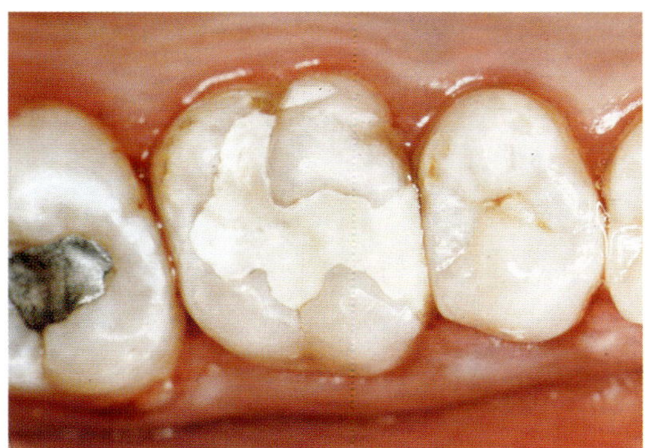

Fig 11-6 Failed Class II glass-ionomer restoration with a palatinal extension. The cervical part of the highly viscous filling is fractured.

Compomers

With the introduction of compomers, the number of restorations in primary dentition using conventional glass-ionomers and cermet decreased dramatically. The same was true for amalgam in Germany and some other European countries. Even though compomers represent the most recent class of material discussed in this chapter, several studies with an observation period up to 3 years exist.[79-83] At present, compomers show the highest success rate of all materials in deciduous molars, more than 90% after 3 years (Tables 11-7 and 11-8). In many cases, compomers are the material of choice (Figs 11-4 and 11-5).

Clinical Results in Mixed Dentition

Restorations in permanent teeth of children show generally better results than those in primary teeth but still shorter longevity compared to adults, possibly due to lack of cooperation during treatment.[62,94] Fillings in permanent teeth of children and adolescents are initial restorations in most cases. This distinguishes them from those in adults, where approximately two thirds of restorations are caused by replacement of existing fillings due to failure (Fig 11-6). If caries is diagnosed early, initial restorations usually can be limited by preserving a maximum of sound tooth structure. This is possible thanks to modern and sophisticated diagnostic and preparation instruments, restorative materials, and application techniques, as well as to appropriate patient motivation and education in good oral hygiene.

With the introduction of Sonicsys, an ultrasonic-driven cavity preparation system, and modern restorative materials (such as low-viscosity light-curing resin composites, or flowable composites), it is possible to prepare even proximal minimally invasive cavities without adversely touching the approximal tooth and to place adhesive restorations.[85] Because small fillings are less stressed by chewing forces and show a greater longevity[64,86,87] (see Table 11-7), maximum preservation and protection of natural tooth tissue should still gain in importance in the future.

Table 11-8 Summary of success rates of restorations in deciduous molars after 1 to 5 years.

	Success Rates by Time			
Material Group	1 y	2 y	3 y	5 y
GICs	55*-84-86	64-77	40-63-68	67
Metal-reinforced GICs	60-77-90-97	59-84	59	–
Highly viscous GICs	94	72	–	–
Resin-modified ionomers	88-92-100	90	–	–
Compomers	97-98-100	95	91	–
Resin composites	98	88	60-84	35-(82**)
Amalgams	100	60-68-85	66-82-92	80

* = ART; ** = after 4 years (Class II); GIC = glass-ionomer cement.

Note: Results can only be compared directly if different materials were assessed within the same study, but regarding all studies a certain trend can be observed. Best results were obtained with compomers.

Summary

In spite of substantial improvements during the 1980s, conventional glass-ionomer cements still have shortcomings with regard to moisture sensitivity, wear resistance, flexural strength, and final polishing. Even though the chemical adhesion to enamel and dentin and the fluoride release are major benefits, conventional glass-ionomers are restricted to special indications (Class III and Class V cavities) in operative dentistry.

The use of conventional glass-ionomer cements and metal-reinforced cements has decreased due to the development of new restorative materials, such as highly viscous glass-ionomers and compomers. However, conventional glass-ionomer cements are still an important alternative filling material for patients suffering from allergies to polymerizable resin monomers.

Resin-modified glass-ionomer cements cover the same indications as conventional glass-ionomers. Both materials have a low resistance to abrasion. Therefore, they should not be employed in stress-bearing areas in posterior teeth. To what extent the more wear-resistant highly viscous glass-ionomers and compomers can be used in these areas, with or without limitations regarding cavity size, is a crucial factor in the planning of future controlled clinical trials.

Given improved measures in oral prophylaxis, significantly fewer and smaller cavities will be found in children and adolescents in the future. These lesions probably will be indicated for filling materials that are currently not qualified for large stress-bearing restorations. In primary dentition, compomers, resin-modified glass-ionomers, and highly viscous glass-ionomers are excellent alternative filling materials.

References

1. BGA (Bundesgesundheitsamt). Amalgame–Nebenwirkungen und Bewertung der Toxiztât Zahnârztl Mitt 82:36, 1992 und Amalgame in der zahnârztlichen Therapie. Eine Informationsschrift des Bundesgesundheitsamtes, 1992.

2. Mjör IA. Problems and benefits associated with restorative materials: Side-effects and long-term cost. Adv Dent Res 1992;6:7.

3. Hickel R. Moderne Füllungsmaterialien. Dtsch Zahnarztl Z 1997;52:573.

4. BMG (Bundesministerium für Gesundheit). Konsensuspapier Füllungsmaterialien. Zahnarztl Mitt 1997;87:1812.

5. Hickel R. Glass ionomers, cermets, hybrid-ionomers and compomers—Long term clinical evaluation. Trans Acad Dent Mater 1996;9:105.

6. Wilson AD, Kent BE. A new translucent cement for dentistry: The glass-ionomer cement. Br Dent J 1972;132:133.

7. McLean JW. Alternatives to amalgam alloys. Br Dent J 1984;157:432.

8. McLean JW, Gasser O. Glass cermet cements. Quintessence Int 1985;16:333.

9. McLean JW. Cermet cements. J Am Dent Assoc 1990;120:43.

10. McKinney JE, Antonucci JM, Rupp NW. Wear and microhardness of a silver-sintered glass-ionomer cement. J Dent Res 1988;67:831.

11. Moore BK, Swartz ML, Phillips RW. Abrasion resistance of metal reinforced glass-ionomer materials. J Dent Res 1985;64:371.

12. Swift EJ. Silver glass ionomers. A status report for the American Journal of Dentistry. Am J Dent 1988;1:81.

13. Simmons JJ. The miracle mixture: Glass-ionomer and alloy powder. Tex Dent J 1983;100:6.

14. Simmons JJ. Silver-alloy powder and glass-ionomer cement. J Am Dent Assoc 1990;120:49.

15. Williams JA, Billington RW. The radiopacity of glass-ionomer dental materials. J Oral Rehabil 1990;17:245.

16. Sarkar NK, El-Mallakh B, Graves R. Silver released from metal reinforced glass-ionomers. Dent Mater 1988;4:103.

17. Berg JH, Donly KJ, Posnicj WR. Glass-ionomer silver restorations: A demineralization-remineralization concept. Quintessence Int 1988;19:639.

18. Forss H, Seppä L. Prevention of enamel demineralization adjacent to glass-ionomer filling materials. Scand J Dent Res 1990;98:173.

19. Kakaboura A, Vougiouklakis G, Mountouris G. The effect of an air powder abrasive device on the bond strength of glass -onomer cements to dentin. Quintessence Int 1989;20:9.

20. Olsen BT, Garcia-Godoy F, Marshall TD, Barnwell GM. Fluoride release from glass-ionomer-lined amalgam restorations. Am J Dent 1989;2:89.

21. Peutzfeld A, Asmussen E. Bonding and gap formation of glass-ionomer cement used in conjunction with composite resin. Acta Odontol Scand 1989;47:141.

22. Staehle HJ. Experimentelle Untersuchungen über die Haftung von drei verschiedenen zahnärztlichen Präparaten am Dentin bei unterschiedlichen Versuchsbedingungen. Dtsch Zahnarztl Z 1986;41:743.

23. Thornton JB, Retief DH, Bradley EL. Fluoride release from and tensile bond strength of Ketac-Fil and Ketac-Silver to enamel and dentin. Dent Mater 1986;2:241.

24. Tjan AHL, Morgan DL. Metal-reinforced glass-ionomers: Their flexural and bond strengths to tooth substrates. J Prosthet Dent 1988;59:82,137.

25. Hickel R, Petschelt A, Maier J, Voß A, Sauter M. Nachuntersuchungen zu Cermet-Zementen. Dtsch Zahnarztl Z 1988;43:884.

26. Lidums A, Wilkie R, Smales R. Occlusal glass-ionomer cermet, resin sandwich and amalgam restorations: A 2-year clinical study. Am J Dent 1993;6:185–188.

27. Wilkie R, Lidums A, Smales R. Class II glass-ionomer cermet tunnel, resin sandwich and amalgam restorations over 2 years. Am J Dent 1993;6:181–184.

28. Krämer NK, Kunzelmann KH, Pollety T, Pelka M, Hickel R. Langzeiterfahrungen mit Cermetzementfüllungen in Klasse-I/-II-kavitäten. Dtsch Zahnarztl Z 1994;49:905–909.

29. Hickel R. Einsatzgebiete und -verfahren von glasionomerzement als Füllungsmaterial. Zahnarztl Mitt 1989;79:914.

30. Hickel R. Aesthetik und Dauerhaftigkeit plastischer Füllungsmaterialien in Abhängigkeit von Topographie, Material und Verarbeitung. In: Bayrische Landeszahnärztekammer: Aesthetik in der Zahnheilkunde. Berlin: Quintessenz, 1990; 43–55.

31. Hung TW, Richardson AS. Clinical evaluation of glass-ionomer silver cermet restorations in primary molars: One year results. J Can Dent Assoc 1990;56:239–240.

32. Qvist V, Laurberg L, Poulsen A, Teglers PT. Longevity and cariostatic effects of everyday conventional glass-ionomer and amalgam restorations in primary teeth: Three-year results. J Dent Res 1997;76:1387–1396.

33. Frencken JE, Sonpaisan Y, Phantumvanit P, Pilot T. An atraumatic restorative treatment (ART) technique: Evaluation after one year. Int Dent J 1994;44:460–464.

34. Karlson S. Personal communication, 1996.

35. Kunzelmann KH. Glass-ionomer cements, cermet cements, "hybrid"-glass-ionomers and compomers—laboratory trials—wear resistance. Trans Acad Dent Mater 1996;9:89–104.

36. McLean JW, Nicholson JW, Wilson AD. Proposed nomenclature for glass-ionomer dental cements and related materials. Quintessence Int 1994;25:587–589.

37. Hickel R. Kompomere. Quintess Zahnarztl Z 1996;47:1581.

38. Gladys S, Van Meerbeek B, Braem M, Lambrechts P, Vanherle G. Comparative physiomechanical characterization of new hybrid restorative materials with conventional glass-ionomer and resin composite restorative materials. J Dent Res 1997;76:883–894.

39. Christensen GJ. Restoration of pediatric posterior teeth. J Am Dent Assoc 1996;127:106.

40. Widstrom E, Forss H. Selection of restorative materials in dental treatment of children and adults in public and private dental care in Finland. Swed Dent J 1994;18:1–7.

41. Oldenburg TR, Vann WF, Dilley DC. Composite restorations for primary molars: Results after four years. Pediatr Dent 1987;9:136–143.

42. Hicks MJ, Flaitz CM, Silverstone LM. Secondary caries formation in vitro around glass-ionomer restorations. Quintessence Int 1986;17:527–532.

43. Svanberg M, Mjör IA, Orstavik D. *Mutans streptococci* in plaque from margins of amalgam, composite and glass-ionomer restorations. J Dent Res 1990;69:861–864.

44. Tyas MJ. Cariostatic effect of glass-ionomer cement: A five-year clinical study. Austr Dent J 1991;36:236–239.

45. Williams B, Laxton L, Holt RD, Winter GB. Fissure sealants: A 4-year clinical trial comparing an experimental glass polyalkenoate cement with a bis glycidyl methacrylate resin used as fissure sealants. Br Dent J 1996;180:104–108.

46. Mjör IA. The reasons for replacement and the age of failed restorations in general dental practice. Acta Odontol Scand 1997;55:58–63.

47. Wilson NHF, Burke FJT, Mjör IA. Reasons for placement and replacement of restorations of direct restorative materials by a selected group of practitioners in the United Kingdom. Quintessence Int 1997;28:245–248.

48. Silverstone LM. The histopathology of early approximal caries in the enamel of primary teeth. J Dent Child 1970;37:201–210.

49. Ripa LW, Gwinnett AJ, Buonocore MG. Prismless outer layer of deciduous and permanent enamel. Arch Oral Biol 1956;11:41–48.

50. Eidelmann E. The structure of the enamel in primary teeth: Practical applications in restorative techniques. J Dent Child 1976;43:172–176.

51. Garcia-Godoy F, Gwinnett AJ. Effect of etching times and mechanical pretreatment on the enamel of primary teeth: An SEM study. Am J Dent 1991;4:115–119.

52. Hosoya Y. The effect of acid etching times on ground primary enamel. J Clin Pediatr Dent 1991;15:188–194.

53. Moll KH, Haller B, Hofmann N, Klaiber B. Phosphoric acid etching and enamel bond of composite/glass-ionomer hybrids. J Dent Res 1996;75:171,1225.

54. Triolo PT, Barkmeier WW, Los SA. Bonding efficacy of a compomer using different conditioning procedures. J Dent Res 1995;74:107,761.

55. Kunzelmann KH, Bauer M, Hickel R. Randdichtigkeit "lichthärtender" Glasiomer-Zemente und Kompoionomere in dentinbegrenzten zervikalen Kavitäten. Poster presentation 118th Annual Meeting of the German Scientific Dental Association, Travemünde 1994 and Med Diss 1998, Munich.

56. Atkinson AS, Pearson GJ. The evolution of glass-ionomer cements. Br Dent J 1985;159:335.

57. Hotz PR. Glasionomer-Zement—Verarbeitung, Antikariogenität. Schweiz Mschr Zahnheilk 1987;97:336.

58. Kullmann W, Triadan H. Die Oberflächenbearbeitung von Glasionomer-Füllungsmaterialien. Schweiz Mschr Zahnheilk 1984;94:634.

59. Qvist V, Thylstrup A, Mjör IA. Restorative treatment patterns and longevity of resin restoration in Denmark. Acta Odontol Scand 1986;44:351.

60. Qvist V, Thylstrup A, Mjör IA. Restorative treatment patterns and longevity of amalgam restoration in Denmark. Acta Odontol Scand 1986;44:344.

61. Mjör IA. The safe and effective use of dental amalgam. Int Dent 1987;37:147.

62. Holland IS, Walls AWG, Wallwork MA, Murray JJ. The longevity of amalgam restorations in the deciduous molars. Br Dent J 1986;161:255.

63. Barr-Agholme M, Oden A, Dahllof G, Modeer T. A two-year clinical study of light-cured composite and amalgam restorations in primary molars. Dent Mater 1991;7:230–233.

64. Östlund J, Möller K, Koch G. Amalgam, composite resin and glass-ionomer cement in class II restorations in primary molars—a three year clinical evaluation. Swed Dent J 1992;16:81–86.

65. Varpio M. Proximoclusal composite restorations in primary molars: A six-year follow-up. J Dent Child 1985;52:435–440.

66. Walls AWG, Murray JJ, McCabe JF. The use of glass polyalkenoate (ionomer) cements in the deciduous dentition. Br Dent J 1988;165:13.

67. Engelsmann U, Kocher T, Albers H-K. Vergleichende Langzeituntersuchung über die Füllungsmaterialien KetacFil und Amalgam an Milchzähnen. Dtsch Zahnarztl Z 1988;43:291.

68. Stratman RG, Berg JH, Donly KJ. Class II glass ionomer silver restorations in primary molars. Quintessence Int 1989;20:43–47.

69. Forsten L, Karjalainen S. Glass ionomers in proximal cavities of primary molars. Scand J Dent Res 1990;98:70.

70. Hickel R, Voß A. A comparison of glass cermet cement and amalgam restorations in primary molars. J Dent Child 1990;57:184.

71. Welbury RR, Walls AWG, Murray JJ, McCabe JF. The 5-year results of a clinical trial comparing a glass polyalkenoate (ionomer) cement restoration with an amalgam restoration. Br Dent J 1991;170:177–181.

72. Andersson-Wenckert IE, van Dijken JWV, Stenberg R. Effect of cavity form on the durability of glass-ionomer cement restorations in primary teeth: A three-year clinical evaluation. J Dent Child 1995;62:197–200.

73. Croll TP, Helpin ML. Class II Vitremer restoration of primary molars. ASDC J Dent Child 1995;62:17–21.

74. Espelid I, Tveit AB. Clinical behavior of glass-ionomer restorations in primary teeth. J Dent Res 1995;74:433 [abstract 264].

75. Kilpatrick NM, Murray JJ, McCalce JF. The use of a reinforced glass-ionomer cement for the restoration of primary molars: A clinical trial. Br Dent J 1995;129:175–179.

76. Qvist V, Teglers PT, Manscher E. Conventional and resin-stabilized glass-ionomer restorations in primary teeth. Preliminary results. J Dent Res 1995;74:440 [abstract 318].

77. Reeka A, Benz C, Loher C, Hickel R. Klinische Studie zur Versorgung von Klasse-I- und -II-

Kavitäten im Milchgebiß mit Kompomer. German Society for Pedodontics, Leipzig, 1995. Dtsch Zahnarztl Z (In press 1998).

78. Donly KJ, Kanellis M. Glass ionomer restorations in primary molars: Two-year clinical results. J Dent Res 1996;75:285 [abstract 2144].

79. Kimura M, Nishida I, Maki K, Ge L. Clinical evaluation of a light-cured glass-ionomer cement for restorative fillings. Pediatr Dent J 1996;6:115–123.

80. Peters TCRB, Roeters JJM, Frankenmolen FWA. Clinical evaluation of Dyract in primary molars: 1-year results. Am J Dent 1996;9:83–87.

81. Roeters J, Frankenmolen F, Burgersdijk R. Two years' clinical evaluation of class I and II compomer restorations in deciduous molars. Int Dent J 1995;45:305 [abstract 112].

82. Roeters JJM, Frankenmolen F, Burgersdijk RCW, Peters TCRB. Clinical evaluation of Dyract in primary molars: 3-year results. Am J Dent 1998; 11:143–148.

83. Frankenberger R, Sindel J, Krämer N. Viscous glass-ionomer cements: A new alternative to amalgam in the primary dentition? Quintessence Int 1997;28:667–676.

84. Vulicevic ZR, Beloica D, Vulovic M. A clinical trial of two compomer systems. J Dent Res 1997;76:165 [abstract 1211].

85. Kitty MY, Wie SHY. Clinical evaluation of compomer in primary teeth: 1-year results. J Am Dent Assoc 1997;128:1088–1096.

86. Council on Dental Materials and Devices: Status report on the glass-ionomer cements. J Am Dent Assoc 1979;99:221.

87. Croll TP. Glass ionomer silver cermet class II tunnel restorations for primary molars. J Dent Child 1988;55:177.

88. Croll TP. Glass-ionomer for infants, children and adolescents. J Am Dent Assoc 1990;120:65.

89. Knibbs PJ, Plant CG. An evaluation of a rapid setting glass-ionomer cement used by general practitioners to restore deciduous teeth. J Oral Rehabil 1990;17:1.

90. Kullmann W, Freers M. Klinische Studie zur Restauration von Milchzähnen mit einem Glasionomerzement im Vergleich zu einem Amalgam. Dtsch Zahnarztl Z 1984;39:333.

91. Plant CG, Shovelton DS, Vlietstra JP. The use of a glass-ionomer cement in deciduous teeth. Br Dent J 1977;143:271.

92. Staehle HJ. Glasionomerzementfüllungen bei Milchzähnen—ein Erfahrungsbericht. Zahnarztl Welt 1984;93:62.

93. Vlietstra JR, Plant CG, Shovelton DS, Bradnock G. The use of glass-ionomer cement in deciduous teeth. Br Dent J 1978;145:164.

94. Qvist J, Qvist V, Mjör IA. Placement and longevity of amalgam restorations in Denmark. Acta Odontol Scand 1990;48:298–303.

Chapter 12

Clinical Applications of Glass-Ionomer Cements: Class III and Class V Restorations

Pierre Jonas, Jean-Jacques Lasfargues, and Michel Degrange

In recent decades, important ongoing developments have progressively changed dental restorative materials. Scientific and clinical requirements have imposed new criteria that take into account not only intrinsic mechanical performance, reliable adhesion to dental substrates, and esthetics, but also biological compatibility and cariostatic potential.

A typical example of such developments is glass-ionomer cements (Figs 12-1a and 12-1b), which originated from polycarboxylates and have been used successfully since the 1970s. They were initially simple acid-base cements, but the sophisticated technology of light-activated monomers yielded a resin-modified version. The addition of resin to glass-ionomer cements led to a wide categorization of materials of different compositions, including hybrid materials such as compomers. The diversity of available materials, as well as the inconsistencies between scientific terminology and commercial advertising, present difficulties for the practitioner in distinguishing a product's actual characteristics and appropriate indications.

When Wilson and Kent's[1] first works were published in 1971 on the special properties of glass-ionomer cements, the dental community realized the importance of these new materials in clinical applications. The cariostatic potential of fluoride is undeniable and the release of fluoride by glass-ionomer cement is a determining prophylactic element in therapeutic choices according to many authors.[2]

Today, with 30 years of hindsight, it is possible to assess the clinical behavior of glass-ionomer cements. They have shown high quality and durability in their spontaneous and direct adhesion to the tooth, even on smooth and nonretentive surfaces.[3–5] This adhesion is easily and quickly achieved and offers a satisfactory sealed restoration. By contrast, the resin bonding technique is more demanding and takes substantially more time to achieve an acceptable result than initially anticipated. However, conventional glass-ionomer cements suffer from several disadvantages (Fig 12-2), which explains their limited indications and the reservations of a number of practitioners. The most common drawbacks are:[6]

Figs 12-1a and 12-1b Glass-ionomers used to restore cervical lesions.

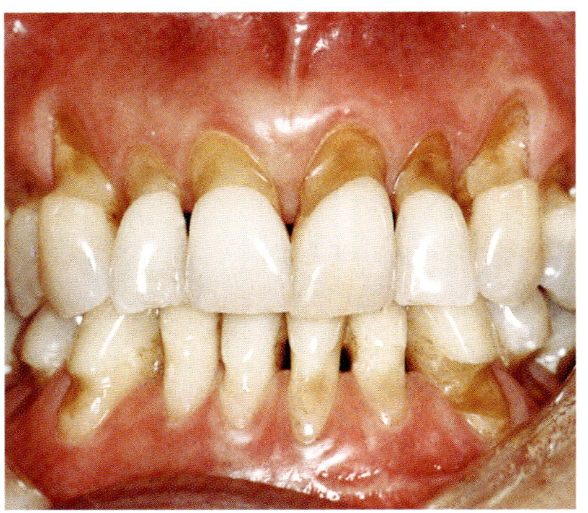

Fig 12-1a Initial situation before restoration.

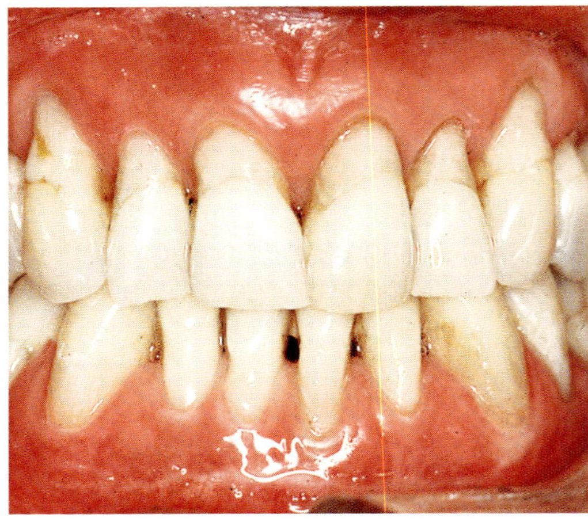

Fig 12-1b Restorations after 10 years.

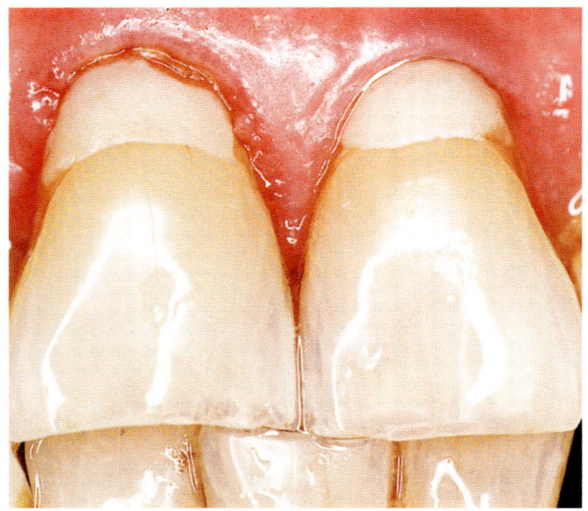

Fig 12-2 Conventional glass-ionomer restoration of a Class V lesion 11 years after placement. The main defects are signs of marginal deterioration (chipping) and poor esthetics. However, restorations are still in place due to the excellent adhesive properties of the glass-ionomers, and there is no secondary caries.

• Modest mechanical performance. Toughness, tensile strength, wear resistance, and hardness are inferior to those of resin composites.
• High initial solubility after mixing. Setting must take place in an area protected from fluid contamination.
• Relatively long setting time (3 to 5 minutes, depending on the product).
• Poor polishability due to the heterogeneous and porous structure of the material.

After a period of stability, and even stagnation, in further development, glass-ionomer cements today benefit from renewed interest among researchers and practitioners, particularly since the introduction of resin-modified glass-ionomers and hybrid cements. In many clinical situations, new glass-ionomer materials have replaced old ones, while they get closer to resin composites in esthetic appearance. Unfortunately, their traditional characteristics and advantages cannot always be maintained.

The scope of recommended indications for conventional glass-ionomers has been extended. Material manipulation is faster and easier and procedures have been simplified, which is beneficial to both the practitioner and the patient. These cements allow the application of two modern strategies in dental treatment: diagnose to prevent and eliminate the need to cure, and consolidate and restore without trauma and destruction.

In this chapter, Class III and Class V restorations are discussed. They deserve particular attention because glass-ionomer materials are very well indicated for these clinical situations.

Class III Restorations

A Class III cavity is a carious lesion on the proximal surface of anterior teeth. This lesion is usually found slightly gingival to the contact area and is located in a site that is favorable to plaque retention. The current literature and manuals of operative dentistry identify different categories of Class III lesions: incipient enamel caries, cavitated enamel caries, and dentinal caries surrounded by enamel, and dentinal caries with margins extending to the root surface.[7,8]

Some authors prefer a classification based on operative access to the cavity. The choice of access to the lesion is important in determining the preservation of the tooth structure. According to Miller,[9] Class III restorations are divided into three types: type 1 has facial access but no lingual access; type 2 has lingual access but no facial access (Figs 12-3a to 12-3e); and type 3 is throughout the tooth (Figs 12-4a to 12-4e).

Incipient enamel caries and cavitated enamel caries can be detected in children and young adults despite systematic or topical fluoride. In addition to patients with medical problems, those with poor oral hygiene and high carbohydrate consumption are candidates for the development and progress of Class III lesions.

When a practitioner determines that the development of a carious lesion does not allow remineralization, operative procedures are required to stop its progression.[10] Class III restorations are among the most frequent and routine operative procedures in dentistry. The treatment rationale, preparation, and choice of restorative material are determined based on several parameters, including the

Figs 12-3a to 12-3e Treatment of a Class III isolated lesion with a compomer. In this young patient, the absence of a high carious risk led to the choice of a compomer to restore this small lesion, which is not subject to occlusal stresses.

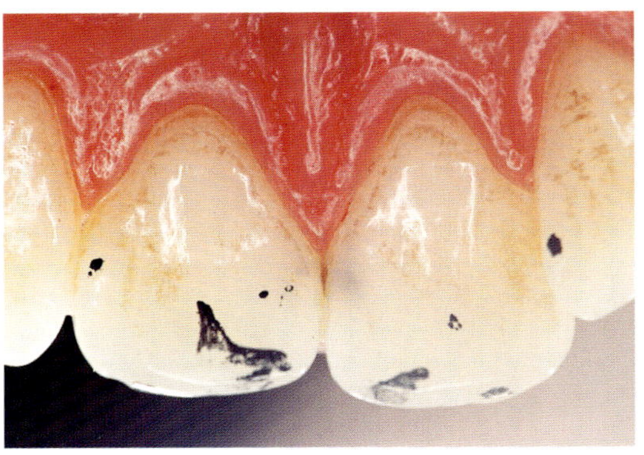

Fig 12-3a Caries is visible through the discolored enamel. The marked occlusion points are not in the restoration area.

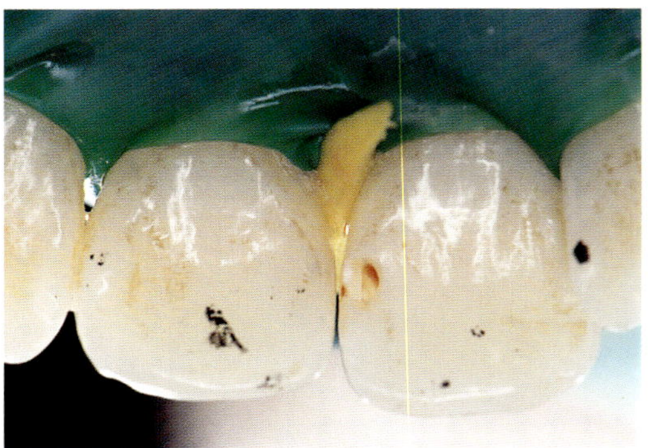

Fig 12-3b After isolation by rubber dam, a round, unbeveled cavity is prepared. A wooden stick is placed to separate the teeth and to prevent any damage to the adjacent tooth. The buccal enamel is kept for esthetic reasons and discolored secondary dentin is also kept on the pulpal wall because it does not affect esthetics.

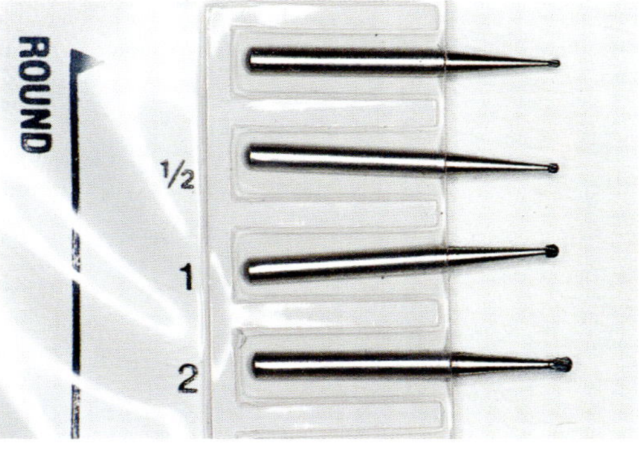

Fig 12-3c A 0.5-mm Tungsten round bur was used.

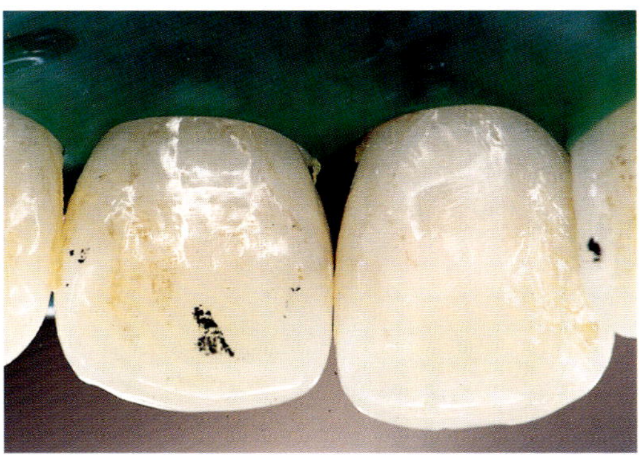

Fig 12-3d After application of a primer adhesive, the compomer restoration is completed.

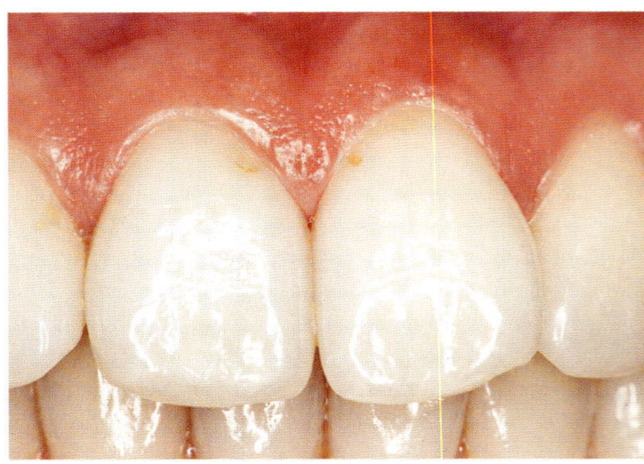

Fig 12-3e The final result preserves previous esthetics.

Figs 12-4a to 12-4e Treatment of proximal caries in a 75-year-old patient. The high carious risk indicated the use of a hybrid glass-ionomer material for its cariostatic potential.

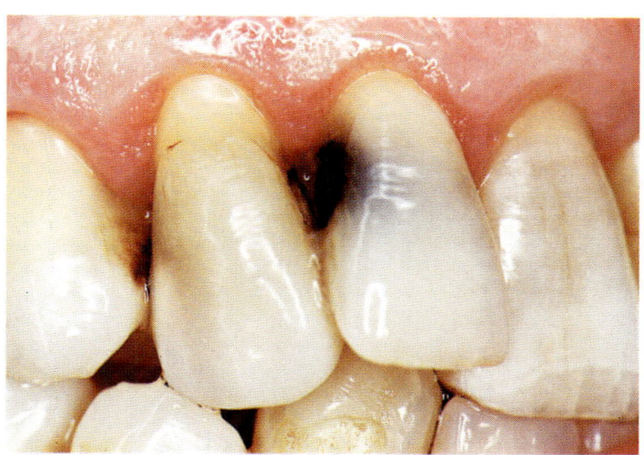

Fig 12-4a Proximal caries is evident in opposing cavities in teeth 12 and 13.

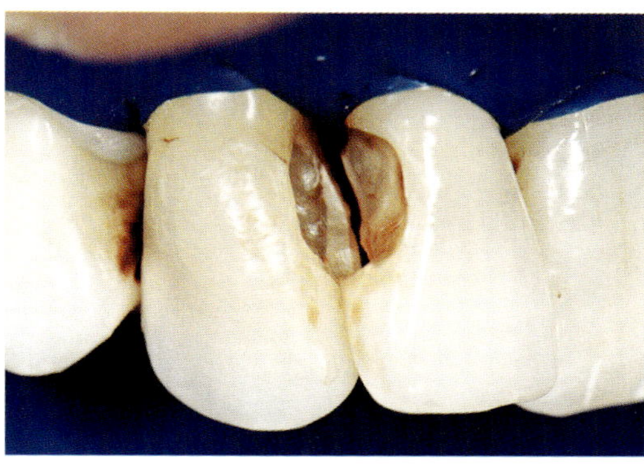

Fig 12-4b After isolation by rubber dam, deep caries is removed. Due to elimination of all cervical enamel, the use of resin composites was not indicated.

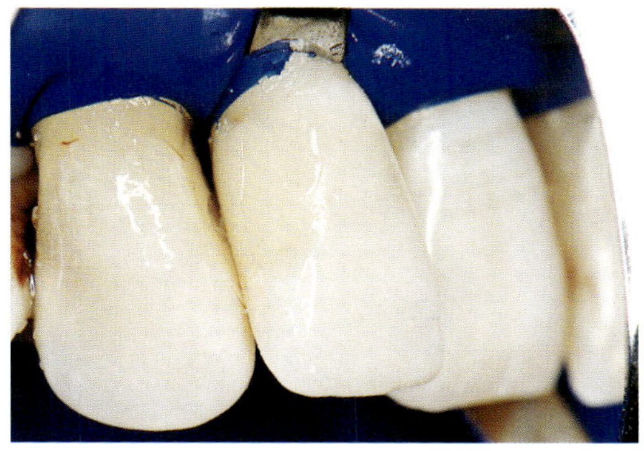

Fig 12-4c After etching with 25% polyacrylic acid for 20 seconds and rinsing, Fuji II LC was injected. The material was light cured and compressed with Mylar tape and polymerized again. The cement was immediately protected with a fluid resin film.

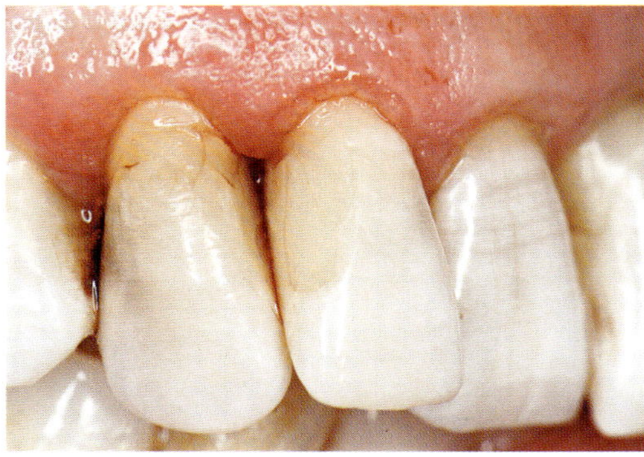

Fig 12-4d Result immediately after removing the rubber dam.

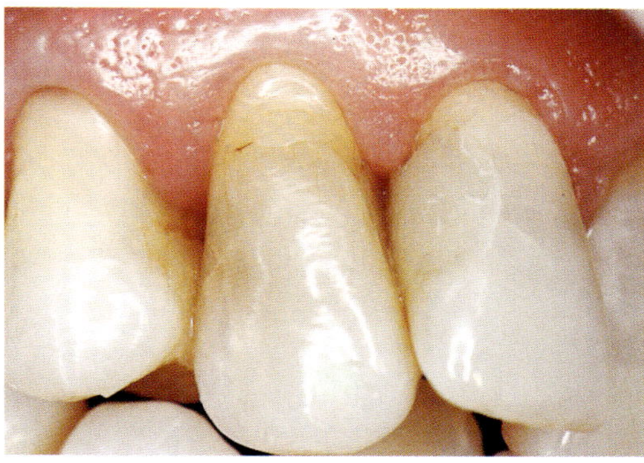

Fig 12-4e The restoration after 2 years. Other lesions have been restored in the same manner. Note the recurrent caries.

Figs 12-5a and 12-5b Proximal caries in teeth 13 and 14 presenting difficult access. Due to low occlusal stresses, the absence of cervical enamel, the small occlusal surface of cavities after elimination of carious tissues, and the high risk of plaque retention, a resin-modified glass-ionomer was chosen to restore these lesions.

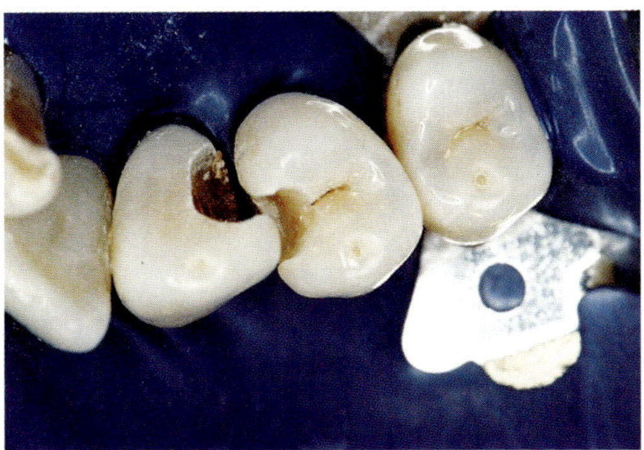

Fig 12-5a Cavities before elimination of caries.

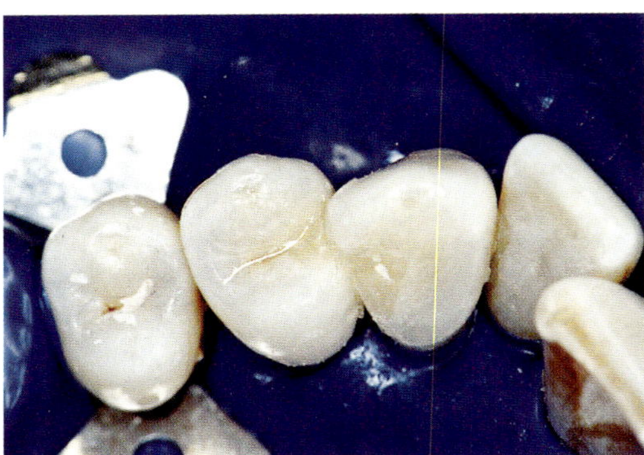

Fig 12-5b Teeth with finished restorations.

topography of the lesion (Figs 12-5a and 12-5b)—that is, extension and depth, access, number of lesions, and the state of the oral environment. An important aspect of treatment planning is the risk, assessment of progression, and recurrence of caries. These factors must be adequately taken into account to achieve successful oral therapy.[11]

A whole range of materials can be used for the restoration of Class III cavities: microhybrids, microfill and flowable resin composites, resin-modified glass-ionomers, or polyacid-modified resin composites (compomers). For patients with a high risk of caries, glass-ionomer cements are preferred because of their cariostatic potential.[12] Their use, along with caries control measures, is helpful in shifting a patient with a high risk of caries to a lower risk category through controlling, stabilizing, and stopping the disease. After this compulsory phase of control and arrest of caries, the dentist can focus on an optimal esthetic restoration, following the rule that health is more important than esthetics. The principles of adhesive dentistry are applied: a minimal, conservative preparation that removes sound tooth structure only to gain access is used; carious tissues are eliminated; and retention grooves are necessary. Mechanical features of the glass-ionomer cement, especially its brittleness, determine the butt joint margins and do not allow bevels.

Clinical procedures

1. Administration of a local anesthetic is optional.
2. The tooth surface is cleaned with nonfluoridated pumice and water on a rubber cup or with an ultrasonic instrument and air flow.
3. The correct shade of cement is selected. Glass-ionomer cements usually are available in several shades according

to VITA standard. The transparency of new glass-ionomer cements is greater than that of former generations.

4. The operative field is prepared. Absolute isolation is only achieved with a rubber dam. Relative isolation can be achieved with cotton rolls.

5. Cavity preparation is the next step. Healthy tooth structure should not be sacrificed unnecessarily. However, for noncavitated lesions, the enamel can be removed with extra-fine diamond burs. In carious lesions, the softened pathologic tissues must be removed, but the deep sclerotic dentin is retained. The dentin and enamel edges must be strong. In all cases, the outline form has to be delineated steadily and plainly.

6. The lesion is covered with a (straight or curved) Mylar strip that extends 1 to 2 mm over the sound tooth structure and is used to compress the restorative material into the cavity. The matrix is selected, tried, adapted, and stabilized before injection of the material. A wedge also is selected if necessary.

7. The cavity is cleansed with a disinfectant such as chlorhexidine. Biofilms, mineralized deposits, and the smear layer need to be removed without demineralizing the intertubular dentin, because glass-ionomer cement reacts chemically with the calcium ions in the dentin.

The surface is etched with 10% to 20% polyacrylic acid for 20 seconds to enhance the bond.

The surface is rinsed copiously and dried gently to avoid desiccation. Excess water should be blotted or wiped off with a cotton pellet. The dentin surface must be kept shiny. If the surface is contaminated at this stage, pretreatment must be repeated.

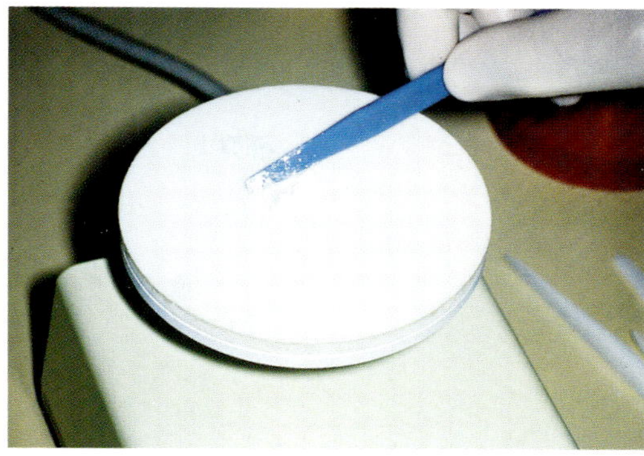

Fig 12-6 A mechanical mixing device (GCMA automixer).

If the resin-modified glass-ionomer Vitremer is used, it contains a combined surface conditioner and primer. After application, the primer is light cured but not rinsed.

8. The preparation of the cement should be executed with a mixture of powder and liquid, according to the manufacturer's recommendations. In some cases, easy, reproductive, and quick mixing can be completed on the nonstick plate of an electric rotary mixer (Fig 12-6). Another approach is to use capsules, triturate and inject directly. The danger of manipulation error is negligible. Nevertheless, capsules still need to be improved with a thinner, more adjustable tip to inject the material with more precision.

9. The material is loaded with a syringe. The matrix is placed to compress the material. A wedge can be inserted on the gingival embrasure if necessary.

10. The restoration is light cured for 45 to 60 seconds. The depth of cure is 3 to 4 mm and provides an appreciable level

of security for setting of the cement. Furthermore, the unreacted cement below 3 to 4 mm cures chemically without diminishing the cement's physical/mechanical properties.

11. According to some researchers, at least 80% of the material is cured at the contouring and polishing stage. The chemical cure can last for approximately 1 day. Therefore, some authors advise starting finishing procedures immediately, but not polishing until 1 or 2 days later. In clinical practice, it is rather difficult to make an appointment only for polishing. Most patients prefer a procedure that is completed in one appointment.

Proximal overhangs are removed with a No. 10 or No. 12 scalpel blade. Contouring is performed with wet finishing burs. Polishing is done with extra-fine diamond burs, finishing discs, and strips under air or water spray without excessive pressure. The major difficulty is to blend the cementoenamel junction.

12. A final application of varnish, bonding, or finishing gloss is required to protect the cement during the first 24 hours of setting. An esthetically pleasing result can be achieved if each detail is carefully handled.

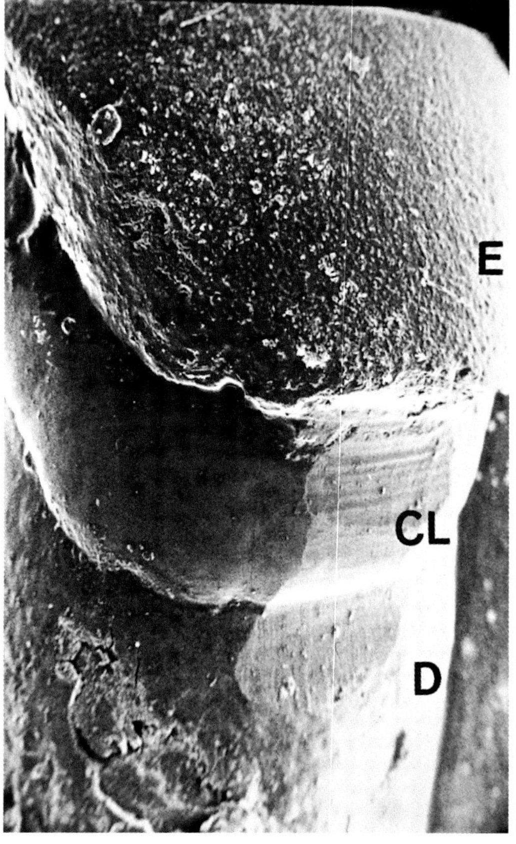

Fig 12-7 Scanning electron micrograph of an extracted tooth with a cervical lesion. The carious lesion (CL) overlaps the cementoenamel junction between the undermined coronal enamel (E) and the radicular dentin (D). The lesion may spread proximally, as shown here, toward embrasures.

Class V Restorations

Class V carious cervical lesions are found in patients of any age with high sugar intake and poor oral hygiene. Cervical caries also can be induced by reduced salivary flow due to radiation (associated with cancer treatment), toxicomania, or neuroleptic drugs.

Root caries especially affects the elderly, because exposed root areas are subject to plaque accumulation if these sites are not brushed and cleaned properly (Fig 12-7). Glass-ionomer cements are particularly indicated for root caries because fluoride release may prevent recurrent caries. Noncarious, wedge- or saucer-shaped cervical lesions are characterized by loss of hard tissue at the cementoenamel junction in the absence

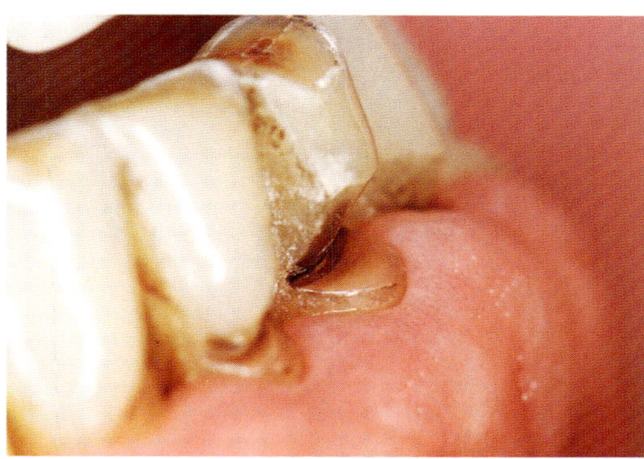

Fig 12-8 An abrasive lesion exhibiting a hard base (due to the presence of translucent sclerotic dentin), sharp outlines, and sharp (notch-shaped) angles.

of caries. The prevalence of these lesions has increased with the improvement of oral hygiene and the aging of the population.

The interaction of several etiologic factors is the source of Class V defects:

- Abrasion associated with mechanical wear (traumatic tooth brushing) often affects groups of teeth unilaterally[13] (Fig 12-8).
- Abfraction associated with stress caused by occlusal forces affects single teeth, most often maxillary first premolars[14] (Figs 12-9a to 12-9g).
- Chemical erosion associated with diet,[15–20] medication, and gastric reflux[21] affects teeth in groups (Figs 12-10a and 12-10b).

Volume and form changes, caused by the mismatch between the restoration and the adjacent tooth structure during setting of the restorative material and during occlusal loading and flexure of the restored tooth, can be factors in debonding and consequent loss of adhesive cervical restorations. Bond strength and stiffness of the restorative material, as well as the configuration factor of the nonretentive cavity, are determining parameters for the success of the restoration.[22] Glass-ionomers initially show elastic behavior and become rigid with time. More than resin composites they have the potential for elastic deformation and thus can compensate for induced strain. It has been shown that flexible materials with a low modulus of elasticity are indicated for Class V restorations, because such materials reduce the risk of failure at the adhesive interface.[23] However, if esthetic and functional results with glass-ionomer cement are unsatisfactory, it is always possible to cover the cement with a resin composite at a later time.

The principles and strategy for treatment of Class V lesions are similar to those for Class III cavities. In the case of noncarious lesions, or when a carious lesion is no longer active, the glass-ionomer can be placed and bonded without pretreatment of the cavity.

When esthetics is a top priority, microfilled resin composite is the material of choice. But when numerous lesions extend to the cementum and spread deeply into dentin, glass-ionomer cement is preferred. In addition to the benefit of fluoride release, the direct bonding ability of glass-ionomers secures a fast and satisfactory seal.

Clinical procedures

The procedures for Class V restorations are similar to those for Class III. Administration of local anesthesia, prophylaxis, and cleaning are as described earlier for Class III restorations.

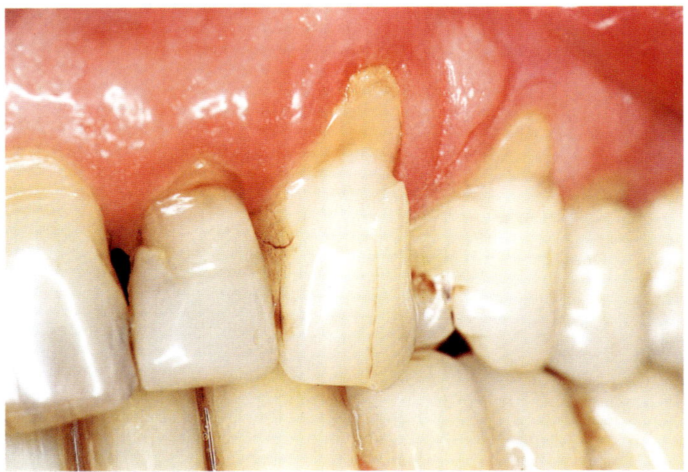

Fig 12-9a Clinical appearance of noncarious cervical lesions.

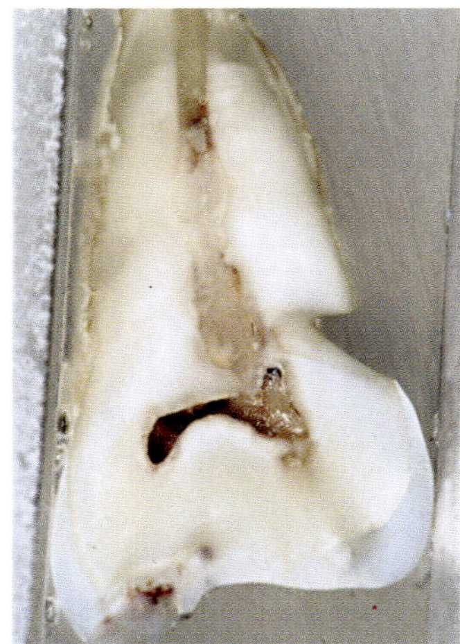

Fig 12-9b Typical lesion on a hemisectioned tooth.

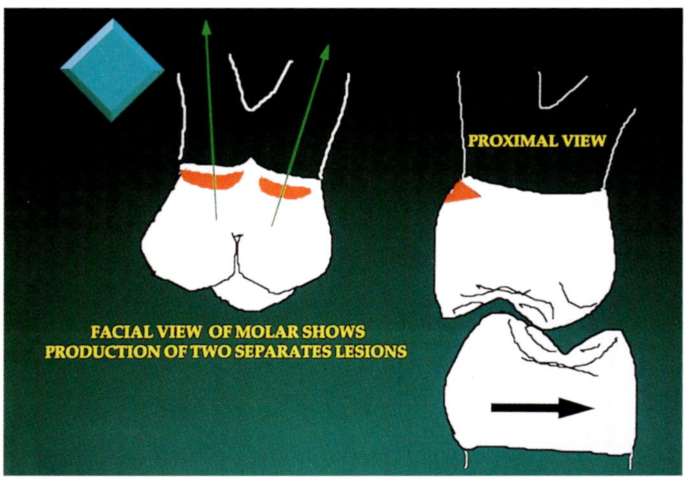

Fig 12-9c Abfraction lesions are caused by dislocation of enamel prisms due to a concentration of stress in the cervical area. (Adapted from Lee and Eakle.[14])

Figs 12-9d and 12-9e The location of abfraction lesions is linked to lateral and propulsive occlusive movement. (Adapted from Lee and Eakle.[14])

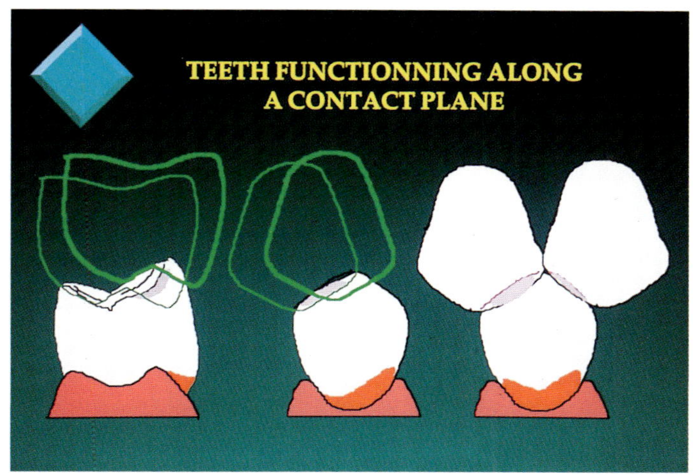

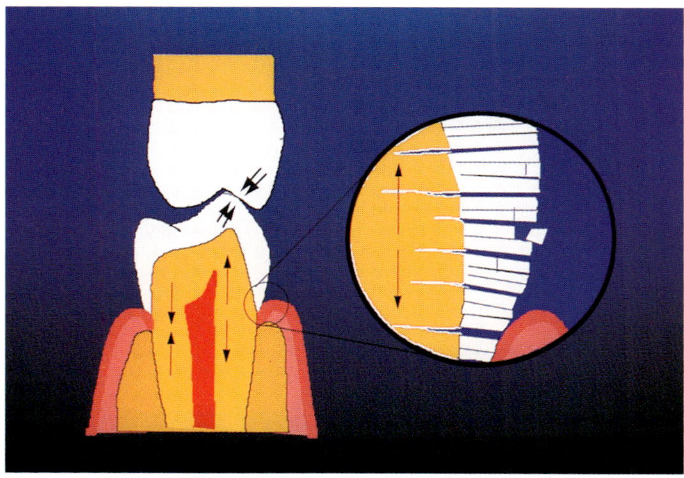

Figs 12-9f and 12-9g The formation of noncarious cervical lesion pathogenesis is not only caused by chemical erosion and traumatic tooth brushing, but cervical flexure of the tooth can also be a contributing factor. Vertical barreling of the tooth due to centric forces (CF) can produce compressive stresses (CS) and lateral deformation (LD) in the cervical restoration (CR), while eccentric occlusal forces (EF) may result in bending of the tooth, causing tensile stresses (TS) in the cervical restoration. (Adapted from Heymann et al.[15])

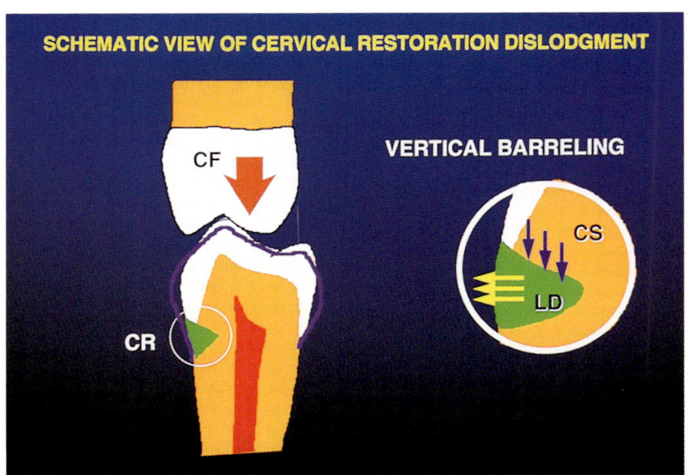

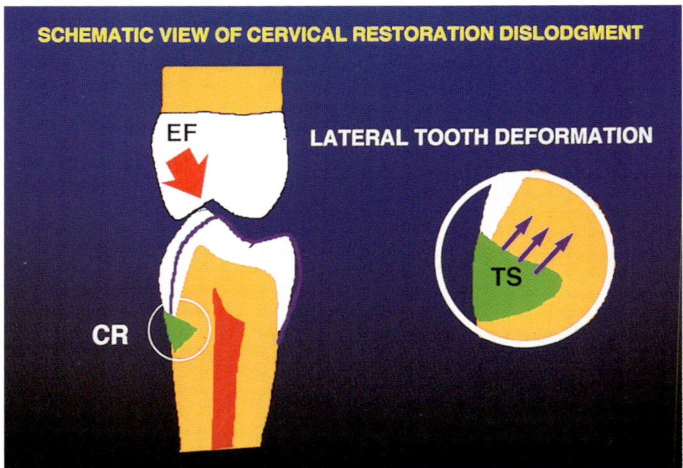

Figs 12-10a and 12-10b Clinical identification of caries.

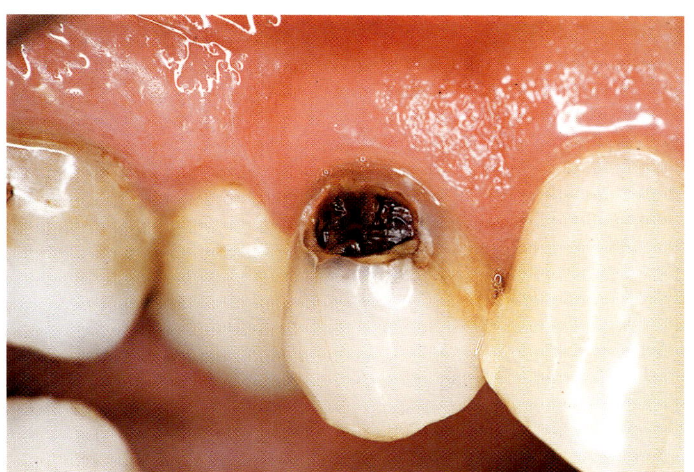

Fig 12-10a Discoloration and softened dentin.

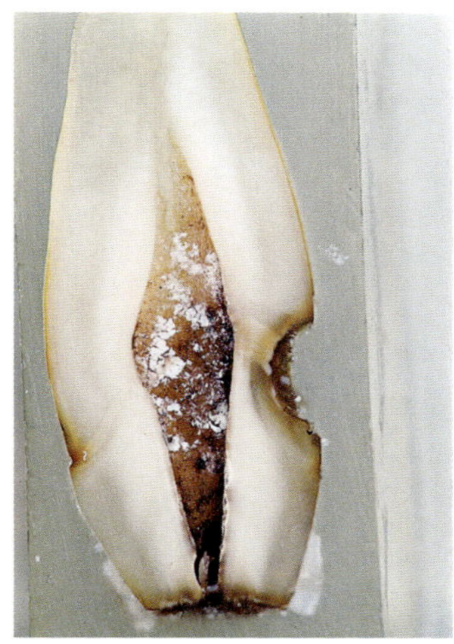

Fig 12-10b Round shape and an absence of sharp (saucer-shaped) outlines in a hemi-sectioned tooth.

1. The correct shade of cement is selected. For cervical lesions, translucency is less important than color. The damaged structure is mainly dentinal. Shades A and B (yellow and dark yellow) can harmonize well with natural tooth structure.
2. The operative field should be isolated from moisture and permit access to the cervical outline as necessary to obtain a good marginal seal. This access is sometimes difficult, when the lesions are partially or wholly subgingival (Figs 12-11a and 12-11b). In some cases, periodontal surgery is required to expose the entire lesion. Glass-ionomer cement is used as a temporary filling before the surgery (Figs 12-12a to 12-12f).
3. Gingival retraction is performed next. When the gingival tissues are healthy, it is possible to expose the gingival margin of the lesion with the help of retraction cords. A surgical silk cord and a second finely knitted cord are packed into the sulcus with a gingival spatula. These cords protect the gingival margin during preparation. After preparation, the finely knitted cord is removed and the rubber dam placed. The remaining silk cord helps prevent sulcular bleeding. When the lesion shows inaccessible subgingival limits, two steps are recommended (Figs 12-13a to 12-13c). An initial filling of resin-modified glass-ionomer is placed. The final restoration is a sandwich of glass-ionomer cement and resin composite.
4. The cavity is isolated with Nos. 9, 211, and 212 retainers. In some cases, rubber dam placement is difficult. The placement of a contour strip in the sulcus provides an alternative to the rubber dam (Figs 12-14a and 12-14b).

Fig 12-11 Overcoming the technical difficulty of isolating the tooth and the lesion in Class V restorations.

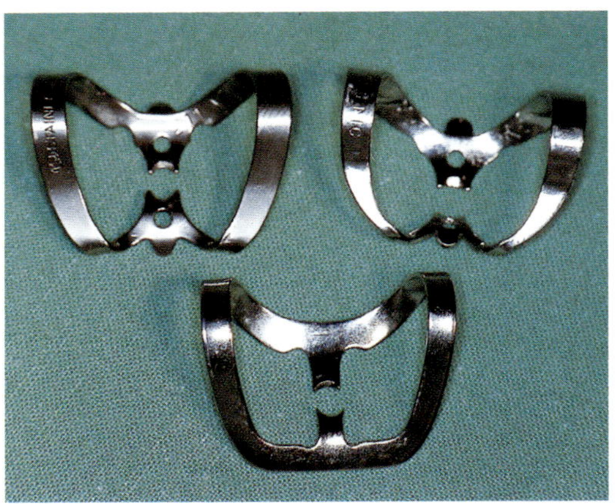

Fig 12-11a Adapted clamps used in isolation.

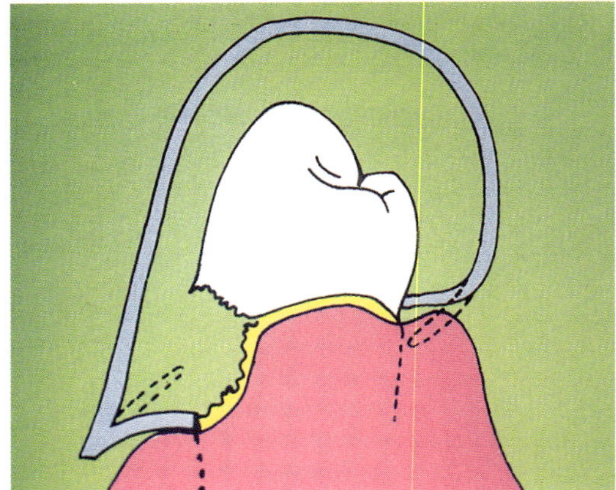

Fig 12-11b Clamps allow a rubber dam to be placed while preserving access to the gingival edge of the lesion.

Figs 12-12a to 12-12f Treatment of radicular juxtagingival caries with glass-ionomer filling.

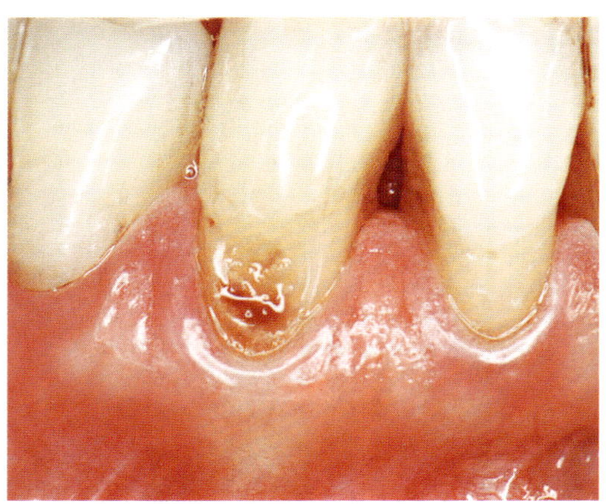

Fig 12-12a Lesion prior to restoration.

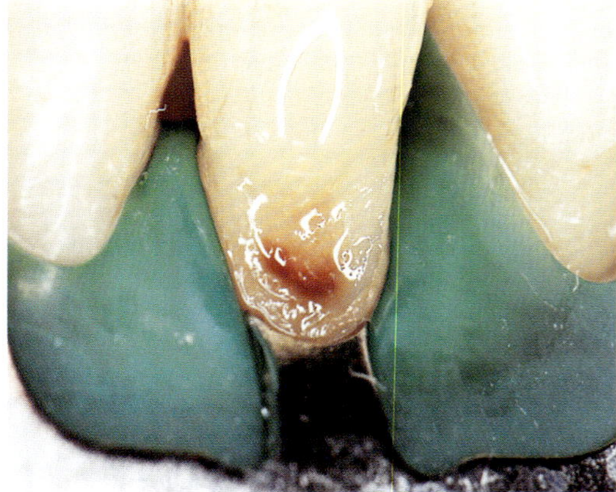

Fig 12-12b The rubber dam is in place and maintained by a No. 212 clamp. The jaws of clamps often need to be sharpened (to a point) with a bur.

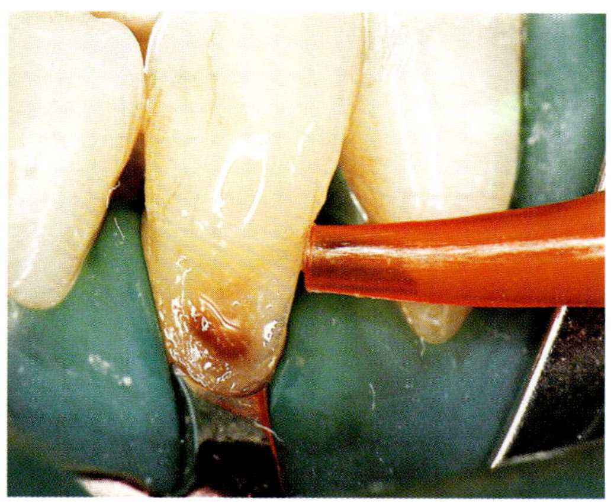

Fig 12-12c The material is injected and adapted without salivary contamination or interference from tongue or cheeks.

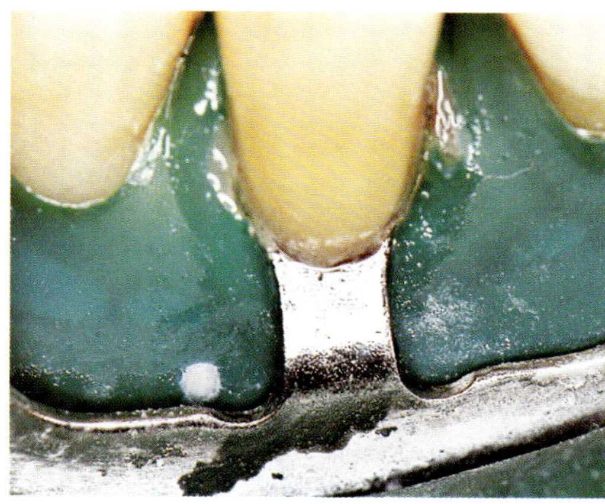

Fig 12-12d After the material is injected, and the excess removed, it is light cured and covered immediately with a fluid resin.

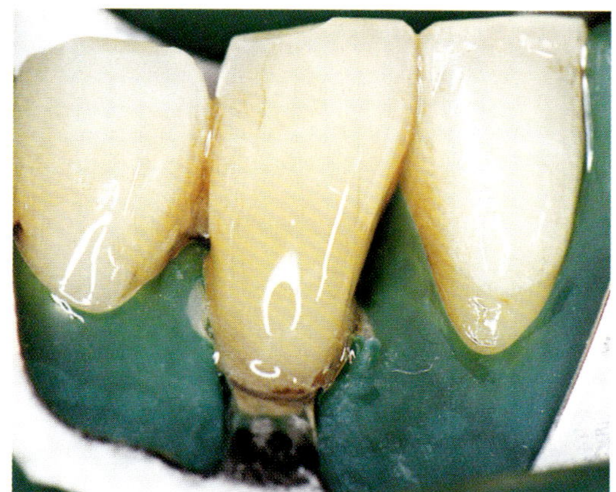

Fig 12-12e After checking the set of the cement, the restoration is outlined and finished following the radicular emergence profile, then the rubber dam is removed.

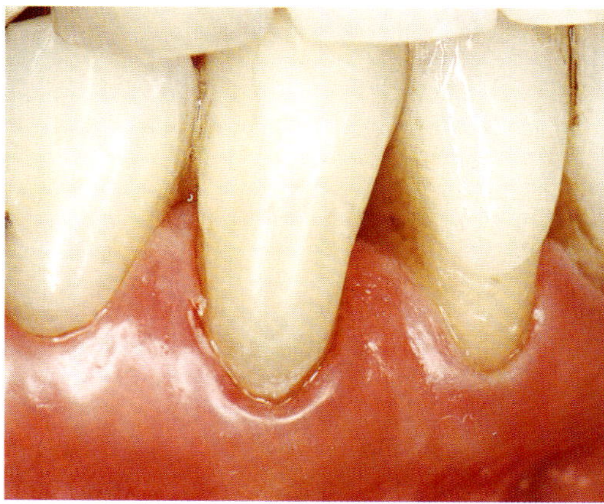

Fig 12-12f Result immediately following the procedure.

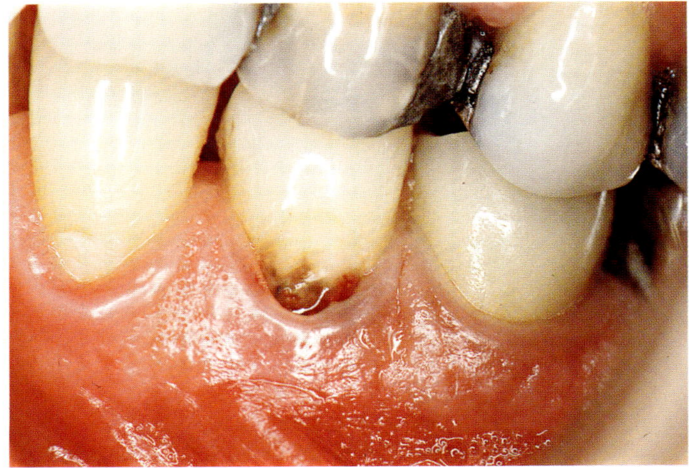

Fig 12-13a Cervical caries associated with the loss of a composite filling.

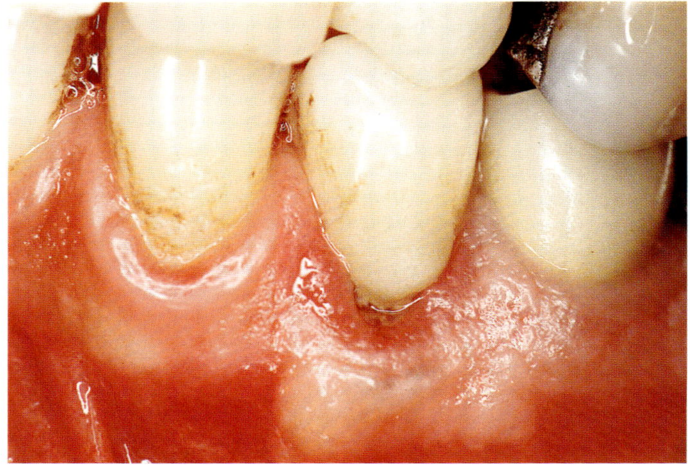

Fig 12-13b Once the gum has been repositioned apically beyond the gingival limit, the cavity is filled with a resin-modified glass-ionomer.

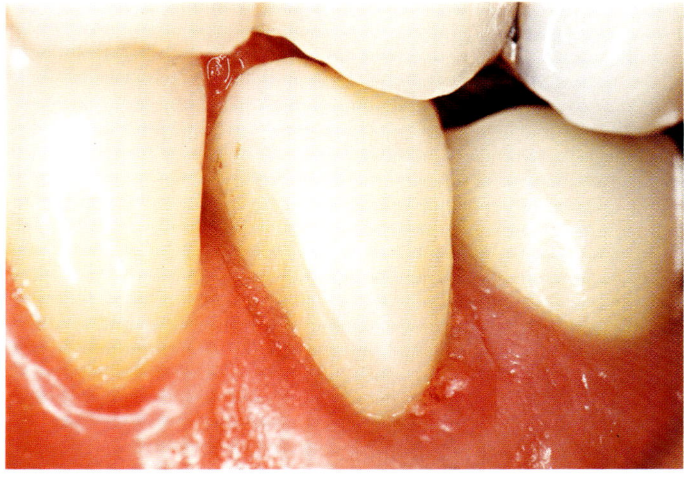

Fig 12-13c When gingival healing is advanced, the glass-ionomer filling is repaired, which allows a better esthetic result.

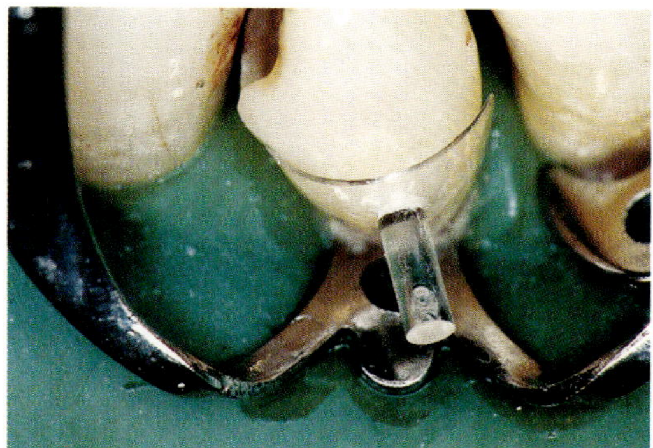

Fig 12-14a The use of Hawe cervical matrix allows a firm compression of the material without oxygen interference.

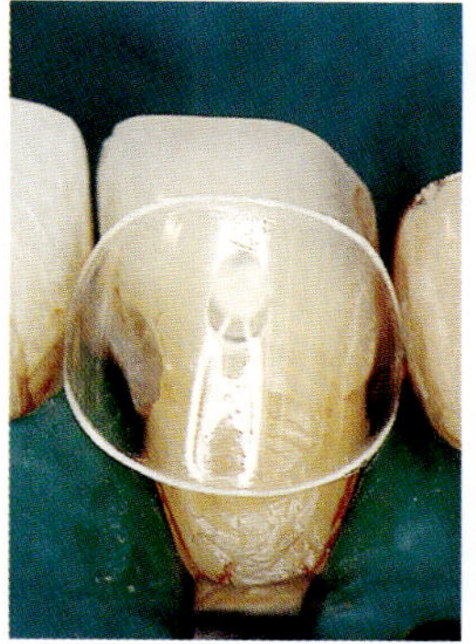

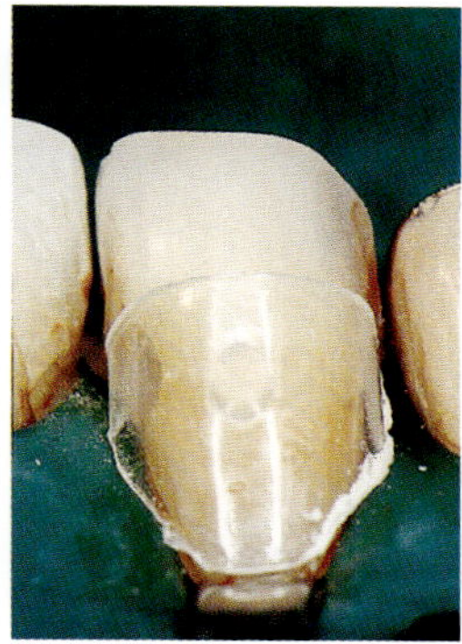

Fig 12-14b These matrices can be trimmed to obtain a precise adaptation to the gingival edge of the cavity.

5. As in preparation of Class III lesions, healthy tooth structure should not be removed unnecessarily. In noncarious lesions, the enamel can be roughened by extra-fine diamond burs. In carious lesions, the softened pathologic tissues are excavated, but the deep sclerotic dentin is retained. The dentin and enamel edges must be strong. In either case, the outline form must be delineated steadily and plainly.

The operative decision regarding the margin varies according to the shape of the lesion. If the lesion is saucer shaped (from erosion), a circumferential groove is cut with a round bur following the outline of the defect to increase the thickness of the filling margins. If the lesion is notch shaped (from abrasion) with a cavosurface angle of about 70 to 90 degrees, the natural butt joint is acceptable without any preparation.

6. A light, permeable matrix is used to compress the restorative material into the cavity. The matrix is selected, tried, adapted, and stabilized before the injection of the material. A wedge also is selected if necessary.

7. Cleansing of the cavity, acid etching, rinsing, and drying, as well as preparation of the cement, are performed as described earlier for Class III restorations.

8. The material is loaded using a syringe with a needle-tube or using a capsule. The injection should proceed slowly to avoid bubbles. Excess filling should be kept to a minimum to make contouring and finishing easier. Resin-modified glass-ionomers are preferred to both conventional glass ionomers and resin composites when there is a minimal risk of caries (Figs 12-15a to 12-15h). The main aim of temporary glass-ionomer fillings is to promote oral hygiene by removing bacterial concentrations and to remineralize the peripheral hard tissues through fluoride release.

9. Placement of the matrix, light curing, contouring, and polishing are executed as for Class III restorations.

Figs 12-15a to 12-15h Glass-ionomers are preferred to compomers and resin composites when there is a high risk of caries. Numerous cervical lesions were identified in this 45-year-old patient. Before placing definitive restorations, lesions were stabilized and peripheral hard tissues remineralized. Because of their ability to release fluoride, glass-ionomers were recommended as caries preventive temporary fillings.

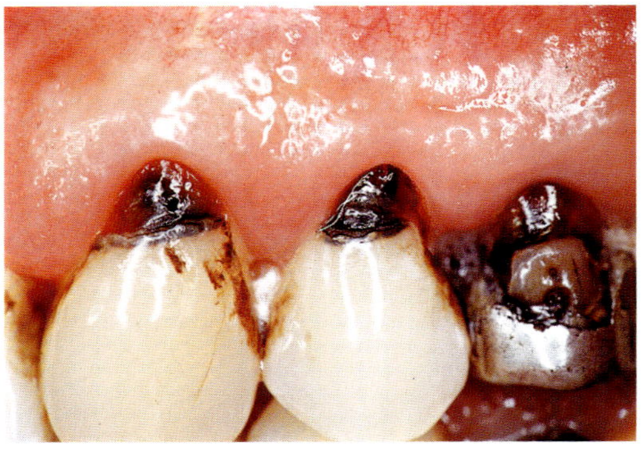

Fig 12-15a Initial lesion.

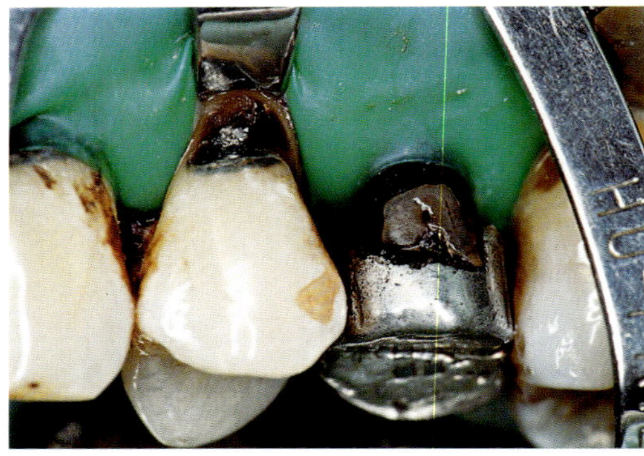

Fig 12-15b Isolation of the operative field for tooth 15 with a No. 212 clamp.

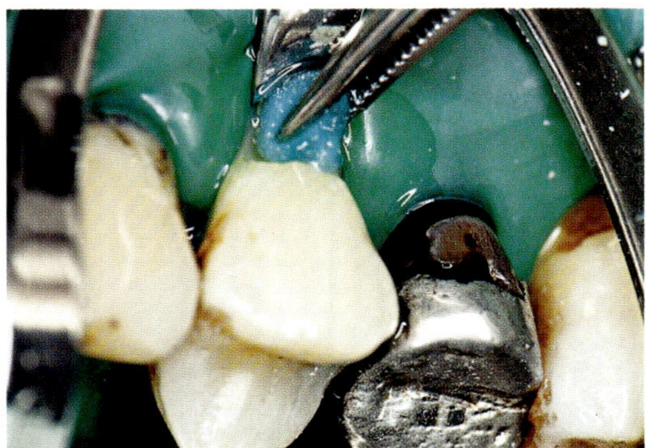

Fig 12-15c Etching of the cavity surface with polyacrylic acid for 20 seconds.

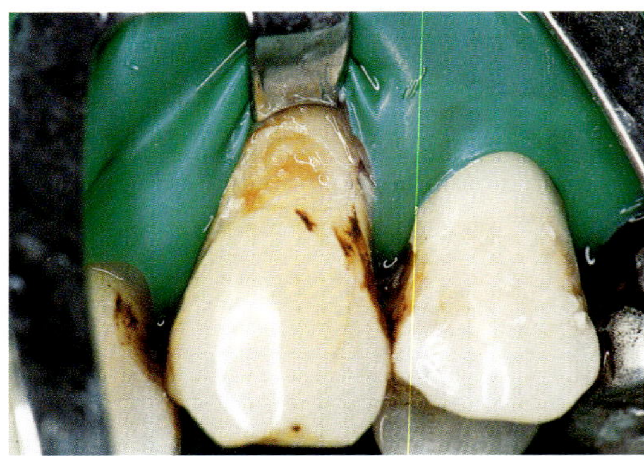

Fig 12-15d Once the restoration of tooth 15 is completed, the clamp is moved to treat tooth 14. The cavity shape depends on the elimination of carious dentin, but the peripheral demineralized enamel is not removed.

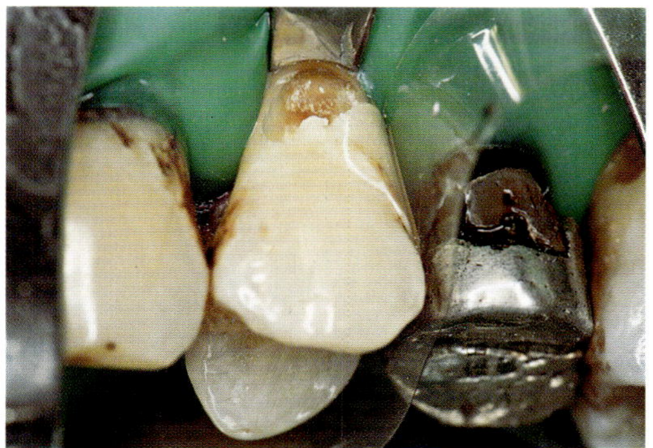

Fig 12-15e Due to proximal extension of the lesion, filling with resin-modified glass-ionomer cement was carried out in two steps. The distovestibular portion, held in place by Mylar tape inserted in the distal embrasure, is first light cured.

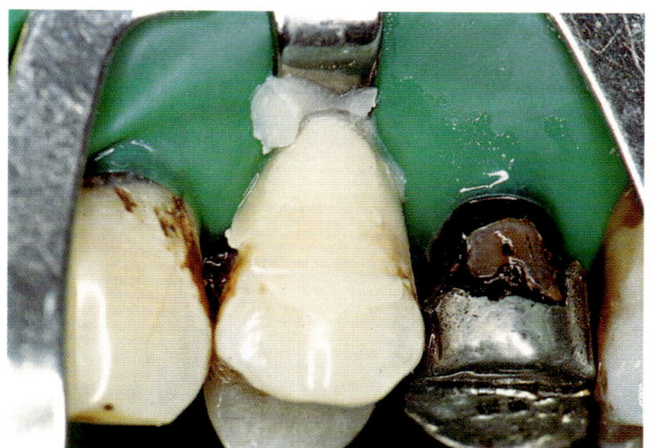

Fig 12-15f The rest of the cavity is filled, compressed by a Hawe matrix, and light cured.

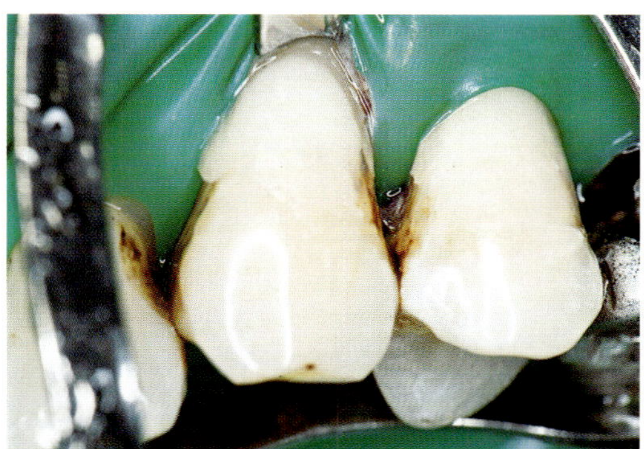

Fig 12-15g Excess is removed with fine, flame-shaped diamond burs, and fillings are polished with silicon points.

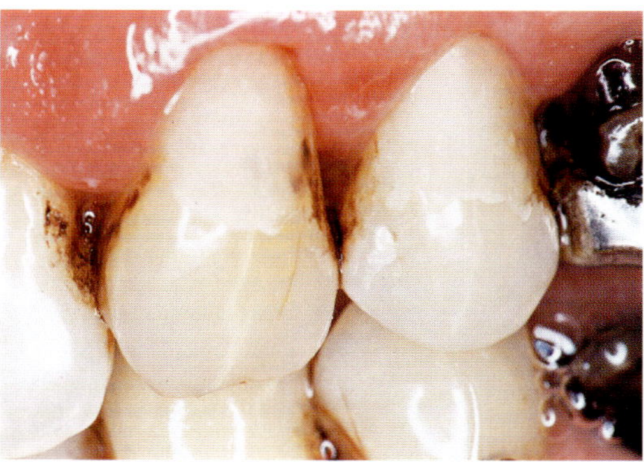

Fig 12-15h The completed restorations are esthetically acceptable although this was not a priority.

Clinical assessment

The use of glass-ionomer cements as Class V cervical restoration materials now benefits from more than 20 years of clinical experience. The results from the few relevant clinical studies conducted since the 1980s were unfavorable, particularly concerning esthetics and wear. The cement became opaque with time and the surface appeared rough and porous (see Fig 12-2).

The need to control moisture when placing the material and during initial setting is acknowledged as the major problem with conventional glass-ionomer cements. When such control is lacking, it causes faster damage to the material and a loss of esthetics, together with deterioration of physical, chemical, and mechanical properties. However, when recommended procedures are followed exactly, it is possible to obtain more satisfactory, long-lasting (up to 15 years) clinical results with glass ionomers than with composites.[24] Until the 1990s, most authors believed glass-ionomer cements had a greater potential marginal seal and retention rate than composite restorations in the long term.[25]

The sealing properties of glass-ionomer cements is due to their spontaneous adhesion capacity, including adhesion to cervical dentin which is often sclerotic and hypermineralized. Filling failures are due more often to cohesive fractures within the filling than to adhesive rupture at the cement–dentin interface. This is not the case with resin composites, which bond poorly to hypermineralized cervical dentin. Before the latest versions of dentin adhesives were developed, it was impossible to achieve an excellent survival rate for composite restorations.[26] It is well established that one of the major factors in adhesive cervical resin composite restoration failure is occlusal stress leading to flexural stress, which is at a maximum in the cervical area. The concentration of stress favors bonding disruption and even ejection of the restoration.[15] This disruption trend is more serious when the material's modulus of elasticity is substantially different than that of the dentin. From this point of view, glass-ionomer cements, which are less stiff than resin composites, work better. This could explain their high retention rate despite low and generally inferior adhesion values to the dentin compared with those of resin composites.

Another reputed advantage of conventional glass-ionomer cement is fluoride release. This release continues for several years after initial placement and can give these materials a cariostatic potential that has been widely demonstrated in vitro. Prevention of recurrent caries around glass-ionomer restorations also has been demonstrated in vivo.[27,28] However, more recently, Mjör[29] and Wilson et al[30] discovered that the main cause for replacement of glass-ionomer cement restorations was recurrent caries. An explanation for such results might be that the glass-ionomers that failed were probably placed in difficult clinical situations, in hostile oral environments, and in unmotivated and uninformed patients, where all other restoration materials had already failed or were inappropriate or unusable. Under these conditions, restoration failure was inevitable. Currently, glass-ionomer cements are victims of their reputation as easy-to-use "miracle materials" that bond well and prevent caries. Clinical procedures are said to be easy, nonrigorous, and nonspecific. These standards are nearly impossible to meet consistently.

Although some authors find the results of current glass-ionomers better than those of resin composites,[31] all authors agree that the esthetic performance of conventional glass-ionomer cements does not meet the requirements of today's patients. To overcome this disadvantage, an initial solution of adapting the "sandwich" technique to Class V restorations has been suggested. This combined glass-ionomer/resin composite technique has two advantages:[32,33]

- The resin composite present on the surface layer prevents wear degradation and improves the marginal quality and esthetics when used with enamel etching (Figs 12-16a to 12-16g).
- The retention rate is higher, equal to that of glass-ionomer cement used alone and better than fillings using only resin composites.

However, the combined use of the two materials is complex and contrary to the need for simplicity in general practice. This is why, during recent years, new materials have been developed from glass-ionomers and light-cured technology: dual-cured glass-ionomer cements, or resin-modified glass-ionomers and compomers. Unfortunately, clinical studies on resin-modified materials are rare and, when they exist, do not have adequate observation time. In the short term (1 to 2 years), the retention rate of cervical fillings with resin-modified glass-ionomer cements and with compomers was nearly 100%, and all other restorations were considered clinically acceptable.[34,35] All tested fillings showed signs of deterioration and marginal discoloration, which are considered clinically unacceptable. In the case of compomers, the discoloration affected the enamel margins more than the dentin in the gingival area.[35] This tends to justify the pretreatment of enamel with phosphoric acid before the placement of a compomer. Today, no restoration system (resin composites, modified glass-ionomer cements, or modified composites) seems able to completely prevent microinfiltrations in either the incisal or the cervical margins of Class V fillings.[36]

Recently, Van Dijken and Hörsted[37] compared the enamel marginal adaptation of resin-modified glass-ionomers, compomers, and resin composites in Class III fillings in vivo. After 1 year, the quality of marginal adaptation of all three restoration systems was evaluated as good, regardless of the nature of enamel pretreatment. Resin-modified glass-ionomers displayed the best adaptation to enamel, followed by composites, then compomers. The difference between resin-modified glass-ionomers and compomers was significant. On the basis of current clinical data, it is not possible to recommend the use of compomers to replace either resin-modified glass-ionomer cements or resin composites.

Additional random, controlled clinical trials (the gold standard of clinical research) are necessary to assess long-term performance of the two hybrid materials in Class V and Class III restorations. More investigations also are needed to confirm their adhesion and sealing potential, wear resistance, and potential to prevent recurrent caries. Preservation of esthetics, color stability, and resistance to staining also have to be established.

The clinical consequences of using compomer in patients whose risk of ca-

Figs 12-16a to 12-16h Treatment of generalized cervical abrasions. Generalized abrasive lesions of all anterior teeth are identified in this 50-year-old patient treated for rapidly advancing periodontitis without caries.

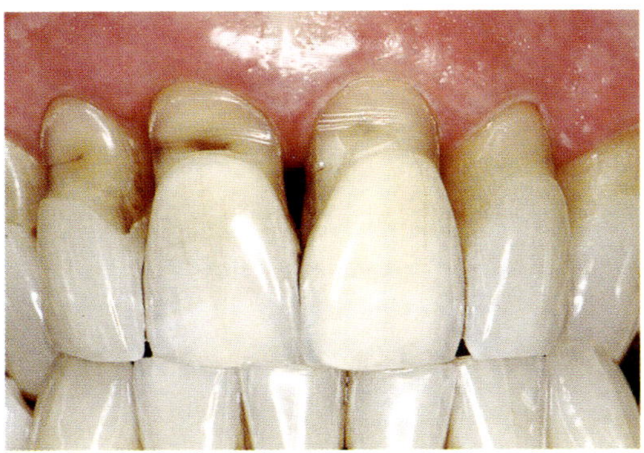

Fig 12-16a Lesion etiology was traumatic tooth brushing. An esthetic, abrasion-resistant material was required, and a compomer was chosen.

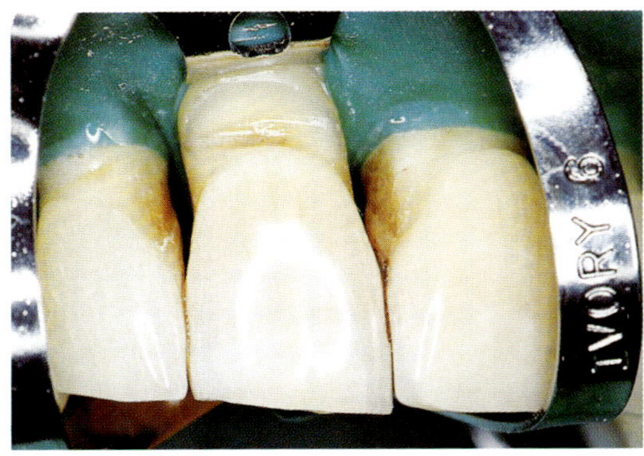

Fig 12-16b All anterior teeth have been isolated by placing a rubber dam from premolar to premolar. A No. 9 clamp is moved from one tooth to another (here to tooth 11) to expose the gingival edge of the cavity.

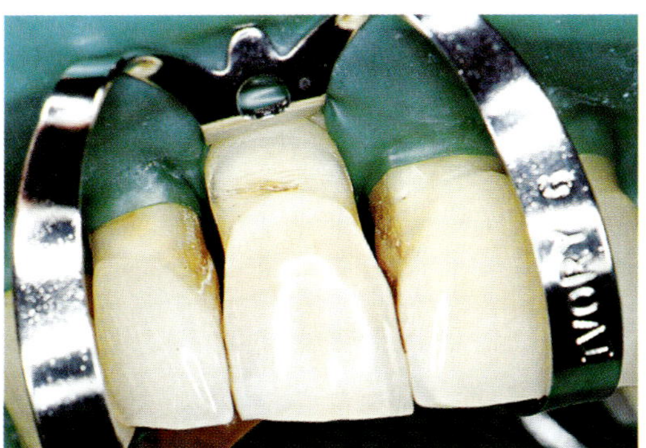

Fig 12-16c Preparations have been etched with 37% phosphoric acid for 20 seconds, rinsed, and dried. This etching, although not recommended by the manufacturer, is indispensable in preventing further risk of marginal infiltration, particularly in the enamel.

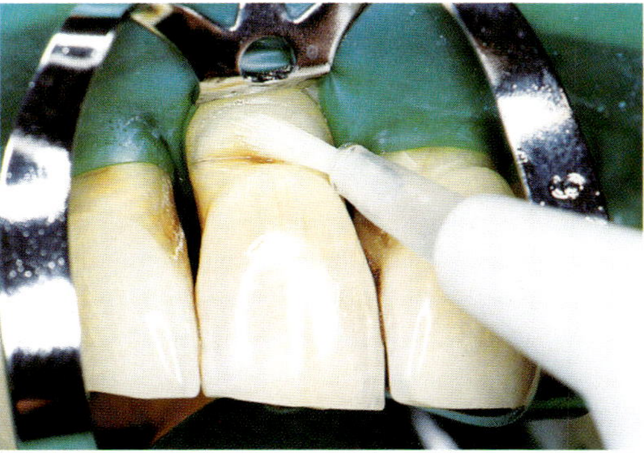

Fig 12-16d The adhesive is applied to the enamel and dentin with a brush to obtain a film of even thickness, air dried, and light cured.

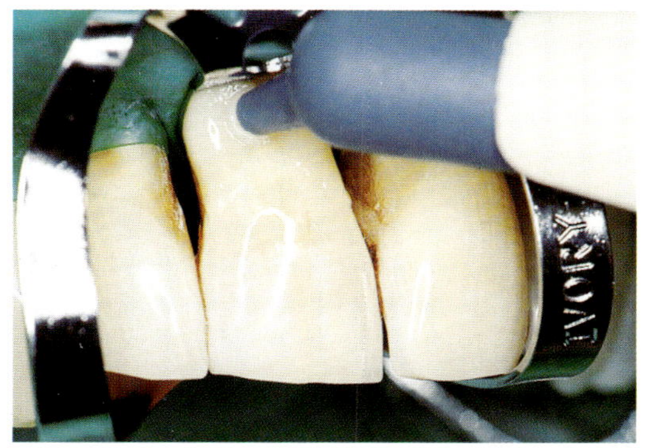

Fig 12-16e The compomer is injected in one or more layers according to the size of the area to be filled.

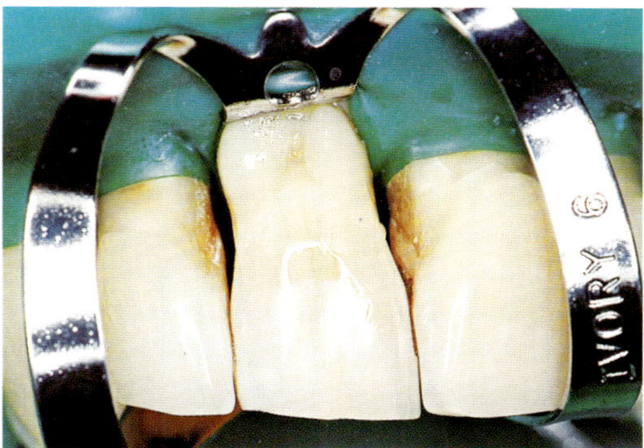

Fig 12-16f Two distinct increments allow mesial and distal faces to be filled.

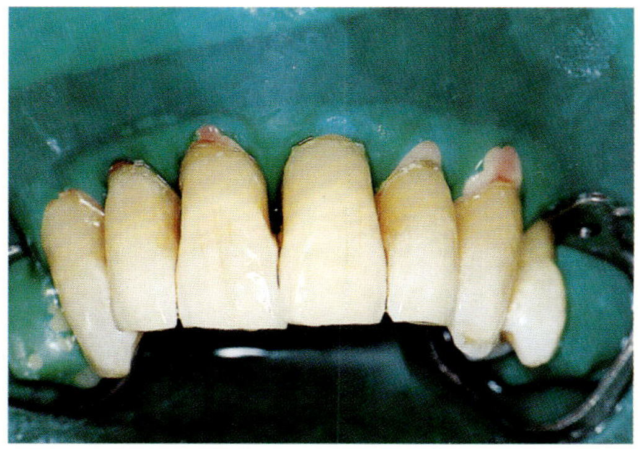

Fig 12-16g Finishing is carried out under the rubber dam.

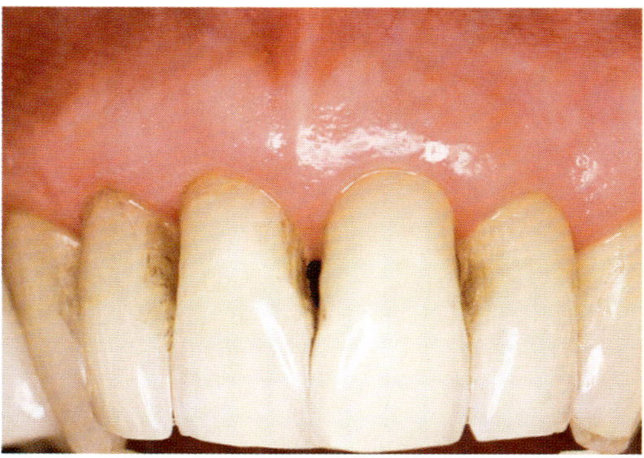

Fig 12-16h The restoration after 1 year.

Figs 12-17a and 12-17b Use of a compomer to repair a defective prosthetic margin.

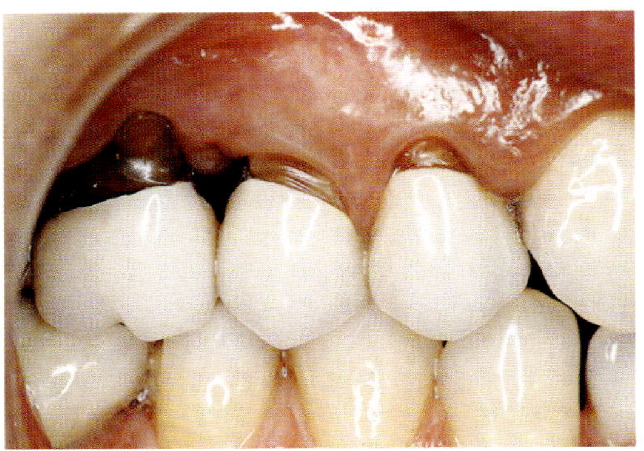

Fig 12-17a Gingival recession has occurred at the margins of ceramic crowns. Abraded sclerotic dentin surfaces are evident.

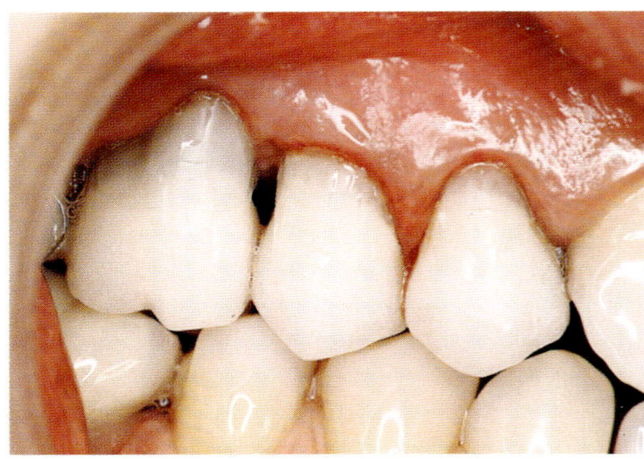

Fig 12-17b Since the crowns were satisfactory, the lesions were treated by bonding a compomer material to the cervical margin. The compomer was chosen for its adhesive properties and its ease of handling in areas that are difficult to access, both in the absence of caries risk.

ries has not been checked are unknown (Figs 12-17a and 12-17b). This material is known to release lower quantities of fluoride than those from conventional or resin-modified glass-ionomer cements.

Summary

Glass-ionomer cements are reliable materials if used correctly. Practitioners can be confident in using these materials and can achieve predictable, satisfactory results that benefit the patient.

Conventional or resin-modified glass-ionomer cements are excellent and useful materials, provided their use is restricted to small restorations that are not directly subject to occlusal forces. A risk of caries should be present, and esthetics should be of secondary importance to the patient. Resin composites associated with modern adhesives remain the favored material for restorations subject to direct occlusal forces and for situations in which the esthetic result is a priority, such as extended Class III and Class V lesions in anterior teeth.

Clinical data currently available do not indicate the use of compomers in the treatment of Class III or Class V cavities as an alternative to glass-ionomer cements or resin composites. Even if the immediate esthetic result is excellent, the long-term preservation of this result is uncertain, particularly due to the high risk of marginal discoloration highlighted recently by several authors.[38]

Compomers are more technique-sensitive than resin-modified glass-ionomers; require a longer handling time; and, above all, do not have the same physical, chemical, and mechanical advantages, such as spontaneous adhesion and fluoride release. The utility of these materials is also questionable when compared to resin composites, which have longer lasting esthetics and greater adhesion potential.

References

1. Wilson AD, Kent BE. The glass-ionomer cement: A new translucent dental filling material. J Appl Chem Biotechnol 1971;21:313.

2. Forsten L. Fluoride release of glass-ionomers. In: Hunt P (ed). Glass-Ionomers: The Next Generation. Proceedings of the 2nd International Symposium on Glass-Ionomers. Philadelphia: International Symposia in Dentistry, 1994;241–248.

3. Hickel R. Les verres-ionomères d'obturation: Applications cliniques actuelles. Real Clin 1991;2:313–324.

4. Wilson AD, McLean JW. Adhesion. In: Wilson AD, McLean JW (eds). Glass-Ionomer Cement. Chicago: Quintessence, 1988;83–106.

5. Erickson RL, Glasspoole EA. Bonding to tooth structure: A comparison of glass-ionomer and composite-resin systems. J Esthet Dent 1994;6:227–244.

6. Meyer JM. Les ciments verres-ionomères. Real Clin 1991;2:281–292.

7. Chan DCN, Cooley RL. Direct anterior restorations. In: Schwartz RS, Summit JB, Robbins JW (eds). Fundamentals of Operative Dentistry. Chicago: Quintessence, 1996;187–205.

8. Alberts HF. Class III-restorations. In: Tooth-coloured-restoratives, 8th ed. Santa Rosa, CA: Alto Books, 1996;8a1–8a7.

9. Miller MB. Class III direct restorations. Reality 1998;12:541–558.

10. Clarkson J. Clinical considerations for restorations. In: Hunt P (ed). Glass-Ionomers: The Next Generation. Proceedings of the 2nd International Symposium on Glass-Ionomers. Philadelphia: International Symposia in Dentistry, 1994;151–160.

11. Elderton RJ. Principles of decision-making to achieve oral health. In: Professional Prevention in Dentistry. Baltimore: Williams and Wilkins, 1994;1–27.

12. Anderson MH. Oral health maintenance by preventive therapy. In: Professional Prevention in Dentistry. Baltimore: Williams and Wilkins, 1994;109–126.

13. Pindborg JJ. Pathology of the Dental Hard Tissues. Copenhagen: Munksgaard, 1970.

14. Lee WC, Eakle WS. Possible role of tensile stress in the etiology of cervical lesions in teeth. J Prosthet Dent 1984;52:374–380.

15. Heymann HO, Sturdevant JR, Bayne S, Wilder AD, Sluder TB, Brunson WD. Examining tooth flexure effects. J Am Dent Assoc 1991;122:41–47.

16. Asher C, Reed MJF. Early enamel erosion in children associated with the excessive consumption of citric acid. Br Dent J 1987;162:384–387.

17. Clark DC. Oral complications of anorexia and/or bulimia: with a review of the literature. J Oral Med 1985;40:134–138.

18. Hällström I. Oral complications in anorexia nervosa. J Dent Res 1977;85:71–86.

19. Levine RS. Fruit juice erosion—an increasing danger? J Dent 1973;2:85–88.

20. Linkosalo E, Markkanen H. Dental erosions in relation to lacto-vegetarian diet. Scand J Dent Res 1985;93:436–441.

21. Xhonga-Oja FA, Valdmanis S. Factor analysis of dental erosion occurrence. J Oral Rehabil 1968;13:247–256.

22. Feilzer AJ, De Gee AJ, Davidson CL. Setting stress in composite resin in relation to configuration of the restoratives. J Dent Res 1987;66:1636–1639.

23. Kemp-Scholte CM, Davidson CL. Marginal integrity related to bond strength and strain capacity of composite resin restorative systems. J Prosthet 1990;64:658–664.

24. Mount GJ. Longevity in glass-ionomer restorations: Review of a successful technique. Quintessence Int 1997;28:643–650.

25. Mathis BA, Cochran M, Carlson T. Longevity of glass-ionomer restorative materials: Results of a 10 year evaluation. Quintessence Int 1996; 27:373–382.

26. VanMeerbeek B, Peumans M, Gladys S, Braem M, Lambrechts P, Vanherle G. Three-year clinical effectiveness of four total-etch dentinal adhesive systems in cervical lesions. Quintessence Int 1996;27:775–784.

27. Wood RE, Maxymiw WG, McComb D. A clinical comparison of glass-ionomer (polyalkenoate) and silver amalgam restorations in the treatment of class 5 caries in xerostomic head and neck cancer patients. Oper Dent 1993;18:94–102.

28. Powell LV, Johnson GH, Gordon GE. Factors associated with clinical success of cervical abrasion/erosion restorations. Oper Dent 1995; 20:7–13.

29. Mjör IA. Glass-ionomer restorations and secondary caries: A preliminary report. Quintessence Int 1996;27:171–174.

30. Wilson NH, Burke FJ, Mjör IA. Reasons for placement and replacement of restorations of direct restorative materials by a selected group of practitioners in the United Kingdom. Quintessence Int 1997;28:245–248.

31. Mount GJ. Glass-ionomer cements: Past, present, and future. Oper Dent 1994;19:82–90.

32. McLean JW, Powis DR, Prosser HJ, Wilson AD. The use of glass-ionomer cements in bonding composite resins to dentine. Br Dent J 1985;158:410–411.

33. Neo J, Chew CL. Direct tooth-colored materials for non-carious lesions: A 3-year clinical report. Quintessence Int 1996;27:183–188.

34. Abdalla AI, Alhadaini HA, Garcia-Godoy F. Clinical evaluation of glass-ionomers and compomers in class V carious lesions. Am J Dent 1997;10:18–20.

35. Tyas MJ. Clinical evaluation of a polyacid-modified resin composite (compomer). Oper Dent 1998;23:77–80.

36. Ferrari M, Davidson CL. Sealing capacity of resin modified glass-ionomer and resin composite placed in vivo in class V restorations. Oper Dent 1996;21:69–72.

37. Van Dijken JW, Hörsted P. Marginal adaptation to enamel of a polyacid-modified resin composite (compomer) and a resin-modified glass-ionomer cement in vivo. Clin Oral Invest 1997;1:185–190.

38. Gladys S. Esthetic performance of hybrid restorative material in cervical class V lesions. In: Gladys S (ed). In Vitro and In Vivo Characterization of Hybrid Restorative Materials. Leuven, Belgium: Leuven University Press 1997;89–97.

Chapter 13

Glass-Ionomer Restorations in Stress-Bearing and Difficult-to-Access Cavities

F. J. Trevor Burke and Nairn H. F. Wilson

Materials for restorations in permanent teeth have many requirements. Apart from favorable biocompatability, sealing ability, and (increasingly) good esthetic qualities, one of the principal requirements is the ability to withstand functional loading in the hostile environment of the oral cavity. There are a number of forces to which a restoration may be subjected. For example, tensile and compressive stress may combine to produce bending forces and shear forces, with the outcome being complex stresses within the restored tooth during loading.[1] The ability of the restorative material, as an integral part of the restored tooth, to resist the many stresses inherent in function largely determines the material's performance in clinical service.

Types of Force

As illustrated in Fig 13-1, when occlusal and bending forces are present, the result may be the formation of tensile stresses. The tensile strength of a dental material has often been considered its most critical physical property, because many clinical failures of restorations have been attributed to tensile failure.[2] Glass-ionomers, cermets, and resin-modified glass-ionomers (all glass-ionomer–derived materials that set by acid-based reaction) possess satisfactory compressive strength, but tend to have a lower tensile strength than resin composite and compomers.[3] This low tensile strength limits the clinical applications of all glass-ionomer materials, notably in stress-bearing situations. In general, when glass-ionomer materials are used in such situations, it is desirable for the material to be protected by the remaining tooth structure or for the restoration to be designed to provide protection of the material in some other way. In this respect, the concept of restoration design (a function of cavity design, location of occlusal contact, and the properties of the restorative material) should be addressed for any given clinical situation and material.

Wear resistance and the associated degradation may be considered a function of many characteristics of a material, including filler loading and type, elasticity of the filler, modulus of elasticity, bonding of filler to matrix, solubility of components in dilute organic acids, hardness, and creep. Although the wear resistance of direct restorative materials has been considered ideal if it is similar to that of

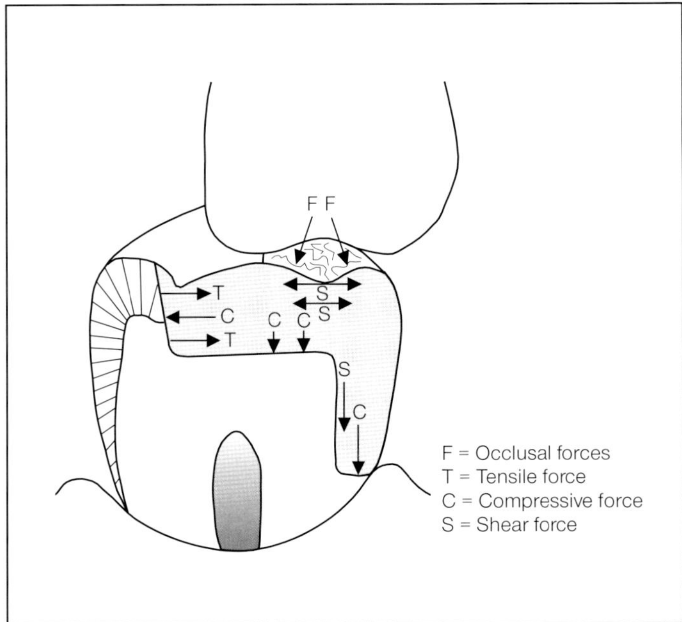

Fig 13-1 Forces applied to restorations.

enamel,[4] current glass-ionomer materials do not satisfy this requirement[5] given their relatively poor resistance to attrition, abrasion, and erosion. This further restricts the use of these materials in situations of direct loading.

Glass-ionomer materials may therefore be deemed to lack the physical properties necessary for satisfactory performance as a substitute for traditional restoratives in load-bearing situations. As a consequence, glass-ionomers, when used in load-bearing teeth with Class I or Class II lesions, may be expected to fail due to fracture and excessive wear. This view is supported by the results of studies of the clinical performance of glass-ionomer restorations in permanent teeth, which indicate a suboptimal rate of success. Hickel and coworkers[6] showed a 50% failure rate of Class II restorations after 2 years, and Mjör and Jokstad[5] reported that after 3 years Class II glass-ionomer/cermet restorations failed more than four times as often as amalgam restorations.

Similarly, Smales and coworkers[7] showed that Class I glass-ionomer restorations did not perform as well as Class I restorations using resin composite or amalgam. Indeed, the latter group of researchers discontinued the use of glass-ionomer/cermet material in their study because of the clinical problems encountered. However, with the growing trend toward preservation in lesion management, the widely reported advantage of fluoride release throughout the life of a glass-ionomer restoration, and a realization of the limitations of traditional restorations in particular situations, glass-ionomer materials may have an expanding range of applications in situations where the material may be protected from damaging occlusal stresses. Among such applications are temporary and interim restorations, sealants and preventive restorations,[8,9] tunnel restorations,[10] "sandwich" (laminate) restorations,[11] atraumatic restorative treatment (ART),[12] and core buildups (foundation restorations).[13] The stresses applied to restorations in children are substantially less than the forces applied in adults, and glass-ionomer materials may be satisfactory substitutes for traditional restoratives in deciduous teeth, as described in Chapter 11.

Types of Restorations

Temporary restorations

A temporary, or provisional, restoration is intended to last for a short period of time, typically a matter of days or, at most, a few weeks. Temporary restorations in glass-ionomer materials may be placed in a wide variety of situations, including:

- Emergency replacement of a lost filling
- Emergency repair of a fractured tooth fragment or cusp, with the adhesion of the material often obviating the need for additional preparation
- Restoration of an endodontic access cavity or "walking bleach" preparation
- Treatment of an inflamed pulp, often in association with a lining of an obtundent material
- A diagnostic procedure, for example, at a failing crown margin or in a chronically sensitive noncarious cervical lesion

Transitional and interim restorations

A *transitional restoration* may be considered a "holding" restoration that remains in situ until circumstances are suitable for placement of a final restoration. Glass-ionomer materials may be used in transitional fillings as

- part of an immediate caries control regimen following excavation of caries in patients with gross, rapid carious destruction of teeth, and
- semipermanent restorations placed while awaiting the outcome of a treatment, such as the effectiveness of root canal therapy or a pulp capping procedure.

Glass-ionomers also may be the materials of choice for transitional restoration of cavities, such as for patients with high caries activity who have begun diet control and initial oral hygiene therapy, for patients receiving radiotherapy treatment to the head and neck, or for patients with xerostomia. Such restorations, although more meticulously executed than temporary fillings, may be placed quickly and cost-effectively, reduce the *Streptococcus mutans* count, and bring caries activity under control. On completion of oral hygiene and diet-control phases, the surface (1.5 to 2.0 mm) of glass-ionomer temporary restorations may be removed, leaving the pulp as the base for an amalgam or a resin composite coating as part of a sandwich technique.

Glass-ionomers also have been preferred for restorations placed under the less-than-ideal conditions common in home care.[14] None of the respondents to a survey on dentists' attitudes to home care in the United Kingdom considered that glass-ionomer cement was the only material appropriate for use in restorations placed as part of such care.[14]

In the case of an interim restoration, the practitioner and the patient agree to place a restoration that lacks the physical properties necessary for ideal longevity, but that may provide a low-cost, esthetic compromise as an expedient. Using this concept with glass-ionomer restorations, it may be possible to employ a more preservative approach to cavity design, thereby retaining as many options as possible for future management of the tooth. For example, this may include resurfacing the restoration with resin composite after a certain period of function. This approach holds the attraction of low initial cost and the provision of a potentially cariostatic restoration, but it can only be useful if it is certain that problems will not arise due to tooth movement following occlusal wear or fracture due to excessive occlusal forces. The concept of interim restorations encompasses a lifelong management strategy for teeth and the overall holistic care of patients who are unable, for whatever reason, to fund or otherwise agree to more definitive care.

Sealants and preventive restorations

Glass-ionomer materials have been suggested for fissure sealing, although there is relatively limited evidence as to the effectiveness of this technique. Results of a study by McLean and Wilson[8] showed a 78% retention of glass-ionomer fissure sealants after 2 years, but others have reported a total or substantial loss of sealants after 6 months.[15–17] It may be relevant that McLean and Wilson[8] recommended that glass-ionomer cements be used only on fissures that were wider than 100 μm.

An extension of the sealant procedure may be the use of glass ionomers in the restoration of occlusally protected or small-access occlusal cavities, with the application of a resin-based fissure sealant to the glass-ionomer surface and remaining fissures. Such a restoration has been termed a "preventive glass-ionomer restoration" by Garcia-Godoy.[9] If radiographic examination of the tooth indicates that the extent of carious attack is limited to the outer third of the dentin and examination of the occlusion reveals a lack of occlusal contact with the proposed restoration, the technique may be considered.

Caries may be removed with a small round bur or with other ultraconservative cavity preparation methods. The glass-ionomer is applied to the cavity and, when set, the enamel margins of the cavity and the fissures are etched as appropriate. The tooth is rinsed and dried and the sealant applied and cured (Fig 13-2).[9] The occlusion should be checked and adjusted as necessary; sealant should be reapplied to any areas of glass-ionomer that have been exposed during adjustment. It is desirable for the type of glass-ionomer material chosen for this application to be among the most wear resistant available; cermets, or metal-reinforced materials, may therefore be most appropriate. Such restorations may from time to time be resurfaced or converted to a sandwich restoration.

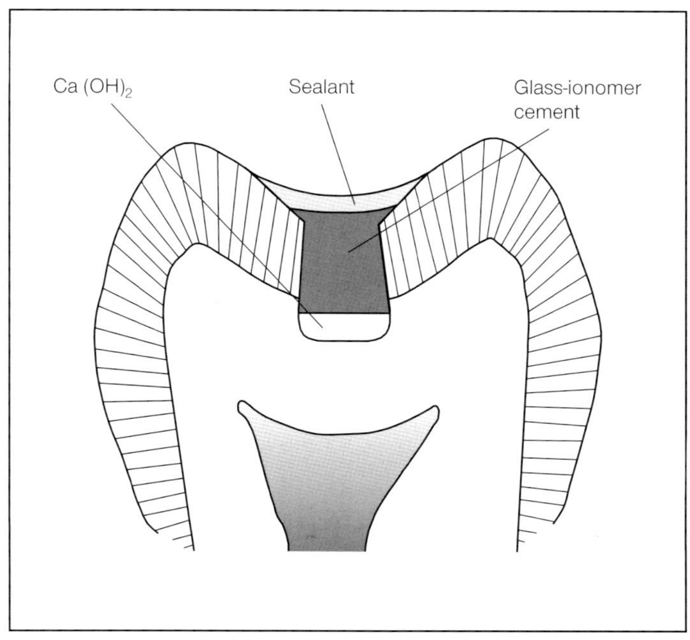

Fig 13-2 A preventive glass-ionomer restoration. (Adapted from Garcia-Godoy.[9])

Occlusal restorations

Early glass-ionomer materials lacked the physical properties of high tensile strength and wear resistance necessary for use in Class I situations. Metal-reinforced glass-ionomer cements were initially considered promising as an alternative to dental amalgam in such situations, but failed to gain popularity or to demonstrate effectiveness in this application.[18,19] Newer, more heavily filled glass-ionomers may possess improved wear resistance. The tensile strength of these materials also is sufficiently improved to permit their evaluation in Class I cavities in limited situations such as the following:

- In small to medium-sized restorations that are protected from occlusal forces by remaining tooth structure
- For patients with a perceived need for fluoride release
- For patients who request a tooth-colored restoration and are prepared to accept a long-term provisional restoration, which may be placed at a lower cost than other tooth-colored restorations such as resin composite
- For nervous, phobic patients in whom the use of materials that require more time to place or are technique sensitive may be precluded
- When an easy-to-place restoration is required, as in atraumatic restorative treatment[20]
- When the margins of large load-bearing restorations require repair

Preparation for occlusal glass-ionomer restorations should first involve careful examination of occlusal contacts, with the occlusal outline being prepared to avoid such contacts if possible. Margins should not be beveled, because this may leave a thin flash of glass-ionomer material that may fracture during function. Following finishing of the restoration, the surface should be cleaned and sealed with a layer of unfilled resin; this may form part of a preventive approach by sealing the remaining fissures.[9] There is an urgent need to evaluate the performance of contemporary glass-ionomer restorations in Class I cavities and to assess the cost-effectiveness of such restorations.

Tunnel restorations

The tunnel restoration was first described by Jinks in 1963 as a conservative alternative to the conventional procedure for Class II cavity preparation in primary molars.[21] He suggested that, following preparation of a Class I lesion in an occlusal fossa, a small round bur could be used to prepare a "tunnel" diagonally under the marginal ridge and into the primary caries. Jinks, who originally suggested the use of a sodium silica-fluoride cement containing silver alloy filings, abandoned tunnel restorations because of a marginal ridge fracture rate of between 12% and 15%.[21]

With the introduction of glass-ionomer materials, tunnel restorations have enjoyed renewed interest, with Hunt,[10] Knight,[22] and McLean[23] independently suggesting the use of glass-ionomers in tunnel restorations in deciduous and permanent teeth. In this application, the glass-ionomer cement is syringed into the proximal lesion prior to the restoration of the occlusal access cavity with a resin-based material (Fig 13-3).[24]

With regard to the performance of tunnel restorations, Croll[25] did not report any cases of marginal ridge fracture or recurrent caries in "dozens" of cases, and the consensus view from laboratory experiments is that the strength of the marginal ridge of teeth restored with tunnel cermet restorations is as great as that of unrestored sound teeth[26] or at least as that of teeth restored with composite.[27] Lumley and Fisher,[28] however, have published data on a long-term pilot study of tunnel restorations stating that 25% of glass-ionomer and 10% of cermet tunnel restorations failed, whereas none of the small Class II amalgam restorations placed as controls required replacement. In a study of tunnel restorations in 27 children, Zenkner and coworkers[29] demonstrated that caries was not eliminated in a large proportion of cases, although the long-term significance of this was not elucidated.

The use of magnification techniques may be considered essential for carrying out tunnel restorations. Caries detection solutions also may be helpful in ensuring complete removal of the lesion. It is suggested that tunnel restorations are most successfully completed when they are prepared using an intraoral video camera in conjunction with a lens that permits accurate viewing of the operative field.

The advantages of the tunnel technique are retention of the marginal ridge and interproximal contacts; disadvantages include the difficulty in locating proximal caries and ensuring its removal. Anecdotal evidence also indicates that practitioners consider tunnel restorations difficult to complete with confidence. For these reasons, the tunnel restoration has

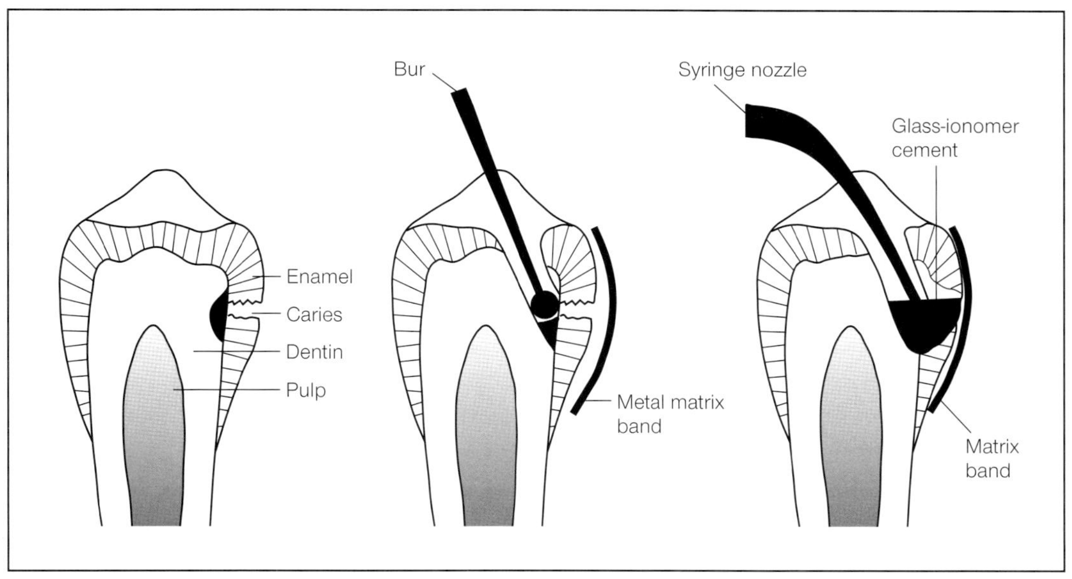

Fig 13-3 A tunnel restoration. (Adapted from Tay and Lynch.[24])

not achieved great popularity, as confirmed by statistics provided by the National Health Service in the United Kingdom.[30] These results showed that only 10,538 tunnel restorations were placed in 1 year, compared to 4.7 million Class II amalgam restorations, although more than half of the latter may have been replacements of defective restorations. The failure of the few clinical evaluations carried out to demonstrate the advantages of tunnel restorations over Class II amalgam and resin composite restorations in permanent teeth tend to indicate that the clinical acceptance of this technique will continue to be limited, at least in the foreseeable future.

An alternative approach to the operative management of small proximal carious lesions may be the "lateral" tunnel, or slot, preparation (Fig 13-4) described by Morand and Jonas[31] and using either a bur or newer ultrasonic means of preparation. In this technique, the proximal lesion is accessed from the lingual or buccal surface, with the preservation of substantial amounts of tooth tissue, including the marginal ridge. Optical aids and fiber-optic illumination are required to view the lesion and its preparation. This technique may be particularly useful for elderly patients who have suffered gingival recession which thereby facilitate access to the lesion. As with the tunnel concept, a radiopaque glass ionomer is most appropriate, so the proximal area may be checked radiographically for recurrent caries. Morand and Jonas[31] have provided guidelines for the success of such preparations. These include the removal of the smear layer prior to application of a resin-modified

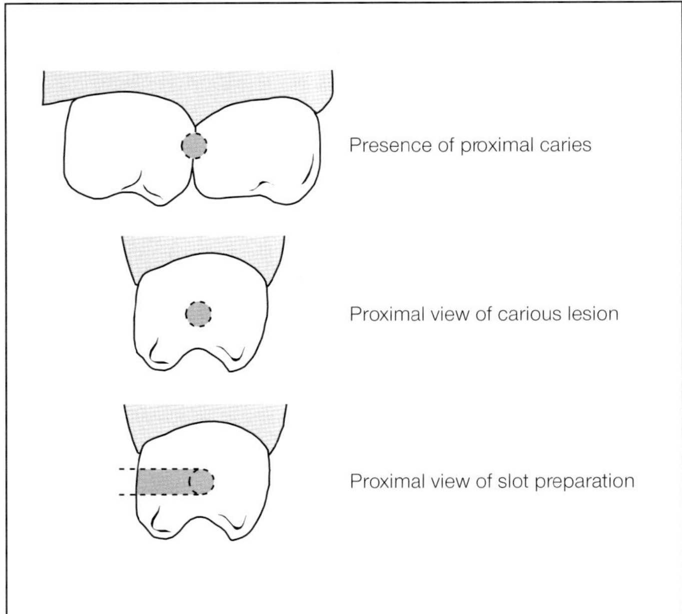

Fig 13-4 A lateral tunnel, or slot, preparation. *(top and middle)* Lateral and proximal views of carious lesions; *(bottom)* Slot preparation from the lingual or buccal aspect of the cavity.

glass-ionomer, placement of the material using a syringe to avoid incorporation of air bubbles or voids, and tight compression of the matrix. As with the use of glass-ionomers in Class I situations, randomized clinical trials are required to investigate the long-term efficacy of lateral tunnel restorations.

Atraumatic restorative treatment

In developing countries, most dental caries is left untreated and, if treated, is managed by extraction. Reasons for the lack of treatment may include the remote locations of the population; inadequate number and distribution of dental personnel; lack of availability of reliable water supplies; and insufficient finances to purchase equipment, materials, the services of oral health professionals, and the premises in which they may operate (if only a mobile surgery unit). Furthermore, most restorative dentistry carried out in industrialized countries is highly dependent on the availability of suitable electrically powered equipment. However, electricity is neither available nor reliable in rural or suburban areas of many less industrialized countries,[20] and contemporary dental procedures are therefore difficult to carry out. As a result, the inhabitants of such countries may not benefit from recent developments in dental materials and techniques.

The atraumatic restorative treatment (ART) was first evaluated in Tanzania in the mid-1980s, along with interested manufacturers of materials, based on manual excavation of caries and the use of an adhesive restorative material and sealant (currently, but not originally, a reinforced glass-ionomer). This makes it an appropriate intervention for people living in underdeveloped countries, other groups such as refugees, and people living in deprived communities who are unable to obtain restorative dental care. This technique, however, is only one component of oral health care that also must include promotion of other messages such as a nutritionally balanced diet, good oral hygiene, and the use of a fluoride-containing toothpaste.[20]

The ART concept need not be confined to less industrialized countries. Because it is based on the concept of minimal intervention and minimal cavity preparation, there is potential for its application in restorative treatment in children. It also may provide a treatment option for groups such as the physically or mentally handicapped, persons living in shelters, and those receiving home care services.

With regard to the success of the technique, results of a study on the longevity of restorations placed under field conditions in rural Thailand using ART with glass-ionomer restorations, based on evaluation criteria that included the absence or presence of restorations and of marginal defects, indicated that the success rate of single-surface restorations in permanent teeth was 93% and 67% for dual-surface restorations after 1 year; in deciduous teeth, the success rates were 79% and 55% for single-surface and dual-surface restorations, respectively.[12] Results of a study in Zimbabwe indicated that 85% of single-surface restorations in permanent teeth were rated good or acceptable after 3 years, and ART has been well received by the majority of patients.[20]

The principal stages in the ART technique are isolating the tooth with cotton rolls, cleaning it with wet cotton pellets, obtaining access to the carious lesion with a hatchet or similar instrument, removing the soft carious material with an excavator, providing pulpal protection if necessary, and placing the restorative material. The occlusion should be checked, any excess material removed before it has hardened, and the restoration coated with varnish or petroleum jelly. Limitations to ART include hand fatigue during instrumentation. The technique takes no less time than an amalgam restoration and works best on minimal cavities in permanent teeth. To allow the glass-ionomer to perform optimally, there must be sufficient tooth substance to surround the restoration. There are no long-term clinical data on its success.

The size of the lesion appears to be of particular importance. Atraumatic restorative treatment is most appropriate to small cavities, because, with the limited treatment availability in such situations, the best treatment of large carious lesions may be to render the cavity self-cleansing in the hope that the caries will be arrested. However, access to a minimal lesion may be difficult without a drill.

Sandwich restorations

It has been shown that it is possible to bond resin composite materials to glass-ionomer cements.[32] Given that glass-ionomer cements bond to both enamel and dentin,[33] it also is possible to bond a

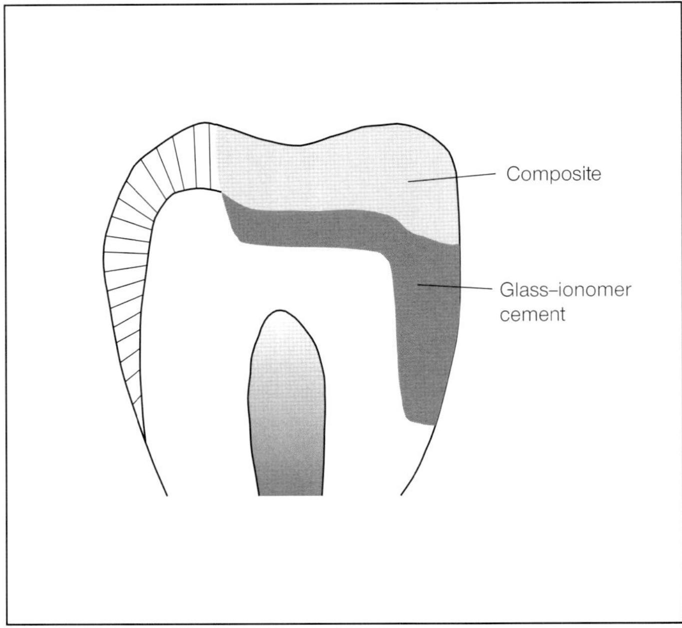

Fig 13-5 An open sandwich restoration.

resin composite restoration to dentin with an intermediate layer of glass-ionomer. This is known as a sandwich, or laminate, restoration. The sandwich restoration may be "open," when the glass-ionomer forms part of the external surface of the restoration (Fig 13-5), or "closed," when the glass-ionomer is completely contained by the overlying composite (Fig 13-6).

Initially, acid etching of the glass-ionomer surface was considered necessary to produce satisfactory bond strengths,[32] but etching during the maturation phase of the cement was found by Taggart and Pearson[34] to adversely affect the material. These researchers concluded, after a series of laboratory tests, that the practice of etching a glass-ionomer was not advisable, but that, if etching were considered, it should be carried out for no longer than 10 seconds and preferably 24 hours after mixing, which is not a clinically viable option.

In the sandwich restoration, a glass-ionomer cement is used to replace the dentin of the cavity, with a resin composite used in conjunction with acid etching of the enamel to provide an esthetic restoration of the remaining cavity. This technique may be applied to Class I, Class II, Class III, and Class V lesions, and the chemical bond and leaching of fluoride optimize the properties of the resin composite and the glass-ionomer.[35]

The sandwich technique also may be employed for posterior restorations, using either an open or closed version. Results from a survey in Australia indicated that 65% of respondent dentists used this technique, but clinical observation of biological problems such as pulp

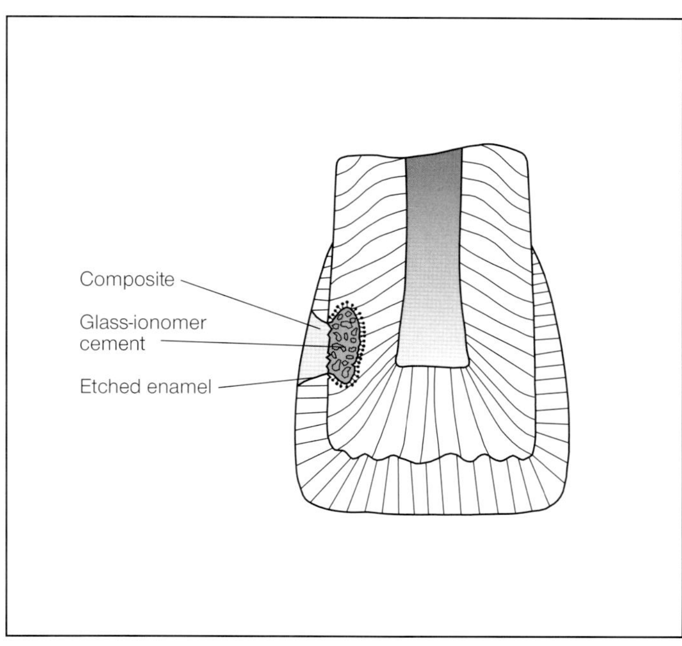

Fig 13-6 A closed sandwich restoration. (Adapted from McLean et al.[32])

symptoms and secondary caries were said to occur "often," with 14% of the respondents also reporting dissolution or wear of the proximal cement.[36] Forsten et al[37] reported similar results from a survey in Scandinavia, with wear or dissolution of the open proximal glass-ionomer cement surface being reported by 17% of respondents. Furthermore, results of a clinical trial using a similar technique, reported by Welbury and Murray,[38] demonstrated the limitations of the technique; the authors concluded that the sandwich technique failed to provide acceptable restorations during their trial. It would therefore appear that the open sandwich technique is not to be recommended. However, the closed technique, using the glass-ionomer as a thick base to replace the dentin, appears to be well liked by operators, although no data are available on the long-term clinical success of the technique in posterior teeth.

Factors dictating the choice of glass-ionomer material for sandwich restorations include the mechanical stress to which the cement-resin union is to be subjected and the desirability of radiopacity in the cement. If mechanical stress is expected to be high, a cement with optimal compressive and tensile strengths should be used, along with a resin composite with low polymerization shrinkage and a bonding agent with high wettability. If the restoration is in a posterior tooth, a radiopaque cement such as a cermet or lining cement should be used.[11]

A clinical routine described by Mount[11] suggests preparing the cavity without beveling, etching the entire cavity with 10% polyacrylic acid for 20 seconds and

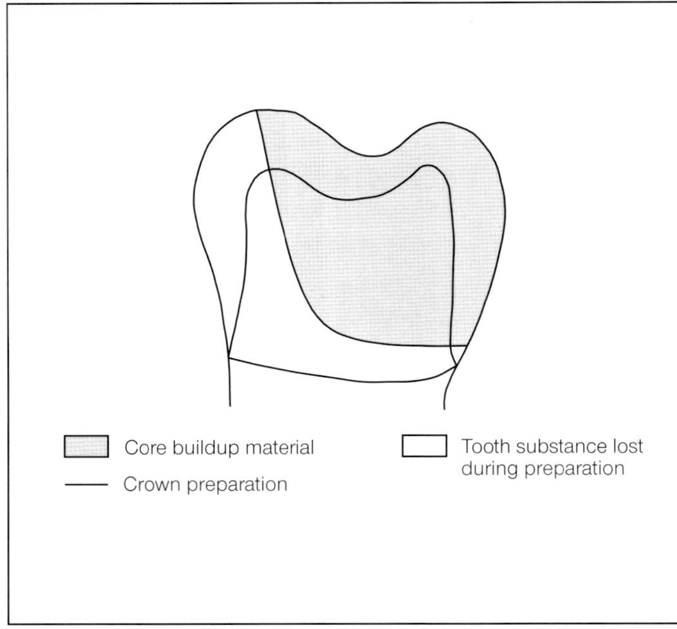

Fig 13-7 A core buildup. Building the core provides resistance and retention form to the crown preparation.

rinsing for 15 seconds, placing matrix and wedge, and inserting the glass-ionomer cement to cover the entire dentin, except at the gingival floor. The cement is trimmed to provide a flat gingival floor and axial wall and the excess removed from the enamel, which is etched with 35% phosphoric acid for 30 seconds and rinsed for 15 seconds. Unfilled resin is then applied to the cement and etched enamel. The composite restoration is then cured and finished.

Core buildup

The construction of a core, or foundation restoration, is often necessary prior to crown preparation in order to give the final crown appropriate resistance and retention (Fig 13-7). By implication, the core should have its own retention by means of retentive features in the buildup cavity, pins or posts, or the use of a material that reliably adheres to tooth structure.

Following placement of a crown, the core becomes an integral part of the load-bearing structure of the tooth; it is therefore essential that the mechanical properties of the core are adequate for this function. Among the properties a core buildup material should possess are adequate compressive, tensile, and flexural strengths; nonirritance to tooth tissue; radiopacity similar to that of enamel; a coefficient of thermal expansion similar to that of dentin; low thermal conductivity; the ability to adhere to or be bonded to tooth structure, pins, and/or posts; ease of mixing and placement; short setting time; lack of adverse reaction to temporary crown materials or cements; and a color that contrasts with that of the tooth.[13]

Until recently, amalgam was thought to afford the most favorable physical characteristics for core buildup procedures. However, amalgam cannot be built up and prepared in one visit, nor does it adhere to tooth tissue unless amalgam bonding techniques are employed. Early glass-ionomer materials lacked the necessary tensile and flexural strengths for anything other than fashioning small core buildups or blocking out undercuts in preparations, but the improved tensile strength and fracture toughness of resin-modified glass-ionomers and heavily filled glass-ionomers make these materials appropriate for core buildups. Furthermore, the coefficient of thermal expansion of these materials approximates that of tooth tissues more than resin composite does, and they therefore may possess many of the properties associated with the ideal core buildup material.

No currently available material appears to possess sufficient adhesion to tooth to permit its use without additional retention by means of pins, posts, or retentive features where there has been extensive loss of tooth tissue. Current thoughts on core buildups negate the use of pins and posts wherever possible, with the foundation material being packed into the pulp chamber in root-filled teeth. In vital teeth, it is essential that efforts be made to conserve all remaining tooth tissue during core buildup and subsequent preparation, including ferruling to limit damaging stresses.

Classification of Proximal Carious Cavities

Mount[39] considered some modification of conventional cavity design appropriate for proximal lesions. These ideas have been further refined and developed, with Mount and Hume[40] suggesting a new classification for cavities that may be particularly appropriate to accommodate the "new" caries situations, such as those seen in gerodontics. These include circumferential cavities at the gingival margin and proximal lesions that are inappropriate for conventional Class II restorations.

The suggested classification takes into account the site, size, and complexity of the lesion. Site 1 lesions are similar to Class I lesions, namely those originating in pits and fissures. Site 2 lesions are those associated with contact areas and are divided into subcategories: size 1 (minimal), size 2 (moderate), size 3 (enlarged), and size 4 (extensive). Site 3 lesions are those originating close to the gingival margin around the full circumference of a tooth. This would include those lesions referred to as Black's Class V lesions and includes cavities occurring on mesial or distal tooth surfaces following gingival recession. Site 2, size 1 (#2,1) lesions would therefore be appropriate for restoration by a tunnel, slot, or other minimal cavity preparation designed to maintain the maximum amount of tooth structure. Glass-ionomer cement may be considered an appropriate material for such cavities, and it therefore follows that this revised classification of carious lesions may be more appropriate to modern adhesive restoratives than the classification suggested by G. V. Black almost a century ago.

Improving the Performance of Glass-Ionomer Materials

Glass-ionomer materials possess many beneficial characteristics. It would therefore be reasonable for manufacturers and researchers to attempt to overcome the negative characteristics in order to expand the indications for use, particularly in load-bearing situations. Increasing the powder–liquid ratio is one method by which the physical properties of glass-ionomer cements may be improved, with a consistency requirement similar to putty being suggested.[41] Newer materials appear to fulfill this requirement, with their improved physical properties due in part to a reduction in size of the glass particles in the matrix. Some of these materials may be condensable, but not to the extent of amalgam. Correct handling of materials and pretreatment of dentin also are valuable in enhancing the properties of glass-ionomer materials, as are delayed finishing and protection of the restorations.[41]

Summary

All types of glass-ionomer materials, despite many favorable properties and attributes, continue to have relatively limited applications in stress-bearing and difficult-to-access situations, especially in locations where restorations would be subjected to direct loading. However, when afforded protection by remaining tooth tissues; when used as temporary, transitional, or interim stress-bearing restorations; and when applied in special circumstances, glass-ionomers perform efficiently and effectively to the benefit of patients.

References

1. Ferracane JL. Materials in Dentistry. Principles and Applications. Philadelphia: JB Lippincott, 1995.

2. O'Brien WJ. Dental Materials. Properties and Selection. Chicago: Quintessence, 1989.

3. American Dental Association Council on Dental Materials and Devices. Status report on the glass-ionomer cements. J Am Dent Assoc 1979;99:221–226.

4. Willems G, Lambrechts P, Braem M, Vanherle G. Composite resins in the 21st century. Quintessence Int 1993;24:641–658.

5. Mjör IA, Jokstad A. Five-year study of class II restorations in permanent teeth using amalgam, glass polyalkenoate (ionomer) cermet and resin-based composite materials. J Dent 1993;21: 338–343.

6. Hickel R, Petchelt A, Maier J. Nachuntersuchung von Füllungen mit Cermet-Zement (Ketac-Silver). Dtsch Zahnartzl Z 1988;43:851–853.

7. Smales RJ, Gerke DC, White IL. Clinical evaluation of occlusal glass-ionomer, resin and amalgam restorations. J Dent 1990;18:243–249.

8. McLean JW, Wilson AD. Fissure sealing and filling with an adhesive glass-ionomer cement. Br Dent J 1974;136:269–276.

9. Garcia-Godoy F. The preventive glass-ionomer restoration. Quintessence Int 1986;17:617–619.

10. Hunt PR. A modified class II cavity preparation for glass-ionomer restorative materials. Quintessence Int 1984;10:1011–1018.

11. Mount GJ. Clinical requirements for a successful "sandwich"—dentin to glass-ionomer cement to a resin composite. Aust Dent J 1989;34:259–265.

12. Frencken JE, Songpaisan Y, Phantumvanit P, Pilot T. An atraumatic restorative treatment (ART) technique: Evaluation after one year. Int Dent J 1994;44:460–464.

13. Burke FJT, Watts DC. Cermet—an ideal core material? Dent Update 1990;17:364–370.

14. Burke FJT, McCord JF, Hoad-Reddick G, Cheung S-W. Provision of domiciliary care in a UK urban area: Results of a survey. Prim Dent Care 1995;2:47–50.

15. Shimokobe H, Komatsu S, Hirota K. Clinical evaluation of glass-ionomer cement used for sealants. J Dent Res 1986;65:812 [abstract 780].

16. Boksman L, Gratton DR, McCutcheon E, Plotzke OB. Clinical evaluation of a glass-ionomer as a fissure sealant. Quintessence Int 1987;18:707–709.

17. Mejare I, Mjör IA. Glass-ionomer and resin-based fissure sealants: A clinical study. Scand J Dent Res 1990;98:345–350.

18. Wilkie R, Lidums A, Smales R. Class II glass-ionomer cermet tunnel, resin sandwich and amalgam restoration over 2 years. Am J Dent 1993;6:181–184.

19. Lidums A, Wilkie R, Smales R. Occlusal glass-ionomer cermet, resin sandwich and amalgam restorations: A 2-year clinical study. Am J Dent 1993;6:185–188.

20. Frencken JE, Phantumvanit P, Pilot T, Songpaisan Y, van Amerongen E. Manual for the Atraumatic Restorative Treatment Approach to Control of Dental Caries. Groningen: World Health Organisation Centre for Oral Health Services Research, 1997.

21. Jinks GM. Fluoride-impregnated cements and their effect on the activity of interproximal caries. J Dent Child 1963;30:87–92.

22. Knight GM. The use of adhesive materials in the conservative restoration of selected posterior teeth. Aust Dent J 1984;29:324–331.

23. McLean JW. Limitations of posterior composite resins and extending their use with glass-ionomer cements. Quintessence Int 1987;18:517–529.

24. Tay WM, Lynch E. Glass-ionomer cements—clinical usage and experience: 2. Dent Update 1990;17:51–55.

25. Croll TP. Glass ionomer-silver cermet bonded composite resin class II tunnel restorations. Quintessence Int 1988;19:533–539.

26. Hill FJ, Halasseh FJ. A laboratory investigation of tunnel restorations in premolar teeth. Br Dent J 1988;165:364–367.

27. Purk JH, Roberts RS, Elledge DA, Chappell RP, Eick JD. Marginal ridge strength of class II tunnel restorations. Am J Dent 1995;8:75–79.

28. Lumley PJ, Fisher FJ. Tunnel restorations: A long-term pilot study over minimum of five years. J Dent 1995;23:213–215.

29. Zenkner JE, Baratieri LN, Monteiro S, de Andrad MAC, Viera LCC. Clinical and radiographic evaluation of cermet tunnel restorations on primary molars. Quintessence Int 1993;24:783–791.

30. Dental Practice Board. Digest of Statistics 1996/97. Part 1. Detailed Analysis of GDS Treatment Items. Eastbourne: Dental Practice Board Dental Data Services, 1997.

31. Morand J-M, Jonas P. Resin-modified glass-ionomer cement restoration of posterior teeth with proximal carious lesions. Quintessence Int 1995;26:389–394.

32. McLean JW, Prosser HJ, Wilson AD. The use of glass ionomer cements in bonding composite resins to dentine. Br Dent J 1985;158:410–414.

33. Wilson AD, Kent BE. A new translucent cement for dentistry. The glass-ionomer cement. Br Dent J 1972;132:133–135.

34. Taggart SE, Pearson GJ. The effect of etching on glass polyalkenoate cements. J Oral Rehabil 1991;18:31–42.

35. Wilson AD, McLean JW. Glass-Ionomer Cement. Chicago: Quintessence, 1988.

36. Forsten L, Mount GJ, Knight G. Observations in Australia of the use of glass-ionomer cement restorative material. Aust Dent J 1994;39:339–343.

37. Forsten L. Clinical experience with glass-ionomer for proximal fillings. Acta Odontol Scand 1993;51:195–200.

38. Welbury RR, Murray JJ. A clinical trial of the glass-ionomer cement—composite resin "sandwich" technique in class II cavities in permanent premolar and molar teeth. Quintessence Int 1990;21:507–512.

39. Mount GJ. Glass-ionomer cements in gerodontics. A status report for the American Journal of Dentistry. Am J Dent 1988;1:123–128.

40. Mount GJ, Hume WR. A revised classification of carious lesions by site and size. Quintessence Int 1997;28:301–303.

41. Naasan MA, Watson TF. Conventional glass ionomers as posterior restorations. A status report for the American Journal of Dentistry. Am J Dent 1998;11:36–45.

Chapter 14

Glass-Ionomers: Advantages, Disadvantages, and Future Implications

Graham J. Mount

Given the discussions in the preceding chapters of this book, it is logical to consider the relative position of glass-ionomers in the practice of modern restorative dentistry. It is not long since amalgam and silicate cement were regarded as the only feasible materials for simple restoration of a carious lesion, with gold as the only alternative. However, during the second half of the 20th century, there has been continuous research into the development of reliable alternatives, particularly related to the use of esthetic materials. The three plastic restorative materials presently in common use should be discussed and put into perspective because each has its strengths and weaknesses. No material should be regarded as universal and combinations of two materials can be used to compensate for perceived weaknesses or shortcomings.

A number of factors must be taken into account in the selection of the most appropriate material for the restoration of any particular lesion, with the most obvious properties being esthetics and longevity. Because replacement of a restoration inevitably means a further loss of tooth structure, it is important to stress the potential life span of each material. This in turns leads to a discussion of resistance to recurrent caries, which is essentially resistance to bacterial colonization and microleakage into the interface between the restoration and tooth structure, as well as physical strength and resistance to wear under occlusal load.

It also is necessary to consider the carious process the restoration is meant to repair. This is now recognized as a simple balance between the demineralization and remineralization of the surface of the tooth structure in the presence of saliva, which is a supersaturated solution of the same calcium and phosphate ions that constitute both enamel and dentin. It is assumed that there is a continuous exchange of ions and, in a healthy mouth, the tooth will remain stable. If the ambient pH of the oral environment is allowed to drop below 5.5 (the critical pH of hydroxyapatite) either frequently or for prolonged periods, demineralization may become the dominant factor and carious degeneration of the tooth will follow. If fluoride is introduced into the environment in small, regular quantities, there will be an increase in resistance to further demineralization because the critical pH of fluorapatite is 4.5. Even more important, the process of remineralization is expedited in the presence of free fluoride ions. This suggests that any source of fluoride within the oral environment is desirable both to slow demineralization and to enhance the process of remineralization.

However, it must be recognized that in the presence of a long-term hostile low pH environment no restorative material can prevent continuing caries activity. In the presence of plaque, which is colonized by *Streptococcus mutans* and frequently inoculated with refined carbohydrate, there is inevitably a sustained reduction of pH with resultant demineralization. The only way to break this cycle is to eliminate one of the three contributing factors—plaque, *S mutans*, or carbohydrate—and it should be the aim of professionals to educate their patients to take responsibility for their own oral condition. It is interesting to note that plaque and the associated pellicle layer, in the absence of either or both *S mutans* and carbohydrate, in fact protects the tooth surface because plaque also is heavily saturated with both calcium and phosphate ions and may contain fluoride ions as well.

The foregoing suggests that no material should be regarded as proof against or a preventive for caries, and this reinforces the contention that it is time the profession moved away from the system promoted by G. V. Black nearly 100 years ago which adopted a surgical approach to the elimination of caries. This approach is unduly destructive, because it is unscientific to remove tooth structure to eliminate the disease and restorative materials cannot be relied on to prevent or eliminate caries. On the other hand, it is well recognized that the process of demineralization occurs some time before the penetration of bacteria into a carious lesion. This suggests that, if the bacteria-laden section of a cavity could be removed and the lesion sealed with a bioactive material, it might be possible to induce remineralization of the remaining softened "precarious" tooth structure, thus leading to a degree of healing.

In this discussion, two surfaces of the restoration are relevant. The outer surface exposed to the oral environment should be esthetically pleasing, physically strong, and resistant to wear. Any bioactivity would be available only to the immediately adjacent tooth structure and most ion release would be lost into the saliva. However, on the assumption that a complete seal develops between the tooth and the restoration, preventing further bacterial penetration, the inner surface could be regarded as a sealed environment in which bioactivity could take place, unimpeded by outer influences. The presence of a positive dentinal fluid flow would provide the fully hydrated environment necessary for ion exchange to occur, and there would be at least a potential for healing wounded tooth structure.

Thus, it seems highly desirable to develop "biomimetic," or "bioactive," restorative materials. Each of the available restorative materials is reviewed here to examine their potential in this area.

Restorative Materials

Amalgam

Amalgam is still regarded as the most reliable and economic material for repair of extensive lesions in posterior teeth where the restoration is under considerable occlusal load. However, it does not have good esthetics and requires removal of additional sound tooth structure beyond the carious lesion, such as occlusal dovetails and retentive grooves, for mechanical retention within the crown of the tooth. It is relatively simple to place and corrodes within the oral environment, thus sealing its own interface with the cavity walls. The corrosion products prevent microleakage of bacteria and help to prevent recurrence of caries, so to this extent amalgam can be regarded as mildly bioactive. As the cavity becomes larger and the occlusal load heavier, amalgam becomes more useful because it is relatively strong and resistant to wear, supporting the remaining weakened tooth structure from occlusal load. However, the use of amalgam as a restorative material is steadily declining and it is certainly no longer the material of choice for restoration of a new carious lesion. Also, once a cavity has been prepared for restoration with amalgam, it becomes more difficult to place an alternative material because the cavity is inevitably larger than ideal for modern adhesive restoratives.

Resin composites

The most popular esthetic restorative material at present is resin composite. The first work on the use of polymers began during the late 1940s, but it was not until the 1970s that new materials reached a degree of sophistication where they could be relied on for relatively long-term restorations. The modern heavily filled hybrid resin composite is now recognized as a relatively reliable material with acceptable esthetics, although placement and proper curing can be time-consuming and demanding.[1] Light activation is the most popular method of curing, leading to excellent color stability with some degree of operator control over the placement of the restoration. However, it poses the problem of controlling shrinkage of the material away from the cavity floor and walls, and limited light penetration can result in incomplete curing in the deeper layers of the restoration.[2] Cytotoxicity studies suggest that resin composite, which has been polymerized as far as possible, probably causes minimal pulpal irritation.[3] However, incompletely cured resin, because of either the unpolymerized monomers or the surface active complexes formed between the low molecular weight components of the light-activated initiator systems, is a potential hazard and an allergen.

One of the advantages offered by resin composites is the micromechanical attachment that can be developed between the resin and enamel. Prior to placement of the restoration, the enamel surrounding the cavity is beveled and acid etched to allow generation of a mechanical bond.[4] Some authorities recommend etching of the dentin as well to develop a further bond. There is considerable evidence that acid etching of dentin does not cause pulpal inflammation because the acid is buffered by dentin and does not reach the pulp tissue.[5] However, etching the dentin removes the smear layer and opens the tubules, allowing a positive dentinal fluid flow which leads to an increase in the wetness of the dentin surface and limits the penetration of a resin bond into the tubules. Also, should subsequent marginal leakage occur, the pathway to the pulp is more open and the pulp more susceptible to irritation. Unless the marginal seal of the restoration is complete, particularly on the root surface, there is a substantial risk of sensitivity, caries, and/or pulpal irritation resulting from microleakage and the ingress of bacteria and their toxins.

Until recently, attempts to achieve a reliable seal to dentin have been unsuccessful over the long term and there have been wide variations in the results of physical testing in vitro and in vivo. The latest improvements in techniques and materials suggest a higher rate of success, although the bond remains a micromechanical interlock rather than a chemical union such as that available with glass-ionomers.[6,7] Bonding to dentin requires the removal of all demineralized affected dentin. This is often undesirable because it means the removal of dentin that could otherwise be remineralized in the presence of a bioactive material. It also must be noted that the deeper the cavity, the greater the total area of open dentinal tubules and, therefore, the greater the problem of a positive dentin fluid flow[8] that is likely to compromise the development of adhesion.

Resin-based materials are being developed that are supposed to release fluoride ions, and there are currently suggestions for similar materials that release calcium and/or phosphate ions. However, in the absence of the hydroxyl ion, it is impossible for ion migration from the restoration to be anything but superficial and transitory. It is therefore unlikely that this class of material will ever be regarded as bioactive.

Compomers

There have been a number of attempts to develop compromise materials with potential biomimetic properties. One particular subgroup comprises "compomers" (derived from *compo*site and ion*omer*). Initially it was claimed that these materials enjoyed both the acid-base setting reaction and the fluoride release of glass-ionomers along with all the esthetic properties of resin composites. However, it is now apparent that they belong properly in the group with resin composites[9,10] and their only property related to glass-ionomers is a small fluoride release that becomes available some time after placement. This release only becomes available following a degree of water uptake from the oral environment and is considerably lower than that available from glass-ionomers.

The method of adhesion between compomers and enamel and dentin is based on a resin bonding agent, and this precludes any opportunity for the development of the ion exchange adhesion which is typical of glass-ionomers. The final limitation of these materials is that they generally are not as heavily filled as the commonly available hybrid resin composites and therefore their resistance to wear is low. They may be a useful material when selected and placed correctly, but they should not be confused with nor placed instead of a glass-ionomer cement. Nor should they be used in an area that is subject to heavy occlusal load as a substitute for resin composite.

Glass-ionomer cements

Since the development of glass-ionomer materials in the early 1970s,[11] they have proved to be of value for the restoration of initial carious lesions, erosion/abrasion/abfraction lesions, and the control of advancing caries, particularly where the occlusal load is not excessive.[12] It is the only material presently available that can be regarded as bioactive, or therapeutic, because it has the potential for encouraging remineralization of surrounding tooth structure and has been shown to be bioactive in relation to bone.[13] It also prevent bacterial microleakage because of the ion exchange adhesion that develops with both enamel and dentin.[14–16] Glass-ionomer cement develops a new ion-enriched material at the interface with tooth structure which consists of phosphate and calcium ions from enamel or dentin and calcium (or strontium), phosphate, and aluminum ions from the cement.[14] It is interesting to note that in some materials the calcium in the glass has been replaced with strontium and, because strontium is also an apatite-forming specie, this has facilitated observation of the ion exchange phenomenon. If there is subsequent failure of a restoration, it occurs within cohesiveness of the glass-ionomer, leaving the ion exchange adhesion layer firmly attached to the cavity wall. This means that the dentinal tubules remain sealed against penetration of bacteria or their toxins.

Clinical observation has led to the conclusion that glass-ionomers both reduce the tendency to demineralization and enhance the remineralization of enamel and dentin that has been subjected to caries.[17] It is assumed that fluoride release is the dominant factor and this release has been well documented.[18,19] Most of the fluoride released is in the form of sodium fluoride, which is not a critical salt for matrix formation, so the continuing release does not represent an ongoing breakdown of the restoration. However, in the presence of transitory low pH values, there may be a notable increase of fluoride flow, probably arising from a breakdown of glass particles. In other words, in the presence of a highly active caries rate, there may be degradation of a glass-ionomer restoration, which emphasizes that no restorative material can be relied on to prevent caries in a hostile oral environment. Also, breakdown has been noted in the presence of serious long-term xerostomia; this can be attributed in part to the lack of hydroxyl ions required for stability in a water-based cement.

Although fluoride has been identified as a catalyst for remineralization, recent research suggests that there is a similar release of both calcium (or strontium) and phosphate ions, all of which could be useful in supporting this process.[20] The pattern of release for all three ionic species is very similar, even to the extent that the release is enhanced in the presence of a low pH.[21]

It is suggested that the biomimetic effects of glass-ionomers should be viewed from two different aspects. The outer intraoral surface of a restoration is subject to continuing variation in its immediate environment. The quality, quantity, and pH of the saliva varies from time to time and between patients, so the activity of glass-ionomer cement varies. There is likely to be some degree of ion exchange with tooth structure at the margin of the cavity, with a certain amount of fluoride uptake and possibly an exchange of other ions.[22] A "halo" effect around such restorations has been noted in vitro, but it cannot be expected to be far reaching or sustained in the presence of a continuing low pH.[23]

Other research has shown that there is a continuing ion exchange on the outer surface of glass-ionomer restorations.[24] In fact, the fluoride release is part of an ion exchange process, because other ionic species are taken up simultaneously to maintain diffusion equilibrium. At least some of the fluoride accumulates within mature plaque on the surface of the restoration,[25] suggesting the mechanism which leads to buffering a low pH in the plaque and a reduction of the *mutans streptococci* count.[26] It also has been shown that, although wear resistance is low during the first 7 days, there is a continuing uptake of ions from the saliva and wear resistance increases steadily over time.

The other area of interest is the inner surface within the cavity which, assuming there is an ion exchange adhesion with the tooth structure, is isolated from the oral environment. Because of the continuing dentinal fluid flow, the environment is wet and therefore conducive to an exchange of ions. Also, dentin is likely to take up more fluoride than enamel because of its greater porosity and increased water content, as well as the presence of the organic phase.[27] This fraction of fluoride is thought to be involved in remineralization activities.[28,29] When the glass-ionomer is first placed, there is, as expected, high release of fluoride, calcium (strontium), and phosphate ions from the cement which combine with similar ions from the dentinal fluid and may well lead to a degree of remineralization in any remaining affected demineralized dentin. Even after the glass-ionomer has set, there is a low-level ion exchange available on a continuous basis. This ion exchange may account for the degree of remineralization that has been shown to occur clinically (Figs 14-1a to 14-1c). Recent laboratory investigations tend to verify this observation (Ngo H, unpublished research).

Recent anecdotal clinical observation has suggested a moderately high level of recurrent caries related to glass-ionomer restorations,[30,31] but this is not necessarily an indictment of the material itself but rather of the environment in which it was placed. There is certainly evidence that it is well accepted by the profession and widely used.[32] The preceding comments suggest that glass-ionomer cement discourages the demineralization of enamel adjacent to a restoration[33] and assists in the remineralization of affected dentin. However, as suggested earlier in this chapter, no restorative material will prevent further caries. All restorative dentistry should be carried out in the presence of a vigorous preventive routine, which is particularly important when using minimal intervention techniques as described briefly later in this chapter.

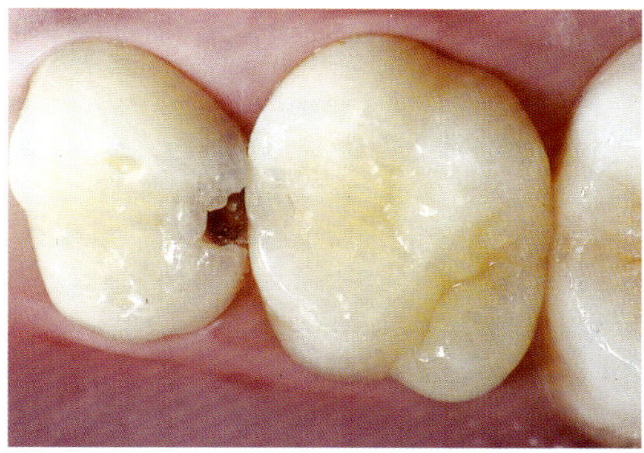

Fig 14-1a A moderate-sized cavity at the distal of a deciduous first molar to be restored with glass-ionomer cement only.

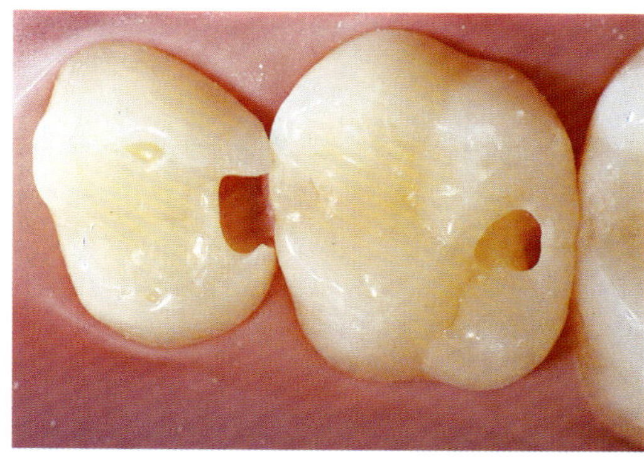

Fig 14-1b The finished cavity after conservative preparation to preserve natural tooth structure. There is still a contact with the adjacent tooth, which will help to maintain a natural contact area, and the axial wall is left as demineralized affected dentin.

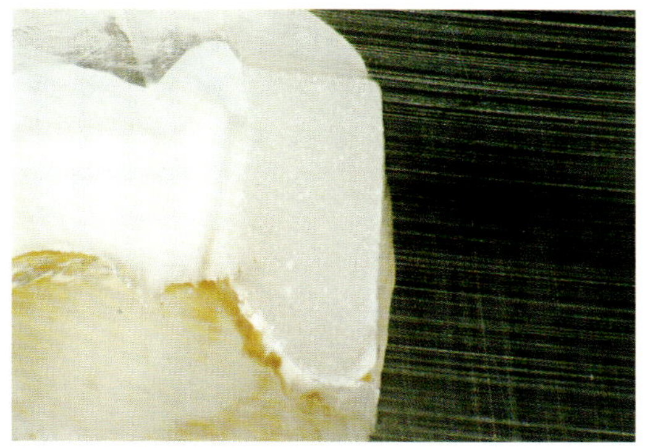

Fig 14-1c The restoration after 3 years. Following exfoliation of the tooth, it was cut mesiodistally to show the remineralization on the axial wall. The dentin appears to be fully mineralized and sound.

Glass ionomers are available in acceptable esthetic forms, and resin-modified materials are quite translucent. The physical properties of the latest autocured materials are close to those of microfilled resin composites,[34] and the wear factor is not a problem once the material has matured. However, fracture resistance is a little lower than that of resin composite, meaning that, unless a restoration is well surrounded and supported by remaining natural tooth structure, it should be covered with another material (the "sandwich" technique) to provide the required strength and ensure longevity. Resin composite is the logical choice for the laminate because it has good esthetics and greater resistance to fracture. There is an additional advantage to the sandwich technique in that the presence of a reasonable bulk of glass-ionomer minimizes the problems of depth of cure and setting shrinkage of the resin composite.[35]

A New Approach to Operative Dentistry

The aforementioned observations suggest that the time has arrived for the profession to reevaluate its approach to operative dentistry, particularly in relation to new carious lesions. In the presence of reliable long-term adhesion with both resin composite and glass-ionomers, and an ion exchange potential in the oral environment with glass-ionomers, cavity designs can be modified safely with the aim of conserving tooth structure. The Black approach to cavity design was based on surgical removal of the carious lesion followed by mechanical interlocking of the restoration so that, by modern standards, any initial lesion treated will be overextended.

If the profession is to adopt new standards and modify its attitude to the treatment of new carious lesions, it would be desirable to develop a different classification for identification. Conservation of as much natural enamel and dentin as possible, including remineralization of demineralized tooth structure, extends the life of the tooth crown and reduces the need for the more extensive and expensive restorative work that has been necessary since the profession learned to save teeth instead of extracting them. A considerable amount of replacement dentistry will be required for several generations, but there is no longer a need, when dealing with a new lesion, to sacrifice tooth structure to prevent further caries or to make room for a restorative material.

The following discussion introduces a possible new classification for carious lesions and identifies early cavities that are not currently recognized under the Black system. However, because of its relatively low fracture resistance, glass-ionomer cement can be used alone in load-bearing areas only where it can be well supported by surrounding tooth structure. The alternative, if there is any doubt of its longevity, is to laminate the restoration with resin composite. The combination of these two materials could herald a new era for conservative operative dentistry.

Proposed classifications

The proposed classification method[36] recognizes that there are only three sites on the tooth crown that are likely to see the initiation of a carious lesion because of accumulation of plaque. These can be listed as follows:

Site 1. Pits, fissures, and enamel defects on occlusal surfaces of posterior teeth or other smooth surfaces, such as cingula pits on anterior teeth

Site 2. Approximal enamel immediately below contact areas with adjacent (anterior or posterior) teeth

Site 3. The cervical third of the crown or, following gingival recession, the exposed root surface

It is logical to classify lesions by these three sites and then to grade them by size, according to the extent of progress of the lesion:

Size 1. Minimal involvement of dentin, but beyond treatment by remineralization alone.

Size 2. Moderate involvement of dentin. Following cavity preparation, remaining enamel is sound, well supported by dentin, and unlikely to fail under normal occlusal load. That is, the remaining tooth structure is sufficiently strong to support the restoration.

Size 3. Enlarged beyond moderate. Remaining tooth structure is weakened to the extent that cusps or incisal edges are split or likely to fail if left exposed to occlusal or incisal load. The cavity needs to be further enlarged so the restoration can be designed to provide support and protection to the remaining tooth structure.

Size 4. Extensive caries with bulk loss of tooth structure.

The principle advantage of using such a classification system is the possibility of 12 variations in the identification of a lesion instead of the present five classes. The resultant precision would facilitate record keeping for patients and epidemiologic studies and would be readily adapted to computer recording.

All three of the basic plastic restorative materials may be used in the restoration of a carious lesion and particularly in replacement dentistry. Logically, the smaller the lesion, the lighter the occlusal load, so the more brittle glass-ionomer is often sufficient by itself. As the occlusal load increases, there is an increased need for strength until the stage is reached in more extensive cavities where amalgam remains the material of choice. However, lamination of two materials together makes possible a satisfactory compromise between physical needs and esthetics.

The following explanations of classifications and techniques are only to emphasize the uses of glass-ionomers and resin composites, either alone or in combination, in relation to the initial lesion. In most developed communities, the majority of operative dentistry is now undertaken following the failure of old restorations and is recognized as replacement dentistry. However, caries rates remain steady or are increasing in many parts of the world and the profession must be encouraged to maintain natural tooth structure as much as possible. Glass-ionomers and composite resins, whether separately or in combination, increase this potential considerably.

It should be noted that size 1 lesions are minimal in extent and cannot be properly recognized within the Black system. The minimal lesion in that classification system has to be extended to a size 2 cavity to take the margins out to "caries-free areas" and to provide mechanical retentive designs, which leads to further tooth loss and weakening of the remaining crown. The following discussion explains the possible design of size 1 cavities in Site 1 and Site 2 and their restoration with glass ionomers, resin composites, or both.

Site 1 lesions

The best example of Site 1, size 1 (#1,1) lesions is in occlusal fissures on mandibular molars (Figs 14-2a and 14-2b). In the Black system, it was necessary to remove the entire fissure system, because it is impossible to successfully complete a cavity partway along a fissure. There would always be a fault, subject to recurrent caries, where the amalgam finished within the unprepared fissure. With adhesive restorative materials, it is possible to enlarge the cavity to a very limited extent, so the infected dentin can be removed

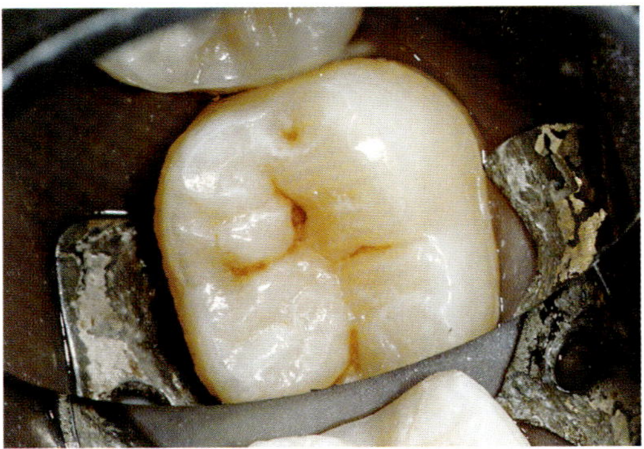

Fig 14-2a Occlusal fissures of a mandibular first molar. The mesial section is obviously carious and needs to be explored. This is classified as a #1,1 cavity.

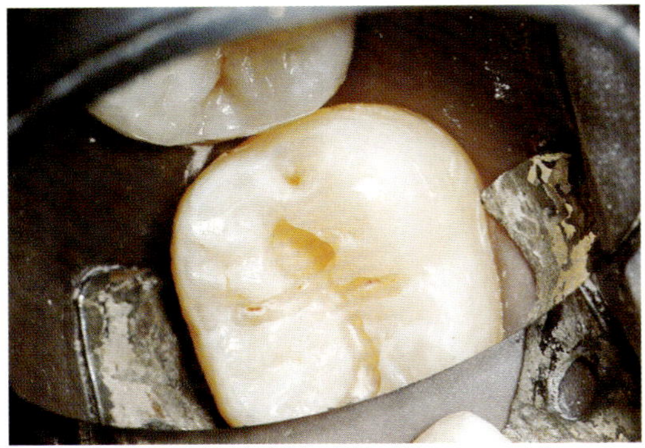

Fig 14-2b The tooth following cavity preparation. Note that only the mesial extension of the fissure system has been opened to any extent and the remaining fissures have been explored conservatively.

and the remainder of the fissure can be sealed with either resin composite or a strong glass-ionomer. Resin composite has been used with success for many years, but glass-ionomer cement should be the material of choice. It releases fluoride and adheres to both the enamel and dentin, and its clinical longevity is well established.

The required cavity preparation[37] should be carried out in a conservative manner, using a very fine tapered diamond bur at intermediate high speed under air/water spray. The opening should be limited to that part of the fissure that is obviously carious and the infected dentin beneath removed carefully with a small round bur. In view of the fact that any remaining affected dentin will be sealed from access to the oral environment, it is not essential to remove all softened demineralized dentin on the floor of the cavity. The remaining fissure system, which is regarded as noncarious, can then be sealed with the restorative material and remineralization can be anticipated.

If the extent of the caries is greater than minimal, the same principles are involved in cavity design in that the fissure system need not be extended beyond the limits of the infected dentin. The cavity is classed as Site 1, size 2 (#1,2)[38] (Figs 14-3a and 14-3b) and a stage may be reached where the ability of a glass-ionomer to withstand the occlusal load is doubtful. Under these circumstances, the glass-ionomer filling should be cut back sufficiently to allow it to be laminated with a 2- to 3-mm layer of resin composite which has superior physical properties, including a higher tensile strength. Once the cement has set, the enamel margin should be exposed around the full circumference of the main cavity to allow for the development of the micromechanical bond between the

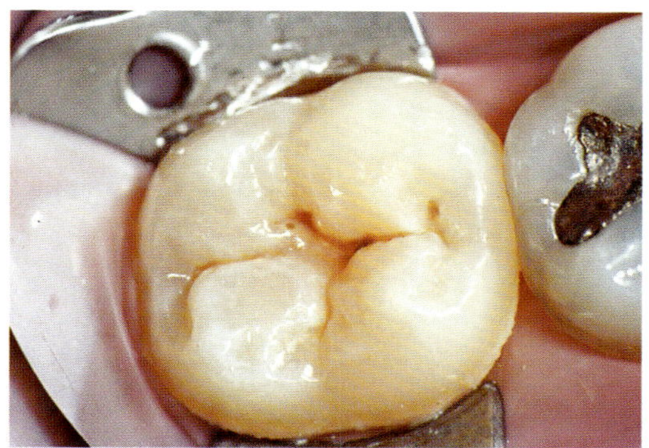

Fig 14-3a Mandibular molar with extensive caries involvement of the mesial fissure.

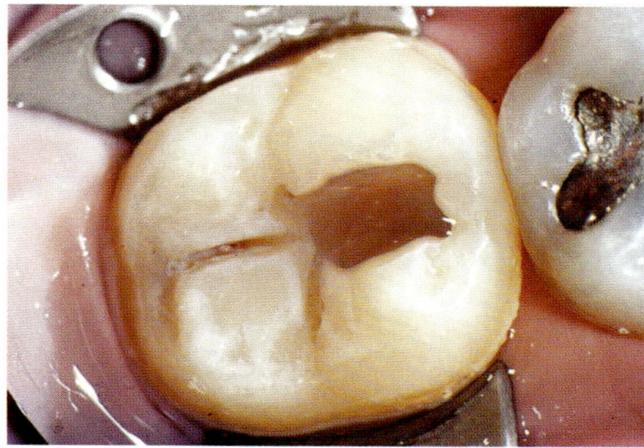

Fig 14-3b The same tooth following cavity preparation. The completed cavity is classified #1,2 but the remaining fissures are explored very conservatively.

enamel and the resin. However, it is unnecessary to extend the cavity outline into the remaining fissures provided they are well sealed with the glass-ionomer.

The principle of minimal extension into uninvolved tooth structure also can be applied in many other situations. The concept of attempting to prevent caries through removal of sound tooth structure is no longer acceptable in the presence of restorative materials that adhere to tooth structure and also release fluoride over a considerable period of time. It is now recognized that isolation of a carious lesion from its only nutritional source—the oral environment—will allow the tooth to heal, at least to a limited degree.[39]

Site 2 lesions

The Site 2 lesion[40] arises from plaque accumulation immediately beneath the contact area between any two teeth, whether anterior or posterior. Black differentiated between the two groups because of the materials that were available for restoration.[41] He recognized that amalgam was unsuitable to restore a cavity in an anterior tooth, and that in restoring a posterior tooth it was necessary to involve the occlusal fissure as well as the entire proximal surface. The contact area cavity in an anterior tooth, however, could be dealt with as a more conservative box form and restored with silicate cement.

The essential elements of the design of the two cavities were therefore quite different, so he classified them as Class II and Class III. In the presence of fluoride-releasing adhesive restorative materials, this variation in classification is no longer necessary.

The principles of minimal removal of tooth structure can again be applied to cavity preparation, at least until the cavity has progressed beyond the early lesion. Initial access can be gained by one of three routes.[42] If the marginal ridge is still reasonably sound and not seriously undermined by the lesion, entry should be through the occlusal surface of the tooth using the tunnel approach. In situations where the lesion is close to the crest of the marginal ridge, it is logical to enter carefully through the outer aspects of the ridge using a slot design. Finally, such a lesion may sometimes be accessed through a more extensive cavity that has already been prepared in the adjacent tooth. This is known as the proximal approach.

Tunnel restorations

In the past, there was doubt about the potential for remineralizing enamel on the proximal surface of a tooth because of limited access and visibility. Modern understanding of preventive dentistry allows greater latitude and it is possible, with a cooperative patient, to stabilize an area to the extent that it may not be necessary to prepare a cavity at all. There are cases, even after a lesion is identified radiographically, where there is no actual cavitation in the enamel. Therefore, it is still possible to control plaque accumulation and thus arrest the lesion and heal it. Of course, the operator may decide that the involvement of the dentin has progressed to the stage where it is desirable to make a limited surgical approach to restore the cavity and support the remaining enamel. However, once the proximal enamel is cavitated it is no longer possible to control plaque accumulation and some form of surgical intervention is essential.

In either of these situations, providing the lesion is more than 2.5 mm gingival to the crest of the marginal ridge, it is possible to enter the lesion from the occlusal fossa immediately above the cavity (Figs 14-4a to 14-4c), using a small tapered fissure diamond bur at intermediate high speed under air/water spray. The bur is set upright and angled buccolingually to develop a triangular entry tunnel. It is then possible to remove remaining infected dentin with a small round bur at slow speed and also to determine the extent of cavitation in the proximal enamel. A short length of metal matrix band is placed interproximally and lightly supported with a wooden wedge to prevent damage to the adjacent tooth. The periphery of any enamel cavitation is cleaned gently, removing only the completely denatured enamel. No attempt should be made to remove remaining demineralized dentin on the axial wall because that will remineralize.

The cavity can now be restored using a strong glass-ionomer. There is no need to place calcium hydroxide on the floor of the cavity because it is relatively shallow and any sublining would interfere with adhesion and remineralization. The cement should be mixed in a capsulated form because the capsule acts as a syringe and permits careful placement in the depths of the cavity. A small plastic sponge may be useful to tamp the cement into place while building the restoration incrementally.

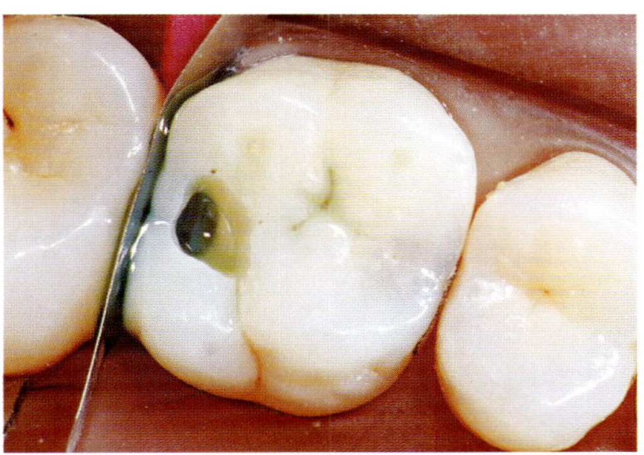

Fig 14-4a A #2,1 tunnel cavity prepared to repair a minimal lesion at the distal of a maxillary first molar. The conditioning etchant has been applied so the dimensions of the cavity can be seen more readily.

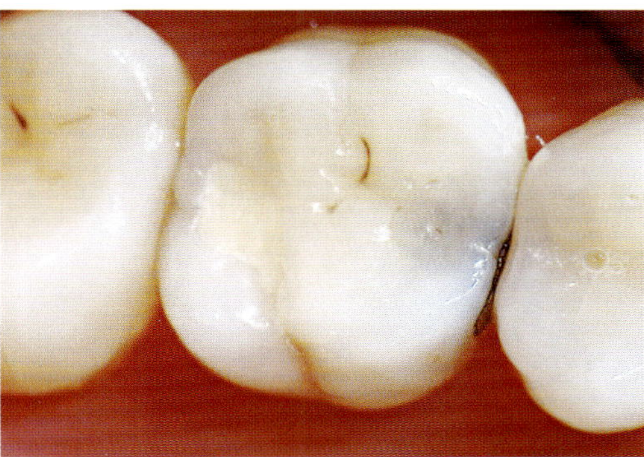

Fig 14-4b The same tooth 5 years following restoration with a glass-ionomer only.

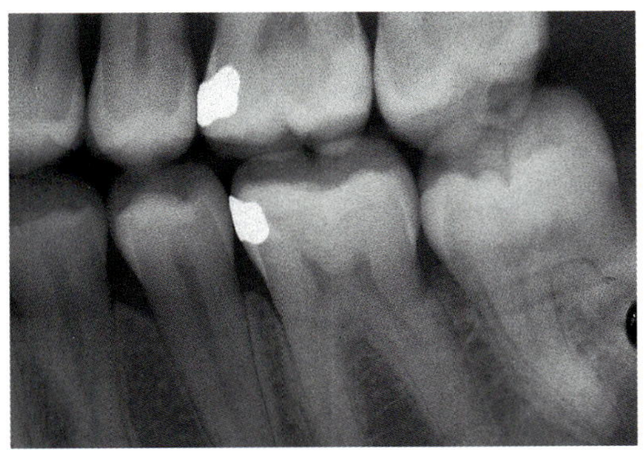

Fig 14-4c A bitewing radiograph taken 5 years following restoration.

In most cases, the restoration will not be subjected to undue occlusal load and the glass-ionomer cement will be sufficiently strong to stand alone as a complete restoration. However, if there is doubt, the cement should be cut back sufficiently to allow it to be laminated with up to 2.0 mm of resin composite, thus reinforcing both the cement and the marginal ridge.

Failure of tunnel restorations can result from either breakage of the marginal ridge or further enamel caries on the proximal surface. Mechanical breakdown can generally be repaired using resin composite. The cavity is extended conservatively, both the enamel and the cement are etched, and the restoration is rebuilt with resin composite. On the other hand, further caries on the proximal surface indicates failure of preventive procedures. The cavity should be restored again as conservatively as possible and the patient counseled carefully on the cause of the

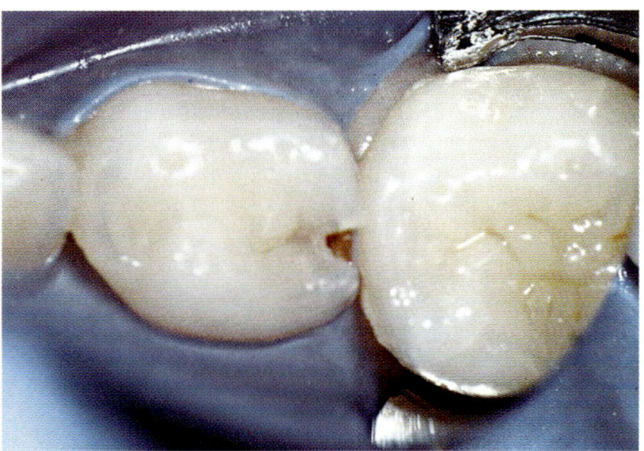

Fig 14-5a A proximal lesion at the distal of a mandibular first deciduous molar, which is considered suitable for a slot preparation.

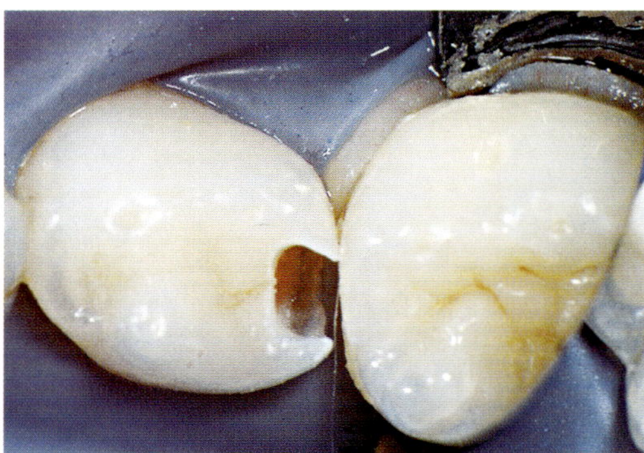

Fig 14-5b The same tooth after cavity preparation. Note there is no occlusal dovetail, and there is still contact with the adjacent tooth.

breakdown. There is no need to extend the cavity to a conventional Black design, because removal of tooth structure is not an acceptable method of preventing further caries.

Slot preparation

A slot preparation[43] should be carried out when a carious lesion has developed close to the crest of the marginal ridge (Figs 14-5a and 14-5b). The lesion is entered through the outer aspect of the marginal ridge using a small tapered diamond bur at intermediate high speed under air/water spray. The cavity is extended buccolingually only as far as the cavitated enamel and the infected dentin is removed conservatively. Because of the ion exchange adhesion of glass-ionomer cement, there is no need to prepare special retentive elements within the cavity, nor is it necessary to include the occlusal fissure unless it is cariously involved. It is acceptable to leave unsupported enamel, because the glass-ionomer will adhere to it and reinforce it to the point where the tooth is approximately as strong as it was originally.

Restoration can be carried out using glass-ionomer alone and a sublining is not required. However, if the occlusal load is expected to be high, it may be wise to laminate the cement as described previously. Failure will again be the result of mechanical breakdown or continuing caries, and the cause must be identified if the restoration is to be successfully repaired. Conservative repair is generally possible without resorting to a more extensive conventional design.

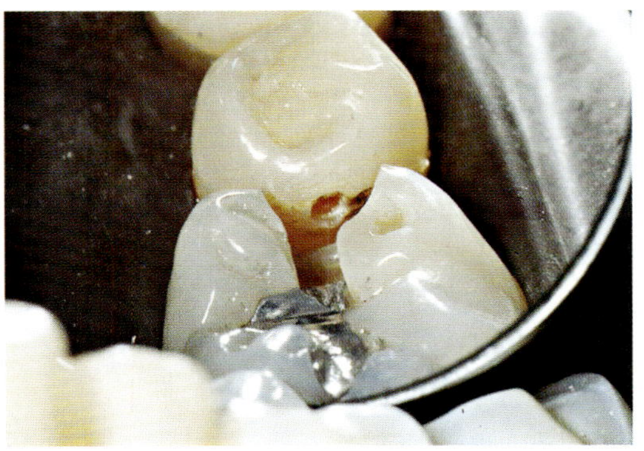

Fig 14-6a A conventional #2,2 cavity on the mesial of a mandibular first molar. Following preparation, a small cavity has become apparent on the distal of the adjacent second premolar.

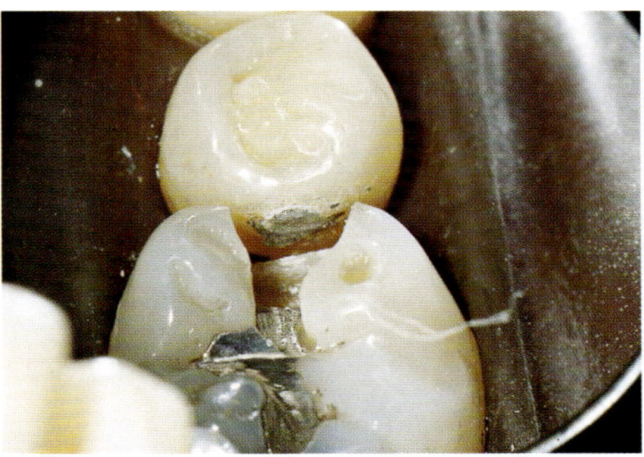

Fig 14-6b The same teeth following restoration of the premolar. A metal-reinforced glass-ionomer was used because there was no esthetic problem and the restoration is radiopaque.

The proximal approach

The situation sometimes arises where preparation of a moderately extensive cavity in one tooth reveals a lesion on the proximal surface of the adjacent tooth (Figs 14-6a and 14-6b). Restoration of the latter is generally straightforward, although access and visibility may not always be simple. The same small tapered fissure diamond bur should be used at intermediate high speed for initial preparation, because it is relatively safe and overextension is unlikely. Care must be taken to preserve as much of the proximal enamel as possible because, if it is not cavitated, it can generally be successfully remineralized. Only the infected dentin is removed, and there is no need to place a sublining because it may interfere with the adhesion of the glass-ionomer. Because the restoration will not be subject to occlusal load, there is no need to laminate the restoration. However, a radiopaque cement should always be used so there will be no confusion with future radiographic examinations.

Site 3 lesions

Site 3 lesions[44] occur around the cervical margin of the tooth crown and are particularly common either as erosion/abrasion/abfraction lesions or as root surface caries. The former are generally simple to restore because access is not a problem and glass-ionomers have been shown to last very satisfactorily. These lesions are classified as size 1 cavities. It is not difficult to obtain acceptable esthetic results,[45] particularly when using a resin-modified glass-ionomer. No cavity preparation is required. In fact, preparation of the eroded surface is contraindicated,

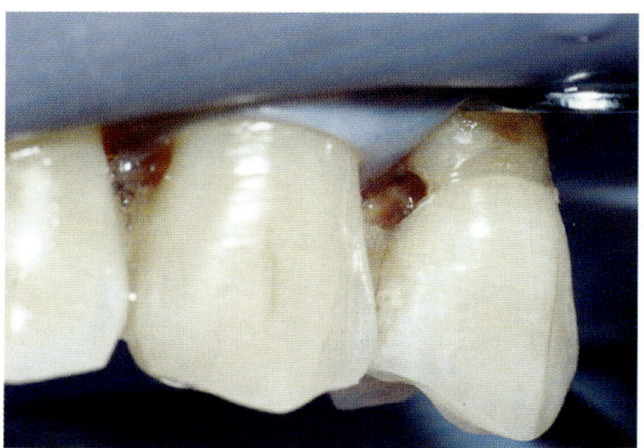

Fig 14-7a A mesial root surface lesion on a maxillary first premolar. This is classified as a #3,3 lesion.

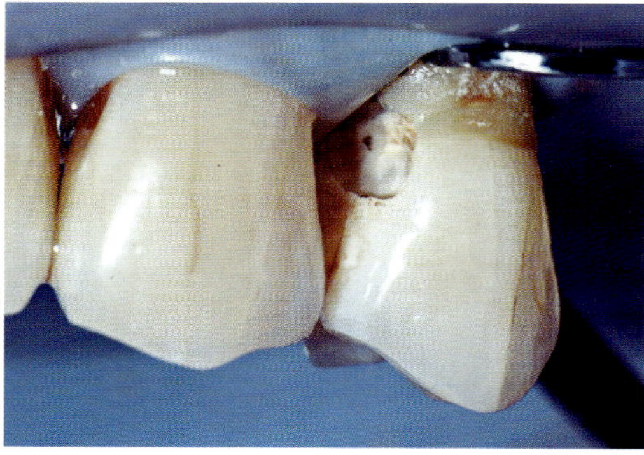

Fig 14-7b The same tooth after cavity preparation. Note the conservative approach, with affected dentin still remaining on the axial wall.

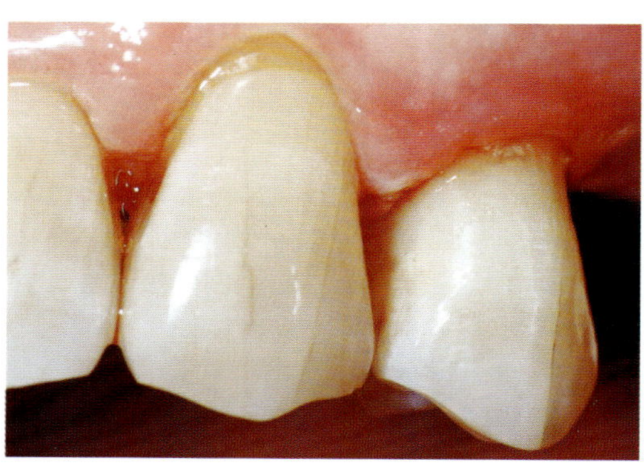

Fig 14-7c The same tooth after restoration with a resin-modified glass-ionomer.

because it will normally be perfectly smooth and adaptation of one material to another is enhanced in the presence of smooth surfaces.

Interproximal root surface caries lesions present a separate problem and it is suggested they be classified Site 3, size 3 (#3,3)[46] because they are relatively difficult to design (Figs 14-7a to 14-7c). They are not identifiable separately in the Black classification, possibly because they were uncommon in the past. Patients tended to lose their teeth at a relatively early age and the average life span was considerably shorter than it is today. However, there has been a recognizable increase in the prevalence of such lesions, and it is desirable that they be identified and the problems of restoration recognized. They are most likely to occur in the elderly patient following gingival recession and are often related to the development of xerostomia. This in turn may be caused or exacerbated by

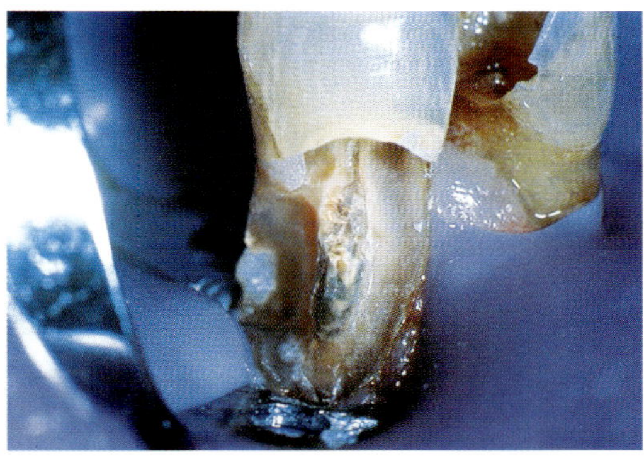

Fig 14-8a An extensive Site 3 lesion on a mandibular canine, extending around more than one surface. The cavity is classified as #3,4.

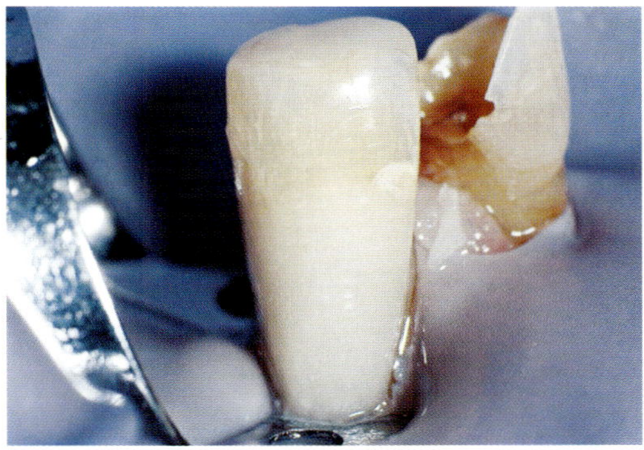

Fig 14-8b The same tooth following restoration with a resin-modified glass-ionomer. Because the restoration will not be under occlusal load, it is not necessary to laminate it unless the esthetic result is not ideal.

multiple medications used to combat the symptoms of disease in this patient population.

Restoration of root surface lesions may pose problems because of difficult access and limited vision. The use of intermediate high speed with diamond burs is desirable, and a short length of metal matrix band should be placed interproximally to protect the adjacent tooth. Access should be dictated by the position of the lesion and its relation to either the buccal or the lingual contours of the crown. The lesion is opened conservatively from its most occlusal aspect and the access cavity enlarged just enough to allow for reasonable vision. A small round bur is used at slow speed to clean the walls of the cavity while maintaining as much tooth structure over the axial wall as possible. There is a considerable risk of exposure of the pulp if all affected dentin is removed and endodontic treatment is not always possible in the elderly patient.

Because the restoration will not be under occlusal load, glass-ionomer cement is the material of choice. The ion exchange adhesion prevents microleakage and the release of fluoride and other ions encourages remineralization with the potential for healing the lesion under the restoration. In the presence of severe xerostomia, however, it may be desirable to laminate the glass-ionomer with a resin composite.

The Site 3, size 4 (#3,4)[47] lesion is similar to the size 3 but extends to two or more surfaces of the crown/root of the tooth (Figs 14-8a and 14-8b). It is therefore more difficult to restore and generally requires the construction of a complex matrix.

Other lesions

The remaining lesions in this classification system mostly come under the heading of replacement dentistry and are not described here because of space limitations. However, many can be restored using a sandwich, or lamination, technique, which is covered briefly. Some lesions, particularly #2,3 and #2,4, may still be restored most effectively with amalgam.

Sandwich technique

One of the advantages of glass-ionomer cement is that it can be laminated with another material and thus reinforced if the occlusal load is expected to be too heavy. This means that in many situations the major advantages of these materials—good adhesion and continuing fluoride release—can be retained. Placement of a strong glass-ionomer as a base for such restorations is clinically simple and effectively overcomes these problems. There has been discussion about the necessity or desirability of bonding the resin composite to the glass-ionomer, but it seems logical to develop adhesion between each layer of material along with adhesion to the tooth structure for a monolithic reconstruction with overall reinforcement of the tooth.

The technique can be applied to the restoration of any cavity but is strongly recommended for restoration of all cavities of moderate or greater size, where resin composite is the primary material of choice. If the entire margin of a cavity lies in sound, well-supported enamel that can be beveled and etched, the strongest bond is that developed between enamel and resin composite. However, if any part of the margin lies in dentin, the sandwich technique is recommended with the possibility of leaving glass-ionomer exposed to the oral environment in the gingival areas.[48] In the presence of a very low pH in interproximal spaces, there is the potential for disintegration of the glass-ionomer. However, under these circumstances, remaining tooth structure is also subject to further caries and this reinforces the suggestion that no restoration can be expected to survive in the absence of good preventive dentistry.

The sandwich technique is straightforward (Figs 14-9a to 14-9d).[36] The cavity is prepared as conservatively as possible and conditioned to allow for the better adhesion.[49] A matrix is constructed as required and the strongest glass-ionomer available used. An encapsulated material is preferred because the capsule becomes a syringe, ensuring proper placement in the depths of the cavity. If hand mixing is performed, a disposable syringe is used for placement and a small plastic sponge in a pair of conveying tweezers is used to tamp the material onto the floor and walls of the cavity. The cavity is overfilled, and the cement is allowed to set or is light cured, depending on the type of glass-ionomer used. Immediately on setting to sufficient hardness, the cavity is prepared again using a small diamond cylinder at intermediate high speed under air/water spray. All enamel walls are cleaned and beveled as required to facilitate acid etching of the enamel and resin composite. Sufficient room must be made for the resin composite, keeping in mind that this is a relatively flexible material and needs to be at least 2 to 3 mm thick to withstand occlusal loading.

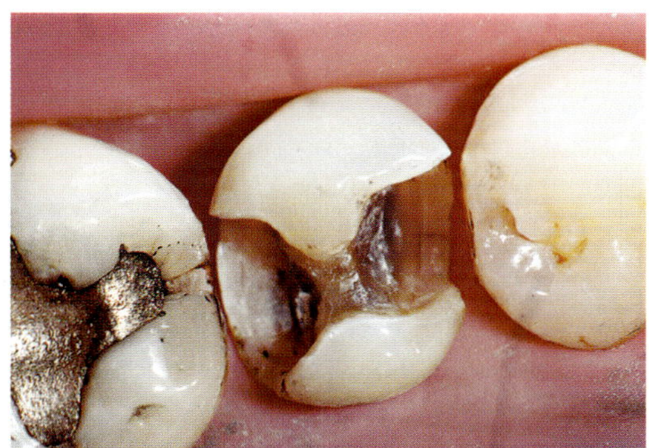

Fig 14-9a A failed amalgam restoration in a mandibular second premolar. Replacement will be with resin composite laminated over a glass-ionomer.

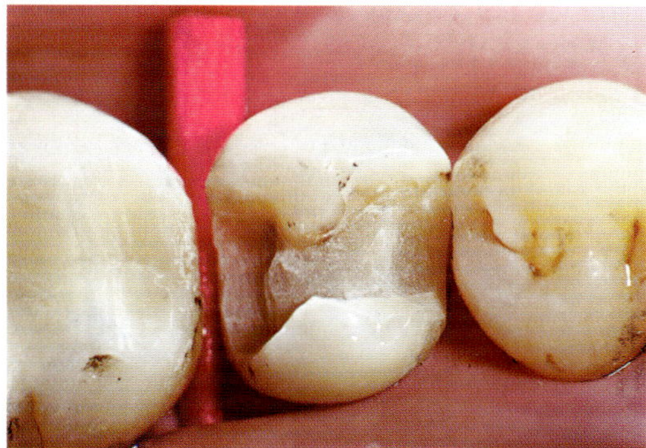

Fig 14-9b The same tooth after the first stage of restoration. The glass-ionomer cement has been cut back to make room for the resin composite. Note that the proximal boxes are still based in the glass-ionomer but the enamel margins have been prepared by etching for adhesion with the resin composite.

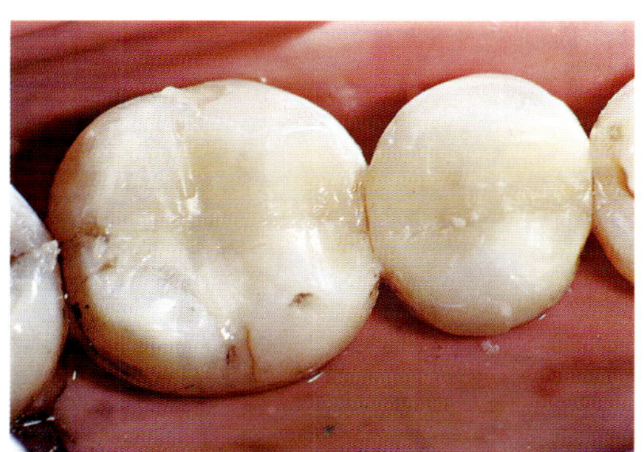

Fig 14-9c The completed restoration.

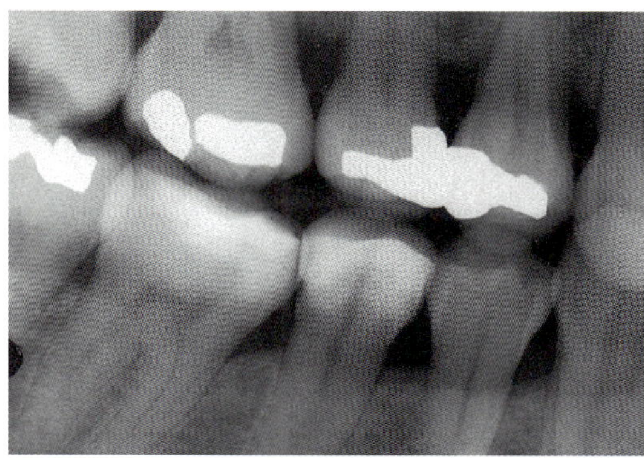

Fig 14-9d A bitewing radiograph 5 years after restoration.

In the absence of sound enamel along the gingival margin, the glass-ionomer is left covering the base of the proximal box almost to the contact area. It is generally safer to build the contact in resin composite even though this is not easy.

The cavity and cement are etched with 37% phosphoric acid for 10 seconds and washed thoroughly.[50] There has been some discussion as to whether the glass-ionomer should be etched, but the consensus suggests that etching is desirable. It may not be essential to etch a resin-modified glass-ionomer, because there is sufficient polymer in the cement to allow for a chemical bond between the two materials. However, it does no harm to etch any glass-ionomer, so there is no need to take undue care to avoid involving the cement. The tooth and cement are washed and lightly dried and the cement and a thin coat of a low-viscosity, unfilled, light-curing bonding resin applied. Clean compressed air is blown gently over the coating to distribute it evenly and it is light cured for 10 seconds.

A matrix is built around the cavity in preparation for incremental buildup of the resin composite. The resin composite is light cured through the tooth structure to encourage shrinkage onto the tooth. The restoration is built in increments of no more than 2.0 mm. Incremental buildup does not necessarily eliminate the shrinkage problem, but it ensures curing throughout the restoration.

There are a number of advantages in the use of the sandwich technique. It overcomes the problem of trying to develop reliable long-term adhesion between resin composite and dentin. There has been a considerable amount of research in this area, but the results remain equivocal. There also is a limit to the actual quantity of resin composite required to complete the restoration, reducing the time taken for placement and total shrinkage. Finally, there is the advantage of fluoride release and strong adhesion available from the glass-ionomer.

Indirect Pulp Capping and Atraumatic Restorative Treatment

The possibility of remineralizing, or healing, demineralized dentin and enamel in conjunction with the placement of glass-ionomer cement has been discussed elsewhere in this book and represents a further significant advance in operative dentistry. Indirect pulp capping using a zinc oxide–eugenol paste as the sealant has been discussed by Massler[51] and others[52,53] over the last 30 years and has been proven effective in arresting caries and easing pulpal inflammation. This technique works because the eugenol is strongly bactericidal and, provided it is not in direct contact with the pulp, will ease inflammation. It has been used extensively for many years to arrest active caries in large cavities by eliminating the superficial infected dentin and sealing the underlying demineralized affected dentin to prevent further bacterial activity and progress. If the seal remains in place for 3 weeks, the dentin is found to be stable and pulpal inflammation eliminated. Remaining softened dentin can then be removed with care and a definitive permanent restoration placed with a high degree of success.

Recent unpublished studies in the author's laboratory have shown that if glass-ionomer is placed instead of zinc oxide–eugenol, the result is even more satisfactory in that there is a degree of demineralization in the affected dentin, as well as the expected stasis in both the carious process and pulpal inflammation. This result is achieved for a number of reasons. First, the adhesion between the tooth structure and cement prevents ingress of further bacterial contamination. There is also evidence that glass ionomers are antibacterial, particularly in relation to *S mutans* and *lactobacillus*-which are both commonly found in active caries. Finally, the ion exchange mechan sm is available, particularly in the enclosed sealed environment created in this system.

Clinical observation over several years suggests that the use of glass-ionomer materials to arrest caries and eliminate pulpal inflammation is a successful technique for dealing with extensive lesions, and recent scientific investigations are beginning to confirm this (Ngo H, unpublished research). The suggested clinical routine is designed to deal with moderate to extensive carious lesions, providing the tooth is free of irreversible pulpitis. Access to the lesion is gained with either hand instruments or conventional rotating drills used only to reveal the extent of the lesion. The superficial infected dentin is removed and the peripheral walls cleaned back to sound dentin to ensure good adhesion around the full circumference of the cavity (Figs 14-10a to 14-10c). Affected dentin is left on the floor, because this is expected to remineralize. It is often difficult to differentiate between infected and affected dentin, but because the cavity will be completely sealed, it is probably not important because any remaining bacteria will become dormant in the absence of normal nutrients. However, a caries disclosing solution may be of assistance, provided it is used with caution. The most significant consideration is to ensure that sufficient room is created to allow for a reasonable thickness of glass-ionomer so it will be strong enough to withstand occlusal load for at least a limited period. The cavity should be acid etched and restored with the strongest glass-ionomer cement available.

Clinical experience suggests that this restoration should be left in place for about 3 months before the cavity is investigated further. If the original lesion is relatively minor, it may be acceptable to leave the glass-ionomer in place as the final restoration or laminate it with a stronger material. However, if there is any doubt about the success of the technique, the temporary restoration should be removed, which would have been done with a zinc oxide–eugenol temporary filling, and a final restoration constructed.

This technique has been successfully adapted to the treatment of caries in disadvantaged countries, where standard clinical dental facilities are not available, and is known as the atraumatic restorative treatment (ART) technique.[52] The object is to retain as many teeth as possible under adverse circumstances where caries rates remain high and the only alternative would probably be extraction. Success rates remain high over relatively short periods of time up to 3 years of observation. Although follow-up with placement of permanent restorations would be the best outcome, the technique is regarded as superior to the alternative of extracting the teeth.

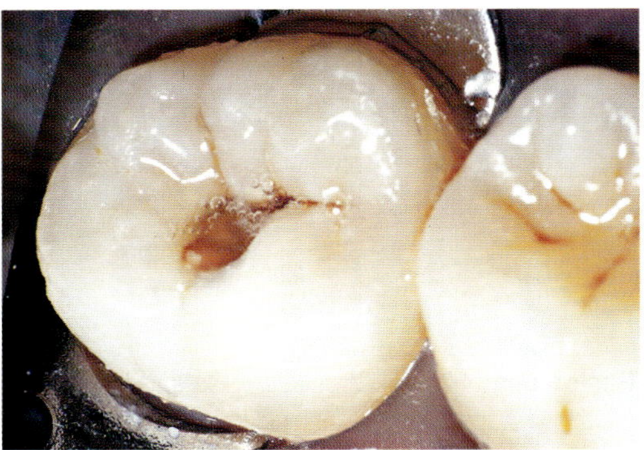

Fig 14-10a A moderately large cavity in a symptom-free mandibular second molar. The ART technique is to be used with a strong glass-ionomer cement.

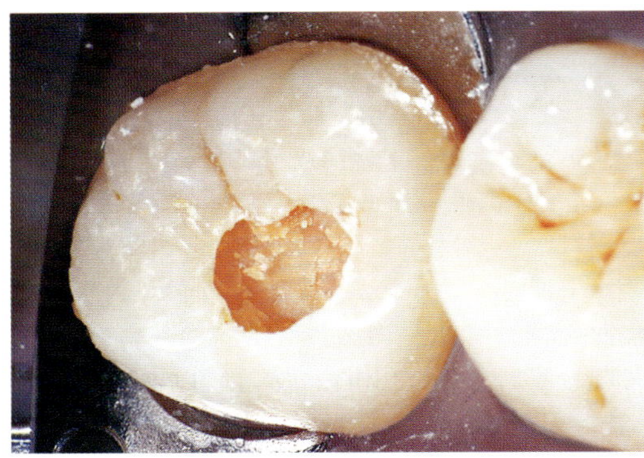

Fig 14-10b The same tooth following cavity preparation. The conservative access cavity has demineralized affected dentin remaining on the floor.

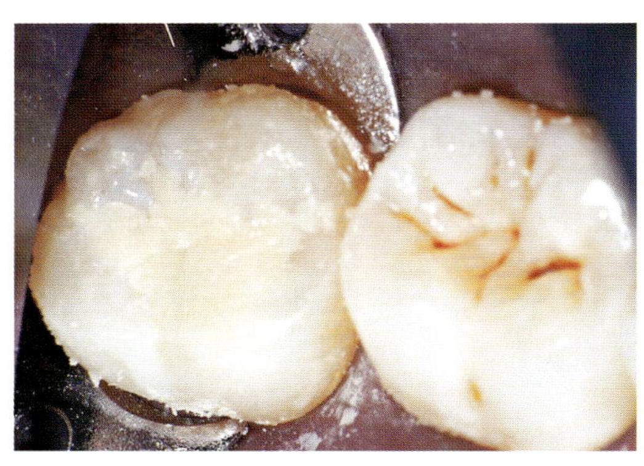

Fig 14-10c The same tooth after conditioning and restoration with the strongest glass-ionomer available. A decision as to the future of this restoration was postponed 3 months.

Summary

It is apparent that glass-ionomers have come of age and should be regarded as moderately biomimetic materials. This chapter has focused mainly on their use as a restorative materials, but they also are useful as both linings and luting cements. The setting reaction, adhesion to tooth structure, and ion release remain the same, but the compressive and tensile strength are reduced because of a lower powder content in the mix.

Resin-modified luting cements are now available and these can also be used to bond amalgam to the cavity wall. Clinical observation has so far been limited, but research continues and there is no doubt their clinical uses will expand. Current investigations into the therapeutic benefits of glass-ionomers show considerable promise but the main limitation of these materials is low fracture resistance. If this can be improved, it is likely their uses will expand still further.

Meanwhile, glass-ionomer cements have reached the stage where they can be regarded as the trigger for the introduction of a far more conservative approach to the treatment of initial carious lesions. Either alone or in combination with resin composites, they make it possible to retain natural tooth structure to a far greater extent than before. The traditional surgical approach to the treatment of caries was dictated, in the absence of adhesion and fluoride, by the need to make room for the placement and condensation of amalgam and always resulted in a cavity that extended well beyond the confines of the lesion itself. All the parameters of this approach should now be abandoned, with preservation and remineralization of tooth structure becoming the driving force behind operative dentistry.

References

1. Jordan RE. Esthetic Composite Bonding: Techniques and Materials, 2d ed. Chicago: Mosby Year Book, 1993.

2. Lutz F. The state of the art of tooth coloured restoratives. Oper Dent 1996;21:237–248.

3. Mount GJ, Hume WR. Preservation and Restoration of Tooth Structure. Chapter 9. London: Mosby International, 1998.

4. Fusayama T. A Simple Pain-Free Adhesive System by Minimal Reduction and Total Etching. Tokyo: Ishiyaku EuroAmerica Inc, 1993.

5. Hume WR, Massey WL. Keeping the pulp alive; the pharmacology and toxicology of agents applied to dentine. Aust Dent J 1990;35:32–37.

6. Tay FR, Gwinnett AJ, Wei SHY. Ultrastructure of the resin-dentin interface following reversible and irreversible rewetting. Am J Dent 1997;10:77–82.

7. Ngo H, Mount GJ, Peters MCRB. A study of glass-ionomer cement and its interface with the enamel and dentin using a low-temperature, high resolution scanning electron microscope technique. Quintessence Int 1997;28:63–69.

8. Pashley DH. Clinical correlations of dentine structure and function. J Prosthet Dent 1991;66:777–781.

9. McLean JW, Nicholson JW, Wilson AD. Proposed nomenclature for glass-ionomer dental cements and related materials. Guest editorial. Quintessence Int 1994;25:587–589.

10. Meyer JM, Cattani-Lorente MA, Dupuis V. Compomers—between glass-ionomer cements and composites. Biomaterials 1998;19:529–539.

11. Wilson AD, Kent BE. A new translucent cement for dentistry: The glass-ionomer cement. Br Dent J 1972;132:133–135.

12. Mount GJ. An Atlas of Glass-Ionomer Cement: A Clinician's Guide, 2d ed. London: Martin Dunitz, 1994.

13. Brook IM, Hatton PV. Glass-ionomers: Bioactive materials. Biomaterials 1998;19:565–571.

14. Mount GJ. Adhesion of glass-ionomer cement in the clinical environment. Oper Dent 1991;16:141–148.

15. Akinmade A. Adhesion of glass-polyalkenoate cement to collagen. J Dent Res 1994;(special issue):181 [abstract 633].

16. Brännström M. Dentin and Pulp in Restorative Dentistry. London: Wolfe Medical Publications, 1987.

17. Frenken JE, Makoni F, Sithole WD. Oral health services and promotion at secondary schools in greater Harare area. Harare, Zimbabwe: Ministry of Health and Child Welfare, 1997.

18. Forsten L. Fluoride release of glass-ionomers. In: Hunt P (ed). Glass-Ionomers: The Next Generation. Proceedings of the 2nd International Symposium on Dentistry. Philadelphia: International Symposia of Dentistry, 1994;241–249.

19. Forsten L. Fluoride release of glass-ionomers. J Esthet Dent 1994;6:216–222.

20. Ferrari M, Davidson CL. Interdiffusion of a traditional glass-ionomer cement into conditioned dentin. Am J Dent 1998;10:295–297.

21. Ngo H, Marino V, Mount GJ. Calcium, strontium, aluminum, sodium and fluoride release from four glass-ionomers. J Dent Res 1998;77:641 [abstract 75].

22. Newbrun E. Cariology. Chicago: Quintessence, 1990.

23. ten Cate JM, van Duinen RNB. Hypermineralisation of dentinal lesions adjacent to glass-ionomer cement restorations. J Dent Res 1995;74:1266–1271.

24. De Moor RJG, Verbeek RM, De Maeyer EAP. Fluoride Release profiles of restorative glass-ionomer formulations. Dent Mater 1996;12:88–95.

25. Forss H, Nase L, Seppa L. Fluoride concentration, *mutans streptococci* and *lactobacilli* in plaque from old glass-ionomer fillings. Caries Res 1995;29:50–53.

26. Loyola-Rodriguez JP, Garcia-Godoy F, Lindquist R. Growth inhibition of glass-ionomer cements on *mutans streptococci*. Pediatr Dent 1994;16:346–349.

27. Melburg JR. Relationship of original mineral loss in caries-like lesions to mineral changes in situ. Short communication. Caries Res 1991; 25:402–405.

28. DeSteno CV, Feagin FF. Effect of matrix bound phosphate and fluoride on mineralisation of dentin. Calcif Tissue Res 1975;17:151–159.

29. Tam LE, Chan GP-L, Yim D. In vitro caries inhibition effects by conventional and resin-modified glass-ionomer restorations. Oper Dent 1997;22:4–14.

30. Mjör IA. The reason for replacement and the age of failed restorations in general dental practice. Acta Odontol Scand 1997;55:58–63.

31. Wilson NHF, Burke FJT, Mjör IA. Reasons for placement and replacement of restorations of direct restorative materials by a selected group of practitioners in the United Kingdom. Quintessence Int 1997;28:245–248.

32. Forsten L. Fluoride release and uptake by glass-ionomers and related materials and its clinical effect. Biomaterials 1998;19:503–508.

33. Serra MC, Cury JA. The in vitro effect of glass-ionomer cement restoration on enamel subjected to demineralisation and remineralisation models. Quintessence Int 1992;23:143–147.

34. Mount GJ, Hume WR. Preservation and Restoration of Tooth Structure. London: Mosby International, 1998;83.

35. Mount GJ. Clinical requirements for a successful "sandwich"—dentin to glass-ionomer cement to composite resin. Aust Dent J 1989;34:159–165.

36. Mount GJ, Hume WR. A revised classification of carious lesions by site and size. Quintessence Int 1997;28:301–303.

37. Mount GJ, Hume WR. Preservation and Restoration of Tooth Structure. London: Mosby International, 1998;128.

38. Mount GJ, Hume WR. Preservation and Restoration of Tooth Structure. London: Mosby International, 1998;130.

39. Brannstrom M, Vojinovic O. Response of the dental pulp to invasion of bacteria around three filling materials. Dent Child 1976;43:15–21.

40. Mount GJ, Hume WR. Preservation and Restoration of Tooth Structure. London: Mosby International 1998;134.

41. Black GV. A Work on Operative Dentistry: The Technical Procedures in Filling Teeth. Chicago: Medico-Dental Publishing, 1917;5.

42. Wilson AD, McLean JW. In: Glass-Ionomer Cement. Chapter 13. London: Quintessence, 1989.

43. Wilson AD, McLean JW. Glass-Ionomer Cement. London: Quintessence, 1989;199.

44. Mount GJ, Hume WR. Preservation and Restoration of Tooth Structure. London: Mosby International 1998;148.

45. Mount GJ. Longevity in glass-ionomer restorations: Review of a successful technique. Quintessence Int 1997;28:643–650.

46. Mount GJ, Hume WR. Preservation and Restoration of Tooth Structure. London: Mosby International 1998;150.

47. Mount GJ, Hume WR. Preservation and Restoration of Tooth Structure. London: Mosby International, 1998;152.

48. Davidson CL. Glass-ionomer bases under posterior composites. In: Hunt P (ed). Glass-Ionomers: The Next Generation. Proceedings of the 2nd International Symposium on Dentistry. Philadelphia: International Symposia of Dentistry, 1994.

49. Mount GJ. Clinical placement of modern glass-ionomer cements. Quintessence Int 1993;24:107–111.

50. Subrata G, Davidson CL. The effect of various surface treatments on the shear strength between composite resin and glass-ionomer cement. J Dent 1989;17:28–32.

51. Massler M. Changing concepts in the treatment of carious lesions. Br Dent J 1967;123:547–548.

52. Frenken JE, Makoni F, Sithole WD, Hackenitz E. Three-year survival of one-surface ART restorations and glass-ionomer sealants in a school oral health programme in Zimbabwe. Caries Res 1998;32:119–126.

Index

C

H

I

L

M

O

P

R

S